Workbook to Accompany

Medical Assisting:
Essentials of Administrative and Clinical Competencies

Lucille Keir, CMA-A

Barbara A. Wise, BSN, RN, MA(Ed)

Connie Krebs, CMA-C, BGS

THOMSON

DELMAR LEARNING   Australia   Canada   Mexico   Singapore   Spain   United Kingdom   United States

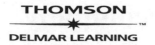

THOMSON

DELMAR LEARNING

Workbook to Accompany

Medical Assisting: Essentials of Administrative and Clinical Competencies

by Lucille Keir, Barbara A. Wise, and Connie Krebs

Executive Director, Health Care Business Unit:
Manager:
William Brottmiller

Executive Editor:
Cathy L. Esperti

Acquisitions Editor:
Rhonda Dearborn

Developmental Editor:
Deb Flis

Executive Marketing Manager:
Dawn F. Gerrain

Channel Manager:
Jennifer McAvey

Editorial Assistant:
Natalie Wager

Executive Production
Karen Leet

Art and Design Coordinator:
Robert Plante

Project Editors:
Sherry McGaughan
Shelley Esposito

Production Coordinator:
Nina Lontrato

ISBN 1-4018-1254-6
Library of Congress Catalog Number
2002031480

NOTICE TO THE READER

CONTENTS

CONTENTS

TO THE LEARNER

This Workbook has been written to help you review the concepts and information presented in the textbook and provide a means for you to achieve competency in performance of various procedures. Each unit in the text is correlated to a unit in this Workbook. The material in the Workbook contains many different types of exercises.

Assignment sheets have been developed to help you review the theory and skill contents, and general technical content. These sheets ask you to answer various types of questions (brief answer, multiple choice, true/false, and critical thinking scenarios), identify correctly spelled words, fill in blanks, match answers, label figures, and word puzzles (unscrambles, word puzzles, word searches, and crossword puzzles). When you have completed the sheets for each chapter, remove them and give them to your teacher for evaluation. Always be sure to fill in your name and the date. (The answers to the questions have been included in your teacher's Instructor's Manual.)

Another feature of your Workbook is Performance Evaluation Checklists. You will find one in the back of this Workbook for each procedure in your textbook. These sheets provide a means for you to achieve a measurement of your ability to perform the procedures. You should practice the procedures following the steps identified in your text, keeping the performance objectives in mind. You will notice procedure competency involves using the correct equipment and materials, accurately performing the procedure steps, and completing the procedure within an acceptable period of time. In procedures where a period of time for completion has not been identified in the objective, it is because of the great amount of variability involved in the task or availabilitiy of equipment and materials. Spaces have been provided on the Performance Evaluation Checklists to document the time required to complete the procedure, as well as the time the procedure began and ended. In procedures where no standards for time and accuracy are provided, your instructor will inform you of the required standards based on the actual classroom situation.

When you feel you have mastered a given skill, ask one of your classmates (if you are in a school situation) to observe your technique following the procedure evaluation requirements. When you are confident of your ability, sign the evaluation form and give it to your teacher. This will inform the teacher that you are ready for evaluation. The teacher will then observe your performance of the procedure (or may delegate the responsibility to another person).

In many units, you will find "situations" to which you are asked to respond. There are no specific right or wrong answers. Think about the things you have read in your text in order to arrive at your answer. You will encounter many similar actual situations both in and out of the office. When family members, friends, and neighbors know you are a medical assistant, they will come to you for information and advice. These simulated situations will be very helpful, but remember, you are not qualified to diagnose an illness or prescribe treatment. Your role is to recognize potential problems, advise, facilitate care and treatment, and provide information within the limits of your knowledge and experience.

It is suggested that you obtain a large three-ring notebook in which to keep your completed assignment and evaluation sheets. Insert the sheets into their original position and maintain your complete Workbook for reference and review.

The authors hope you will find the Workbook to be both challenging and interesting. It is our desire that you master the content of the text to the best of your ability, and we believe this Workbook will assist you in that process. We wish you success as you complete your assignments and prepare to be a medical assistant.

ASSIGNMENT SHEET

Section 1: MEDICAL HEALTH CARE ROLES AND RESPONSIBILITIES

Chapter 1: HEALTH CARE PROVIDERS

Review the objectives and text for each unit before completing the assignment sheet for that unit. When you have completed all sheets for the chapter, remove them from this Workbook and give them to the instructor for evaluation.

Unit 1: A BRIEF HISTORY OF MEDICINE

A. Spelling: Each line contains three different spellings of a word. Underline the correctly spelled word.

1. anesthesha   anesthesia   anethesha
2. aprenticeship   apprentiship   apprenticeship
3. aceptic   aseptic   aseptec
4. caughtery   cauterey   cautery
5. disease   desease   deseace
6. epedemic   epidemic   epidemik
7. ethere   ether   ethir
8. gilds   guelds   guilds
9. infectious   infectuous   enfectuous
10. physican   psychian   physician
11. plaque   plage   plague
12. practitioners   practioners   practitoners
13. scintific   scientific   sientific
14. surgeon   sirgin   sergeon
15. vakcination   vaccination   vacsination

B. Matching: Match the pre-19th-century medical pioneer in column II with his or her correct description in column I.

COLUMN I

___ 1. Father of modern medicine
___ 2. A physician in Rome who wrote over 500 books
___ 3. First reported studies of circulation of blood by heart
___ 4. Built over 200 microscopes and first to see RBCs
___ 5. Founder of scientific surgery
___ 6. Developed the smallpox vaccine
___ 7. Early female physician; author of *Diseases of Women*
___ 8. Greatest French surgeon, who served four kings
___ 9. Developed first mercury thermometer

COLUMN II

a. Anton van Leeuwenhoek
b. William Harvey
c. Edward Jenner
d. Galen
e. Pare
f. Hippocrates
g. John Hunter
h. Gabriel Fahrenheit
i. Trotula Platearius

C. Matching: Match the 19th- or 20th-century medical pioneer in column II with his or her correct description in colunm I.

COLUMN I

_____ 1. Invented the stethoscope
_____ 2. First successful heart transplant
_____ 3. Discovered a red dye that resulted in sulfa drugs
_____ 4. Determined cause of yellow fever
_____ 5. Developed oral polio vaccine
_____ 6. Developed the pap test
_____ 7. Introduced the use of ether as an anesthesia
_____ 8. Discovered the process of pasteurization
_____ 9. Developed the foundation for aseptic technique
_____ 10. Discovered X-rays
_____ 11. Nobel Prize in 1912 for joining blood vessels
_____ 12. Nurse who founded the American Red Cross
_____ 13. First woman to qualify as Physician in the US
_____ 14. Founder of modern nursing
_____ 15. Discovered polio and developed a vaccine
_____ 16. Woman scientist whose work led to radium treatments for cancer
_____ 17. Instituted first nutrition program for medical students in the world.
_____ 18. Discovered a mold that later led to penicillin
_____ 19. Used tubing to replace arteries

COLUMN II

a. George Papaniolaou
b. Wilhelm Roentgen
c. W.T.G. Morton
d. Alexis Carrel
e. Louis Pasteur
f. Sir Alexander Fleming
g. Elizabeth Blackwell
h. A.B. Sabin
i. Christian Bernard
j. Jonas Salk
k. Rene Laennec
l. Marie Curie
m. Gerhard Domagk
n. Walter Reed
o. Clara Barton
p. Michael DeBakey

q. Joseph Lister

r. Grace Goldsmith
s. Florence Nightengale

D. Brief Answer

During the ancient medical history period, several things were believed responsible for illness and some unusual treatments were used.

1. What was credited as the cause of disease? _____

2. How were migraines, epilepsy, insanity, and head injuries treated? _____

3. How did the Egyptians solve "clogged" body canals? _____

4. The Greeks believed in a god of healing. What did they use for treatments? _____

_____

In medieval history, other beliefs and methods of treatment were prevalent.

5. What did Anglo-Saxons in Britain believe caused illness? _____

_____

6. How did the priests cure the sick in about 400 AD? _____

_____

7. In 1277 AD, how was tuberculosis treated? _____

8. In 1352, what different things were believed to be the cause of the plagues? _____

_____

9. The practice of medicine at the beginning of the 17th century was divided among three guilds. Name and briefly describe their education and area of practice.

a. _____

b. _____

_____

c. _____

_____

10. As late as the 1600s, what were some of the old practices still being used in the colonies and what was the unusual prescription ordered for Queen Anne? _____

    _____

11. What sciences aided medical science in making rapid advances in the 18th century? _____

    _____

12. Name the two people who developed polio vaccine and identify the type they developed. What are three reasons the second type was more desirable? _____

    _____

    _____

13. During the 1950s, what changed the way human bodies could be seen inside? _____

14. Name eight types of "artificial" body parts that have been developed.

    a. _____ b. _____ c. _____ d. _____

    e. _____ f. _____ g. _____ h. _____

15. Congress has enacted several laws concerning health care. What did the following laws provide?

    a. Hill–Burton Act: _____

    b. What did the combined Public Health Services and the Food and Drug Administration originally and then later become? _____

    _____

    c. What did the National Cancer Institute and the Public Health Services Hygienic Lab become? _____

    _____

    d. What two health programs were enacted in 1965? _____

16. Women had a difficult time being accepted as physicians. Briefly identify the major contribution of the following female physicians.

    a. Trotula Platearius _____

    b. Elizabeth Garrett Anderson _____

    c. Elizabeth Blackwell _____

    _____

    d. Aletta Jacobs _____

    e. Elsie Strang L'Esperance _____

    f. Dorothy Hansine Anderson _____

    g. Grace Arabell Goldsmith _____

    h. Dorothy Hodgkins _____

17. What did *Ebony* Magazine report in 1993 regarding the accomplishments of Drs. Alexa Canady and M. Deborah Hyde-Rowan? _____

    _____

18. Refer to the Role Delineation Chart in Appendix A of the textbook. Within the area of *Instruction*, which role relates to the content of this unit? _____

After your instructor has returned your work to you, make all necessary corrections and place in a three-ring notebook for future reference.

ASSIGNMENT SHEET

Chapter 1: HEALTH CARE PROVIDERS

Unit 2: THE HEALTH CARE TEAM

A. Multiple Choice: Place the correct letter on the blank line for each question.

_____ 1. One whose primary duty is obtaining a medical history and other important information from patients in the hospital is termed a(n)

    a. registered nurse   c. dietitian

    b. admissions clerk   d. office manager

_____ 2. A _____ performs specialized chemical, microscopic, and bacteriological tests of blood, tissue, and other body fluids.

    a. nurse practitioner   c. laboratory technician

    b. physician assistant   d. accessioning technician

_____ 3. One who practices skills most often in the hospital setting to assist patients in many ways through purposeful activity is called a(n)

    a. physician assistant   c. physical therapist

    b. pharmacist   d. occupational therapist

_____ 4. A member of the health care team who helps patients with their diets, usually in a hospital or clinic, is called a

    a. nurse practitioner   c. dietitian

    b. pharmacist   d. nutritionist

_____ 5. One who is trained by physicians, instructed in certain aspects of medicine, and practices under their direct supervision is called a

    a. registered nurse   c. physician assistant

    b. licensed practical nurse   d. paramedic

_____ 6. The _____ is trained in the art of drawing blood for diagnostic purposes.

    a. paramedic   c. physician assistant

    b. physical therapist   d. phlebotomist

_____ 7. A qualified person who has been trained in assisting patients in rehabilitation programs following accident or injury is called a(n)

    a. occupational therapist   c. registered nurse

    b. physical therapist   d. podiatrist

_____ 8. One who is a licensed specialist in formulating and dispensing medications is a

    a. pharmacist   c. registered nurse

    b. paramedic   d. physician

_____ 9. A professional who is highly trained and skilled in mechanical manipulation of the spinal column is a(n)

    a. occupational therapist   c. licensed practical nurse

    b. chiropractor   d. physical therapist

_____ 10. A member of the health care team who performs procedures to improve the ventilatory functions of a patient is a(n)

    a. phlebotomist   c. radiology technician

    b. electrocardiogram technician   d. respiratory therapist

_____ 11. A _____ provides testing and counseling services to patients in private or group practice.

      a. podiatrist   c. paramedic

      b. dietitian   d. psychologist

B. Spelling: Each line contains four different spellings of a word. Underline the correctly spelled word.

1. dietitian	dietician	deititian	dietision
2. phlebatomist	plebotamist	phlebotomist	pflebotomist
3. therapast	theirapist	therapist	tharapist
4. technicien	technician	technision	tecnician
5. chiropractor	chiropracter	chyroprakder	chirupractor
6. nutricionist	nutrionist	nutritionist	newtritionist
7. ocupational	occupattional	occupational	occupationale
8. licensed	licenced	licensced	licensead
9. professional	preffessional	profesional	professionel
10. physiciaan	physichian	pysican	physician

C. Matching: Match the subspecialty in column I with the correct description in column II.

COLUMN I

_____ 1. Immunology

_____ 2. Preventive medicine

_____ 3. Acupuncture

_____ 4. Hypnosis

_____ 5. Rheumatology

_____ 6. Nutrition

_____ 7. Surgery

_____ 8. Cardiovascular disease

_____ 9. Hypertension

_____ 10. Aerospace medicine

COLUMN II

a. Mainly used in psychotherapy

b. Treats high blood pressure

c. How the body utilizes nutrients

d. Deals with allergies

e. Originated in the Far East

f. Stresses keeping healthy

g. Research effects of space environment

h. Treats inflammatory disorders

i. Many specialized areas

j. Heart and circulatory problems

D. Fill in the Blank

1. The podiatrist or _____ deals with diseases and disorders of the _____

2. The business office manager should have good _____ skills.

3. The licensed practical nurse may perform basic nursing skills under the direct supervision of a physician or _____

4. The _____ is one who specializes in the microscopic identification of cells and tissues.

5. Emergency Medical Technicians must _____ every two years.

6. An R.N. is defined as a _____ nurse who has completed a school of nursing and passed the NCLEX-RN.

7. A _____ is sometimes called an administrative specialist or a ward secretary.

8. A registered nurse who has acquired expert knowledge in a special branch of practice is called a nurse _____

9. The _____ acts as an assistant to, or in place of, the physician, especially in the military and in emergency services.

10. The _____ of the X-ray technician must be proved by the American Registry of Radiologic Technologists.

11. A _____ has graduated from a school with CAAHEP approval and has successfully passed the certification exam of the AAMA.

12. The _____ assists women throughout pregnancy, childbirth, and the postpartum period.

13. The _____ must have met pre-med requirements and successfully completed a two-year program, and works under the direct supervision of the physician.

14. A degree in business administration is desirable to be a _____

After your instructor has returned your work to you, make all necessary corrections and place in a three-ring notebook for future reference.

ASSIGNMENT SHEET

Chapter 1: HEALTH CARE PROVIDERS

Unit 3: MEDICAL PRACTICE SPECIALTIES

A. Fill in the Blank

1. _____ dedicate their lives to the practice of medicine or to acquiring skills in the art and science of treating disease and maintaining health.

2. A physician may have an area of special interest that may be referred to as a _____

3. The term _____ is derived from the Latin word meaning "to teach."

4. Persons who hold _____ or _____ are entitled to be addressed as "doctor."

5. A _____ contributes specific expert skills and knowledge in serving patients.

6. The type of practice that covers the broadest spectrum is called _____

7. Three types of medical specialties that are hospital based are _____ _____ and emergency or traumatic medicine.

8. In the practice of _____ manipulation therapy may be used to alleviate illness.

9. Refer to the Role Delineation Chart in Appendix A of the textbook. Within the area of *Allied Health Professions and Credentialing*, which two roles relate to the content of this unit? _____

   _____

B. Matching: Match the specialty in Column II with the correct abbreviation in column I.

COLUMN I
COLUMN II

_____ 1. OD
a. Doctor of Osteopathy

_____ 2. PhD
b. Doctor of Dental Surgery

_____ 3. DPM
c. Doctor of Medicine

_____ 4. DC
d. Doctor of Divinity

_____ 5. DO
e. Doctor of Optometry

_____ 6. DDS
f. Doctor of Veterinary Medicine

_____ 7. MD
g. Doctor of Philosophy

h. Doctor of Chiropractic

i. Doctor of Podiatric Medicine

C. Multiple Choice: Place the correct letter on the blank line for each question.

_____ 1. One who specializes in the treatment of diseases and disorders of the stomach and intestines is a(an)
    a. gerontologist   c. gastroenterologist
    b. endocrinologist   d. allergist

_____ 2. The field of medicine that deals with diagnosing and treating diseases and disorders of the female reproductive tract is
    a. gerontology   c. nephrology
    b. gynecology   d. obstetrics

_____ 3. Measuring the accuracy of vision to determine if corrective lenses (eyeglasses) are needed describes the field of
    a. orthopedics   c. optometry
    b. oncology   d. obstetrics

_____ 4. A specialty that deals with the diagnosis and treatment of diseases and disorders of the CNS (central nervous system) is
    a. psychology   c. nuclear medicine
    b. neurology   d. nephrology

_____ 5. Treatment and diagnosis of acute illnesses or injuries is a specialty called
    a. surgery   c. pathology
    b. physical medicine   d. traumatic medicine

_____ 6. One who specializes in the treatment and diagnosis of pronounced manifestation of emotional problems or mental illnesses that may have an organic causative factor is called a
    a. psychiatrist   c. neurologist
    b. psychologist   d. podiatrist

_____ 7. Analysis of tissue samples to confirm diagnosis is performed by a
    a. urologist   c. pathologist
    b. hematologist   d. nephrologist

_____ 8. One who specializes in the diagnosis and treatment of the foot is called a
    a. surgeon   c. pathologist
    b. podiatrist   d. chiropractor

_____ 9. Sports medicine is a medical specialty that deals with diagnosing and treating
    a. emotional problems   c. disorders and diseases of the urinary system
    b. injuries sustained in athletic events   d. conditions of altered immunological reactivity

_____ 10. A radiologist specializes in diagnosing and treating diseases and disorders
    a. by manual or operative methods   c. with roentgen rays and other forms of radiant
    b. with the use of radionuclides   energy
                                          d. with manipulative treatment

_____ 11. Dermatology is the specialty of medicine that deals with diagnosis and treatment of diseases and disorders of the
      a. glands of internal secretion   c. teeth and gums
      b. skin   d. kidneys

_____ 12. Nephrology is the medical specialty that deals with the diagnosis and treatment of
      a. blood and blood-forming tissue   c. stomach and intestines
      b. the internal organs   d. the kidneys

_____ 13. One who is a specialist in the diagnosis and treatment of problems in conceiving and maintaining pregnancy is a(n)
      a. pediatrician   c. endocrinologist
      b. family practitioner   d. infertility specialist

_____ 14. A hematologist specializes in the diagnosis and treatment of disorders and diseases of
      a. the internal organs   c. blood and blood-forming tissue
      b. bones   d. the central nervous system

_____ 15. The field of medicine that provides direct care to pregnant females during pregnancy, childbirth, and immediately thereafter is called
      a. obstetrics   c. pediatrics
      b. infertility   d. gynecology

_____ 16. Anesthesiology is the medical specialty that deals with
      a. manual or operative methods   c. administering anesthetic agents prior to and
      b. the use of radionuclides   during surgery
                                           d. altered immunological reactivity

_____ 17. A cardiologist specializes in the diagnosis and treatment of abnormalities, diseases, and disorders of the
      a. glands   c. heart
      b. aging   d. central nervous system

_____ 18. One who specializes in diagnosing and treating diseases and malfunctions of the glands of internal secretion is called a(an)
      a. cardiologist   c. endocrinologist
      b. chiropractor   d. otorhinolaryngologist

D. Crossword Puzzle

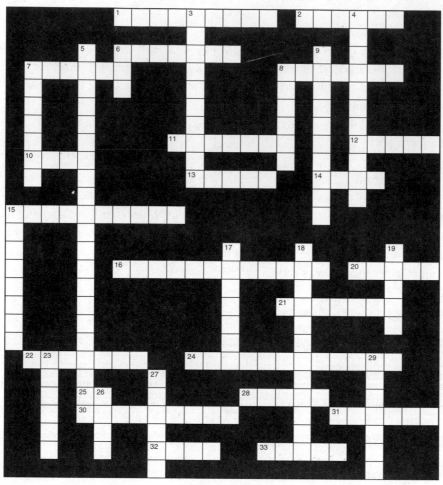

ACROSS

1. Urgency
2. Responsibilities
6. Altered immune reaction
7. Common name for physician
8. Branch of medicine that uses radionuclides
10. A dermatologist treats problems of the _____
11. Renewed periodically
12. Pulmonary specialists treat diseases and disorders of the _____
13. Expertise in a certain area
14. A surgeon cuts _____ skin
15. Field of medicine dealing with small children
16. Deals with pregnancy/childbirth
20. Anesthetics make you _____
21. Pathology is the study of _____
22. Operation
24. Commonly known as a counselor
25. Abbreviation for symptoms
28. Opposite of chronic
30. _____ medicine is practiced in the emergency room
31. Prefix that refers to the heart
32. The health care _____ works together
33. Orthopedics

DOWN

3. Field of medicine that deals with senior citizens
4. Specialist who helps childless couples
5. ENT specialist
6. Practicing medicine is an _____ and science
7. Deals with problems of the teeth and gums
8. A neurologist is expert in this specific anatomical area
9. Career/work
15. Branch of medicine that treats problems of the feet
17. Field of medicine that treats genitourinary problems
18. Chiropractic
19. From general practice to a specialist
23. Emergency
26. Radiologists use these in diagnosing
27. Prefix that refers to blood
29. Endocrinologists study about what glands _____

E. Spelling: Each line contains four different spellings of a word. Underline the correctly spelled word.

1. allargist	allergest	<u>allergist</u>	alergist
2. <u>anesthesiology</u>	annesthesiology	anesthisology	anasthesiology
3. gastrointerologist	<u>gastroenterologist</u>	gastronterologist	gastranologist
4. geriatricks	gariacktrics	giractrics	<u>geriatrics</u>
5. <u>ophthalmology</u>	opthalmology	optamology	ophthalamalagy
6. obstitrician	<u>obstetrician</u>	obstatrician	obstetrecian
7. <u>psychiatrist</u>	psychiotrist	psyciatrist	psychatrist
8. pediatrist	padiatrist	<u>podiatrist</u>	podatrist
9. pediatician	<u>pediatrician</u>	peditrician	pedeatrician
10. <u>urologist</u>	uriologist	urologest	urolgist

CRITICAL THINKING SCENARIOS: What would your response be in the following situations?

1. Your neighbor asks you the difference between an internal medicine specialist and an endocrinologist.

_____

_____

_____

2. You are attending a family reunion and overhear a discussion where there is an obvious uncertainty about the use of the title "Doctor" _____

3. A female patient, whom the physician has never seen before, phones to ask about the possibility of having a food allergy. This patient tells you that she has a fine red rash all over her body. _____

_____

_____

After your instructor has returned your work to you, make all necessary corrections and place in a three-ring notebook for future reference.

ASSIGNMENT SHEET

Chapter 2: THE MEDICAL ASSISTANT

Review the objectives and text for each unit before completing the assignment sheet for that unit. When you have completed all sheets for the chapter, remove them from this Workbook and give them to the instructor for evaluation.

Unit 1: TRAINING, JOB RESPONSIBILITIES, AND EMPLOYMENT OPPORTUNITIES

A. Brief Answer

1. Why did health care occupations develop? _____

2. Name the fourteen fastest-growing occupations in the health service industry. _____
_____
_____
_____
_____

3. Why have health occupations grown? _____
_____

4. Looking at Table 2-2 on page 31 in the textbook, identify the following:
   a. Which occupation showed a surplus in 1998 and is projected in 2008? _____
   b. Which occupation shows the greatest number of job openings? _____
   c. How many projected new medical assistants will be needed by 2008? (Remember, the listings are in thousands.) _____
   d. How many medical secretaries were employed in 1998 and how many more will be needed by 2008? _____
   e. What is the most significant source of training for medical records technicians? _____
5. Where can training for medical assisting be obtained? _____
_____

6. In the discussion of jobs under Career Laddering in the textbook, determine the amount of training and licensure (if needed) required to obtain the following jobs:
   a. Licensed practical nurse _____
   b. Emergency medical technician _____
   _____
   c. Recreational therapist _____
   _____
   d. Respiratory therapist _____
   _____
   e. Dental hygienist _____
   _____
   f. Nuclear medicine technologist _____
   g. Physician assistant _____
   h. Pharmacy technician _____
   i. Occupational therapy assistant _____
7. Refer to the CAAHEP Standards in Appendix B of the textbook. Within the area of *Professional Components,* which curriculum standards are discussed in this unit _____
_____

B. Fill in the Blank: **For each task below, identify if it is considered administrative or clinical by placing an "A" or "C" in the space provided.**

_____ 1. Complete insurance forms

_____ 2. Maintain medical records

_____ 3. Take vital signs

_____ 4. Schedule appointments

_____ 5. Take medical histories

_____ 6. Prepare and give injections

_____ 7. Assist with medical procedures

_____ 8. Prepare medications

_____ 9. Handle mail

_____ 10. Prepare correspondence

_____ 11. Perform ECGs

_____ 12. Handle telephone calls

C. Matching: **Match the definition in column II with the correct term in column I.**

COLUMN I

_____ 1. Administrative

_____ 2. Analysis

_____ 3. Clinical

_____ 4. Competency

_____ 5. Compliance

_____ 6. Confidential

_____ 7. Methodical

_____ 8. Professional

_____ 9. Proprietary

_____ 10. Technologist

_____ 11. Therapist

_____ 12. Therapeutic

COLUMN II

a. Conformity to formal or official requirements

b. Following a plan or method

c. One trained and skilled in the methods of a profession

d. A person trained in the technical aspect of an area of study

e. Business and management tasks of a practice

f. Non-public educational institutions

g. An examination to determine something's content

h. Tasks dealing with patient examination and treatment

i. Having medicinal or healing properties

j. A person who provides restorative treatments

k. Being capable, able to perform at an acceptable level

l. Held in strict confidence, secretive

D. Word Puzzle: Use the clues below to spell out these health occupations.

1.   _ _ O _ _ _ _ _ _ _
2.   _ _ _ _ _ C _ _ _
3.   _ _ C _ _ _ _
4.   _ _ _ U _
5.   _ _ _ _ P _ _ _ _ _ _
6.   _ _ A _ _ _
7.   _ _ _ _ _ T _ _ _
8. _ _ _ _ _ _ I _ _
9.   _ _ _ _ _ O _ _ _ _ _ _
10.   N _ _ _ _
11. _ _ _ _ _ _ S _ _ _ _

1. Individual responsible for maintaining financial records
2. A doctor
3. Legal permit to engage in a certain activity
4. AAMA occupational analysis
5. A person who greets or welcomes
6. A state of freedom from disease
7. Individual responsible for office correspondence
8. An individual who provides a remedy
9. A person who applies scientific or mechanical methods
10. A person who provides care for the sick or injured
11. A person trained and skilled in a profession

After your instructor has returned your work to you, make all necessary corrections and place in a three-ring notebook for future reference.

ASSIGNMENT SHEET

Chapter 2: THE MEDICAL ASSISTANT

Unit 2: PERSONAL CHARACTERISTICS

A. Matching: Match the definition in column II with the correct term in column I.

COLUMN I

_____ 1. Accuracy
_____ 2. Adaptable
_____ 3. Conservative
_____ 4. Courteous
_____ 5. Dependable
_____ 6. Discreet
_____ 7. Empathy
_____ 8. Enthusiasm
_____ 9. Honesty
_____ 10. Initiative
_____ 11. Patience
_____ 12. Perseverance
_____ 13. Punctual
_____ 14. Reliable
_____ 15. Respectful
_____ 16. Self-control
_____ 17. Tact

COLUMN II

a. Can be relied upon, responsible
b. Ambition, hustle; set something in motion
c. Detailed correctness, exactness
d. Trustworthy, the quality of being truthful
e. Show restraint
f. Calmness in waiting; tolerant
g. Delicate skill in saying or doing the right thing
h. In exact agreement with appointed time
i. Zeal, intense interest
j. The ability to adjust
k. Showing regard for, considerate
l. Trying to identify one's feelings with those of another
m. To be cautious, handle with care, not wasteful
n. Prudent, cautious, especially in speech
o. To be polite, well-mannered
p. Trustworthy, dependable, responsible
q. Persistent effort, prolong

B. Brief Answer

1. Five personality qualities were identified in the text. List each one and give a brief definition.

   a. _____
   b. _____
   c. _____
   d. _____
   e. _____

2. Refer to the Role Delineation Chart in Appendix A of the textbook. Within the area of *Professionalism*, which role relates to your appearance? _____

C. True or False: Place a "T" for true or "F" for false in the space provided. For false statements, explain why they are false.

To be perceived as a professional, you must look like a professional. The following statements apply to your image. Indicate if they are true or false.

_____ 1. A skin rash on your body should not cause concern to a patient.

_____ 2. Being grossly overweight is beneficial when dealing with dieting patients who need to identify with a role model.

_____ 3. Personal illness requires prompt attention.

_____ 4. Deodorant will cover the odor from old perspiration.

_____ 5. Refrain from using hand cream because it attracts organisms.

_____ 6. Care should be taken to keep your hands out of your hair.

_____ 7. Chewing gum while working is unprofessional.

_____ 8. It is best to wear white underwear under a white uniform.

_____ 9. Your posture affects your energy level.

_____ 10. Chapped, cracked hands may allow organisms to enter the body.

_____ 11. Wearing a fragrance with a strong aroma helps soften the medicinal environment in the physician's office.

_____ 12. For women, vivid cosmetics and nailpolish are nice accents to a white uniform.

D. Word Puzzle: Use the clues below to spell out these terms.

```
 1.              _ _ C _ _ _ _ _
 2.        _ _ _ _ _ H _
 3.  _ _ _ _ _ _ A _ _ _
                _ _ R _ _ _ _ _
 4.        _ _ _ _ A _ _ _
 5.          _ _ _ C _ _ _ _
 6.          _ _ T _ _ _ _ _
 7.      _ _ _ _ _ E _ _ _
 8.      _ _ _ _ _ _ R _ _ _
 9.        _ _ _ _ I _ _ _ _ _
10.    _ _ _ _ _ S _ _ _ _
11.          _ _ T _ _ _ _ _
12.        _ _ _ _ I _ _ _
13.      _ _ _ _ _ C _ _ _ _
14.        _ _ _ _ S _ _
```

1. Correct
2. Identify with the feelings of another
3. Visible presence
4. Dependable
5. Prudent, cautious
6. Show tolerance
7. Polite

8. Act together
9. Set in motion
10. Intense interest
11. Feelings toward
12. Willing to adjust
13. Show regard for
14. Trustworthy

After your instructor has returned your work to you, make all necessary corrections and place in a three-ring notebook for future reference.

ASSIGNMENT SHEET

Chapter 2: THE MEDICAL ASSISTANT

Unit 3: PROFESSIONALISM

A. Fill in the Blank

1. The pioneers in medicine often were paid with a family's goods or valuables, which is called _____

2. _____ of every transaction between physician and patient is a must.

3. In _____ medical assistants from _____ states met in Kansas City, and adopted the name _____

4. The primary purpose of the AAMA was to raise the standards of the medical assistant to a _____
   _____

5. The Maxine Williams Scholarship fund was established to assist those interested in pursuing a career in medical assisting; scholarships are based on _____

6. The American Registry of Medical Assistants (ARMA) was established in _____ and operates with continual support and guidance from the _____

7. The purpose of the ARMA is to advance the standards and profession of medical assisting and to
   _____

8. A _____ year revalidation process has been developed through the American Medical Technologists Institute for Education (AMTIE) for ARMA members.

9. One who interprets and transcribes patient information from oral to printed form by typing or with the use of a word processor is known as a _____

10. In _____ the American Association for Medical Transcription (AAMT) was incorporated in _____ for the advancement of medical transcription.

11. _____ is the registered service mark for the rating that has become the recognized standard of measurement of secretarial proficiency.

12. The American Medical Technologists outline the requirements of professionalism in their
    _____

13. Both the AAMA national certification exam and the ARMA registry exam are designed to evaluate _____ competency in medical assisting.

14. Continuing education is available through professional medical assistant organizations that offer _____ to those who successfully complete seminars, workshops, publications, and home-study programs.

B. Matching: Match the definition in column II with the correct term in column I.

COLUMN I

_____   1. Evaluation

_____   2. Competent

_____   3. Professionalism

_____   4. Accreditation

_____   5. Registry

_____   6. Revalidation

_____   7. Certification

_____   8. Reputation

_____   9. Initiative

COLUMN II

a. Process of evaluating competency in a specific area of expertise

b. Reconfirmation of one's competency in a specific area of expertise

c. To start on one's own; to begin

d. Assessment; judgment concerning worth of a person

e. The assignment of credentials; approval given for meeting established standards

f. What is generally believed about one's character

g. One who is trained and skilled in the methods of the profession

h. Place where the listing of competent individuals is kept

i. Fit, able, capable in a specific area

C. Brief Answwer

1. When, where, and why did the medical assistant profession begin? _____

_____

_____

2. a. Write the AAMA-approved definition of medical assisting: _____

_____

_____

    b. Write the ARMA approved definition of medical assisting: _____

_____

_____

3. State the purpose of the AMT Standards of Practice and what members must recognize in themselves. _____

_____

_____

_____

4. List the nine competencies outlined in the AAMA Role Delineation Chart that demonstrate professionalism.

_____

_____

_____

5. Explain why it is important for professionals to certify or recertify according to the guidelines set by the professional medical assistant organizations. _____

_____

_____

6. List the professional organizations that would be beneficial to the medical assistant.

    a. _____

    b. _____

    c. _____

    d. _____

D. True or False: Place a "T" for true or "F" for false in the space provided. For false statements, explain why they are false.

_____ 1. The AAPC *Coding Edge* is the professional magazine of the AAMA.

_____ 2. Many employers require current certification or registration for medical assistants to be considered for employment.

_____ 3. To stay current with the field of medicine, medical assistants should participate in continuing education programs to earn CEUs toward recertification.

_____ 4. Medical assistants as well as physicians have a code of ethics to follow in their professions.

_____ 5. The competency of medical assistant programs is determined by the accrediting board of the American Medical Association.

After your instructor has returned your work to you, make all necessary corrections and place in a three-ring notebook for future reference.

ASSIGNMENT SHEET

Chapter 3: MEDICAL ETHICS AND LIABILITY

Review the objectives and text for each unit before completing the assignment sheet for that unit. When you have completed all sheets for the chapter, remove them from this Workbook and give them to the instructor for evaluation.

Unit 1: ETHICAL AND LEGAL RESPONSIBILITIES

A. Multiple Choice: Place the correct letter or letters on the blank line for each question.

_____ 1. Which item is *not* a requirement for a physician to be licensed?
  a. be of good moral character   c. be of legal age
  b. completed approved residency program   d. has no allergies

_____ 2. The exceptions to the need for a license to practice medicine are
  a. an emergency situation   c. treating family members
  b. physician in military   d. school physician

_____ 3. The two basic elements that constitute the practice of medicine are
  a. diagnosis   c. prescribing
  b. scheduling   d. accounting

_____ 4. Areas of medical ethics that are of concern to the medical assistant are
  a. honesty   c. competency
  b. confidentiality   d. all of these

_____ 5. When the medical assistant improves skills and acquires additional knowledge in the field of medicine, who benefits?
  a. the medical assistant   c. the patient
  b. colleagues   d. all of these

B. Brief Answer

1. How can DRGs cause ethical issues for physicians? _____

_____

2. What is the most common transplant? _____

3. Explain what the term emancipated minor means. _____

_____

4. What is the recommended statement that should be made to the patient by the medical assistant responsible for obtaining a signature on the consent form for invasive, experimental, and high-risk medical services?

_____

5. What does *privileged communication* mean? _____

_____

6. Describe the conditions for revocation or suspension of a medical license. _____

_____

7. Describe unprofessional conduct. _____

_____

_____

B. Matching: Match the definition in column II with the correct term in column I.

COLUMN I

_____ 1. Offer
_____ 2. Contract law
_____ 3. Reciprocity
_____ 4. Ethics
_____ 5. Tort
_____ 6. Implied consent
_____ 7. Civil laws
_____ 8. Endorsement
_____ 9. Acceptance
_____ 10. Consideration

COLUMN II

a. Deals with what is morally right and wrong
b. Deals with findings of negligence; most common basis for lawsuits against physicians
c. Takes place when appointment is given and the doctor examines the patient
d. Written consent for medical services
e. Pass exam administered by the National Board of Medical Examiners
f. Takes place when a competent individual indicates desire to be a patient
g. Payment given in exchange for services
h. License granted in new state because of equal requirements of original license
i. Patient enters into agreement by coming to see physician
j. Patient-physician relationship considered contract
k. Defines powers of government and its citizens
l. Deals with laws governing property ownership, corporation, and inheritance

D. Fill in the Blank

1. A medical license may be revoked for _____

2. A license may be revoked because of proven _____ in the application for the license.

3. Physicians who are found to be incompetent to practice because of _____ may have their license revoked.

4. The ethical standards established by a profession are administered by _____

5. The physician must release patient information when the patient authorizes the release or if the release of information is _____

6. With proper documentation, any person of sound mind and legal age may give any part of the body after death for _____

7. Human organs should never be _____

8. Copies of the living will document should be filed with the _____

9. Every member of the medical care team should be currently certified in _____

10. Under the _____ patients must receive written information explaining their right-to-die options according to their state laws.

11. A _____ is defined as any number of actions done by one person or group of persons that causes injury to another or others.

12. The negligent causing of an injury, when committed by a physician in the course of professional duties, is commonly referred to as _____

13. Libel and slander are two forms of _____

14. A deliberate attempt or threat to touch without consent is called _____

15. _____ is the unauthorized touching of another person.

E. Word Puzzle: Use the clues below to spell out these terms.

1.   __ __ **P** __ __ __ __ __
2.   __ **R** __ __ __ __
3. __ __ __ __ __ __ __ **O** __
4.   __ __ **C** __ __ __ __ __
5.   __ __ __ __ __ **R** __ __ __
6.   __ __ __ **A** __ __ __ __ __ __
7. __ __ __ __ __ __ __ **S** __
8. __ __ __ __ __ __ __ **T** __
9.   __ __ __ **I** __ __ __ __
10.   **N** __ __ __ __ __ __ __ __ __
11.   __ __ **A** __ __ __ __ __ __ __
12.   __ __ __ **T** __
13.   __ **I** __ __ __ __ __ __ __
14.   __ __ __ **O** __ __ __ __ __
15.   __ __ __ __ **N** __ __ __ __

1. Definite, specific
2. Violation of a law, contract, or other agreement
3. A standard of criticism or judgment
4. The principles of any branch of knowledge
5. To count separately; name one by one
6. Injury done to a person's reputation by or through slanderous statements
7. To surround, enclose
8. To bind legally or morally
9. Feebleness of body or mind caused by old age
10. Malpractice
11. Characterized by cheating and deceit; obtaining by dishonest means
12. An injurious, harmful action, not involving a breach of contract, for which a civil action can be brought
13. Anything to which a person is liable, responsible, legally bound
14. To cancel; withdraw; take back
15. A legal permit to engage in an activity

After your instructor has returned your work to you, make all necessary corrections and place in a three-ring notebook for future reference.

ASSIGNMENT SHEET

Chapter 3: MEDICAL ETHICS AND LIABILITY

Unit 2: PROFESSIONAL LIABILITY

SUGGESTED RESPONSES TO CRITICAL THINKING CHALLENGE IN TEXTBOOK

1. What should Lisa have done? _____

_____

2. Who is responsible for the patient's record? _____

_____

_____

3. What would you have done? _____

4. Should the supervisor, physician, or office manager be called about this? If so, why? _____

_____

_____

A. Brief Answer

1. Describe the correct procedure for terminating the physician-patient contract.

_____

_____

_____

_____

_____

2. Explain the term *abandonment,* and give an example.

_____

_____

_____

3. What is professional negligence? Give an example.

_____

_____

4. In what situations could a medical assistant be charged with malpractice?

_____

5. What is the purpose of the Good Samaritan Act?

_____

6. List the reasons for keeping medical records.

_____

7. Who owns medical office records?

_____

8. Do patients have the right to the information in their medical records?

_____

9. What special precautions should be taken when giving written instructions to a patient?

_____

10. What kinds of notes are inappropriate in a patient's chart? Why?

_____

_____

11. Describe the acceptable method for making changes in medical records.

_____

_____

12. List and discuss the guidelines for reducing the number of forged prescription orders.

_____

13. Discuss with other class members the issue of manipulated stem cell and cultivated donor tissue
    experimentation and research. Then write your concerns and your opinion about this controversial topic.

_____

_____

**B. True or False: Place a "T" for true or "F" for false in the space provided. For false statements, explain
    why they are false.**

_____ 1. Physicians have no right to determine whom they will see as patients.

_____ 2. Patients have the right to receive care equal to the standards of care in the community as a
           whole.

_____ 3. A physician may choose to withdraw from the care of a patient who does not follow
           instructions for treatment or follow-up appointments or who leaves a hospital against advice
           to stay.

_____ 4. The medical assistant has the right to be free from sexual discrimination.

_____ 5. The victim of sexual harassment must be of the opposite sex.

_____ 6. The testimony of a physician as an expert medical witness is never necessary in a case of
           negligence.

_____ 7. The doctrine, *res ipsa loquitur,* means the thing speaks for itself.

_____ 8. The physician's liability is expressed in the doctrine of *respondeat superior.*

_____ 9. The medical assistant is considered an agent for the physician under the law of agency.

_____ 10. The Good Samaritan law covers physicians even if they receive compensation for the
           emergency care given.

_____ 11. An implied agreement is considered to be a legal contract in a medical office.

_____ 12. The medical assistant should never attempt to perform a procedure without having been
           properly trained.

C. Fill in the Blank

1. Derogatory statements regarding patients may be considered _____ of character and a breach of confidentiality.

2. An attorney may agree to take the testimony of the physician by _____

3. A medical assistant may receive a _____ to appear in court with patient records.

4. A _____ is a law that designates a specific time limit during which a claim may be filed in malpractice suits or in the collection of bills.

5. _____ cannot be tolerated in handling medical records.

6. Each office should have a _____ regarding the release of information from a medical record.

7. The requirement of confidentiality regarding the medical record is no longer recognized when the patient _____ against the physician.

8. When in doubt about disclosing patient information, _____ by not disclosing rather than by disclosing.

9. The _____ to disclose information should be placed in the patient's chart with a copy of the information released.

10. Corrections in the medical record should appear in _____

After your instructor has returned your work to you, make all necessary corrections and place in a three-ring notebook for future reference.

ASSIGNMENT SHEET

Chapter 4: INTERPERSONAL COMMUNICATIONS

Review the objectives and text for each unit before completing the assignment sheet for that unit. When you have completed all sheets for the chapter, remove them from this Workbook and give them to the instructor for evaluation.

Unit 1: VERBAL AND NONVERBAL MESSAGES

SUGGESTED RESPONSES TO CRITICAL THINKING CHALLENGE IN TEXTBOOK

1. What is going on here? _____

2. Does Jackie have a reason to be upset? _____

_____

_____

3. What should Kelly and Sabrina have done to alleviate the brewing situation? _____

_____

A. Unscramble

1. _ _ _ _ _ _ _ _ _ _ _ _   RTMINTRSIEPE
2. _ _ _ _ _ _ _ _ _ _   TIAGBELNN
3. _ _ _ _ _ _ _   SDRTOIT
4. _ _ _ _ _ _ _ _   IUINONITT
5. _ _ _ _ _ _ _ _ _   OIPPETNREC
6. _ _ _ _ _ _ _ _ _ _   ICOGOUNNRSU
7. _ _ _ _ _ _ _ _ _ _ _   UOUSSRUCLLYP
8. _ _ _ _ _ _ _ _ _   NDTICARTCO
9. _ _ _ _ _ _ _ _ _ _   PIEMRIYLALC
10. _ _ _ _ _ _ _ _ _   CUETLTIARA
11. _ _ _ _ _ _ _ _ _ _ _ _   ENZCEOPCUTALI

B. Labeling: Add labels to each boxed section of this communication process model. Refer to Figure 4-1 in the textbook.

C. Brief Answer

1. Describe the basic pattern of communication. _____

_____

_____

2. Give examples of nonverbal communication. _____
_____

3. Explain how verbal and nonverbal communication can sometimes be misinterpreted. _____
_____

4. How can tone and speed of speech affect a message? _____
_____

5. Why is it important to wear appropriate attire when working with patients? _____
_____
_____

6. Explain what perception is. _____

7. Why is it important to develop the skill of perception? _____
_____

8. Why is silence such a powerful nonverbal message (communication)? _____
_____

9. What benefit does the communication of touch provide to patients? _____
_____
_____

D. True or False: Place a "T" for true or "F" for false in the space provided. For false statements, explain why they are false.

_____ 1. The medical assistant can be instrumental in providing comfort and compassion to patients in need.

_____ 2. A harmonious team effort makes for an efficient and pleasant work environment.

_____ 3. Becoming perceptive can only be attained by reading.

_____ 4. Your overall appearance sends out messages to anyone who looks at you.

_____ 5. Setting a good example is not part of your responsibility in the care of others.

_____ 6. Your attitude has nothing to do with your overall appearance.

_____ 7. Gestures are body movements that can help the receiver understand the message being communicated.

_____ 8. Studies show that a caring touch can elicit better response in treatment of patients.

_____ 9. It is possible to contradict a verbal message by an inappropriate facial expression.

_____ 10. Your attitude shows in your facial expression.

_____ 11. Active listening during triage involves repeating back to the patient what was said to you to verify the problem.

_____ 12. There are some expressions, remarks, and hand gestures that may be offensive to those who are from different cultures, backgrounds, or countries.

_____ 13. The proper distance between people who are having a personal conversation is from 10 to 18 feet.

_____ 14. It is very important to be courteous with patients when communicating information to them.

E. Crossword Puzzle

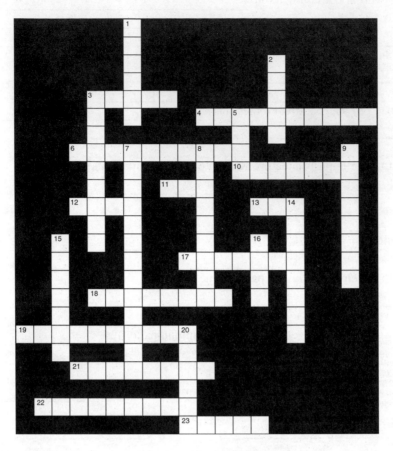

ACROSS

3. How you project this is of utmost importance
4. You must speak this way if you are to be understood
6. Being aware of your own and others' feelings
10. You should set a good _____
11. Effective communication is an _____
12. _____ work
13. Conveys feelings of affection
17. To twist or mess up
18. Efficient use of time comes from _____
19. Good rapport
21. To send a message
22. Unspoken
23. Conveys a positive message

DOWN

1. Spoken
2. Gives patients a sense of security and caring
3. To come between
5. You should speak in a pleasant _____
7. Exchange of information
8. Perception
9. Everyone has them
14. Body movements that send messages
15. What a team gives each other
16. A strong communication (language)
20. You must continually strive to master _____

CRITICAL THINKING SCENARIOS: What would your response be in the following situations?

1. A 25-year-old female patient arrives a half hour early for her appointment. You notice that she is sitting off by herself and is sobbing. _____

_____

2. A middle-aged male patient has just finished a consultation with the doctor. The patient tells you that it is getting harder all the time taking care of his invalid father. _____

_____

3. You notice that a co-worker has made several charting errors in the past few days. It bothers you, for you are worried about quality patient care and the legal ramifications. _____

_____

4. Your physician-employer asks you to help an elderly patient overcome procrastination about taking his medication and eating regularly. _____

_____

5. A young mother of four (ranging in age from 6 months to 5 years) complains to you that she has no time for herself, is always exhausted, and is a nervous wreck. _____

_____

_____

After your instructor has returned your work to you, make all necessary corrections and place in a three-ring notebook for future reference.

ASSIGNMENT SHEET

Chapter 4: INTERPERSONAL COMMUNICATIONS

Unit 2: BEHAVIORAL ADJUSTMENTS

A. Matching: Match the definition in column II with the correct term in column I.

COLUMN I

_____ 1. Adjustment
_____ 2. Analytical
_____ 3. Ardently
_____ 4. Displacement
_____ 5. Intellectualization
_____ 6. Malinger
_____ 7. Projection
_____ 8. Rationalization
_____ 9. Repression
_____ 10. Stratagem
_____ 11. Sublimation
_____ 12. Unobtrusive
_____ 13. Procrastination

COLUMN II

a. To keep down or hold back
b. Devotedly
c. To pretend to be ill
d. To settle or bring into accord
e. Below the threshold of consciousness
f. Rationalism; reasoning without regard to feelings
g. A plan to deceive
h. Question/examine
i. Unconsciously blaming another for one's own inadequacies
j. putting things off
k. Modest; unpretending
l. Transfer of feelings about another to an innocent person
m. Devising a socially acceptable explanation for inadequate behavior
n. Discord; confusion

B. Brief Answer

1. List the commonly used defense mechanisms and give an example of each. _____

_____
_____
_____
_____
_____
_____
_____
_____
_____
_____
_____
_____

2. What could happen to a person who habitually uses one or more of the commonly used defense mechanisms?

_____
_____
_____
_____

3. Why is it necessary to know oneself before one can relate effectively with others? _____

_____

_____

_____

_____

4. What are the problem-solving steps outlined in this unit?

   a. _____

_____

   b. _____

   c. _____

   d. _____

_____

5. Apply the problem-solving steps to a particular problem you may have. _____

_____

_____

_____

6. Explain the importance of one's mental and emotional status to overall health. _____

_____

_____

_____

C. Fill in the Blank

1. Problem-solving skills can help one eliminate _____

2. How we view ourselves is our _____

3. Our response to others is dealt with by our _____

4. Unfortunately, many of us never come close to reaching our true _____

5. Making a list of our strengths and weaknesses is a good way to begin a _____ of ourselves.

6. Two good times to take a look at ourselves for evaluation and renew our goals and aspirations are _____ and _____

7. _____ is a complex process in which one has to be aware of all facets for complete information exchanges to occur.

8. The perceptive medical assistant should be able to decide what _____ to ask a patient to determine whether the look on that patient's face matches the patient's demeanor.

9. The medical assistant must impart a genuine _____ for the patient's well-being.

10. Patients may open up about their problems or preoccupations if the medical assistant shows an _____ and takes the _____ with them that they need.

11. _____ take the blame away from the person you are speaking to and places it on the thing being discussed.

D. Word Search: (1) Find the following words hidden in the puzzle. (2) Use each even-numbered word in a sentence.

1. ACTS
2. AVOID
3. DEFENSE MECHANISMS
4. SELF
5. REGRESSION
6. ACCEPT
7. MALINGER
8. BLAME
9. KIND
10. INFLUENCE

11. ANXIETY
12. RATIONALIZATION
13. CONCERN
14. BEHAVIOR
15. PROBLEM
16. DENIAL
17. PATIENTS
18. EMOTIONS
19. CARE
20. EXPRESS

```
A N L V A Z E S P T V O F T K Q P R O E N
O B S O A C T S A C P S R T L Z M Y M R Y
D R W Z V T A L T S G W L P T O A A B A L
P Z E A O P N S E Q R O A E E S L Z Q C G
A Q R N I N T L Q S R Z P C L B I L R A B
N O V E D E F E N S E M E C H A N I S M S
T D D I O E P G T P G S M A D N G O T Z X
I N F L U E N C E D R A O D L M E B N W O
N I V A L B F I Y Z E D B H M E R L E B T
D K N X C W L T A A S L E F E L A A I L S
I S W A F B E O J L S M H T J B O M T F V
S Z R A T I O N A L I Z A T I O N Z A K A
O P R O X G Z C Q A O T V K B R P F P I L
P C O N C E R N L Z N H I A H P O E R N R
D A A X O W B J E K S N O S S E R P X E Q
Z M B E M O T I O N S A R S S R D M S C B
```

1. _____
2. _____
3. _____
4. _____
5. _____
6. _____
7. _____
8. _____
9. _____
10. _____

After your instructor has returned your work to you, make all necessary corrections and place in a three-ring notebook for future reference.

ASSIGNMENT SHEET

Chapter 4: INTERPERSONAL COMMUNICATIONS

Unit 3: PATIENTS AND THEIR FAMILIES

A. Matching: Match the definition in column II with the correct term in column I.

COLUMN I

_____ 1. Marginal
_____ 2. Holistic
_____ 3. Terminal
_____ 4. Absurd
_____ 5. Incomprehensible
_____ 6. Nonchalant
_____ 7. Hostility
_____ 8. Inevitable
_____ 9. Devastate
_____ 10. Plight

COLUMN II

a. Cannot be understood
b. Showing no interest
c. A sad situation
d. Certain to happen
e. Overwhelm
f. Close to a limit
g. Pertaining to whole
h. Apprehension
i. Ridiculous
j. Antagonistic
k. Final

B. Brief Answer

1. Why is it important to develop good rapport with patients? _____
_____

2. How can the medical assistant safeguard the patient's right to confidentiality? _____
_____
_____
_____

3. What are the patient's options in relation to the physician's treatment plan? _____
_____

4. Describe the stages that patients experience following the diagnosis of terminal illness. _____
_____
_____

5. What is the medical assistant's role in dealing with terminally ill patients? _____
_____

6. What is the purpose of the living will (also referred to as advance directives)? _____
_____
_____

7. What is the purpose of the hospice movement? _____
_____
_____

8. List the services the hospice movement provides. _____
_____
_____
_____

C. Fill in the Blank

1. The first responsibility for the medical professional is to the _____

2. Facing unfamiliar surroundings and unfamiliar medical language adds to the patient's _____

3. Tact and good communication skills help promote _____ with patients.

4. The patient's _____ must be obtained to release information about him or her to unauthorized persons.

5. The physician must be informed of a patient's _____ for it may have some bearing on the condition of the patient.

6. The medical assistant plays an integral part in _____ the physician's orders.

7. _____ is the key in helping patients accept and comply with treatment.

8. By being a good _____ the medical assistant reinforces the physician's advice.

9. A copy of the living will is filed with the physician, the _____ and the family of a terminally ill patient.

10. Terminally ill patients and their families may need _____ guidance more at this time than ever before in their lives.

11. When communicating with patients who speak a different language than you do, an _____ should be scheduled for the time of the patient's appointment.

12. A defense mechanism that protects one from reaching a set goal because it seems too difficult to complete is called _____ behavior.

13. Patients who have documentation stating they do not wish for extreme life-saving efforts should have _____ or _____ written in their chart.

After your instructor has returned your work to you, make all necessary corrections and place in a three-ring notebook for future reference.

ASSIGNMENT SHEET

Chapter 4: INTERPERSONAL COMMUNICATIONS

Unit 4: OFFICE INTERPERSONAL RELATIONSHIPS

SUGGESTED RESPONSES TO CRITICAL THINKING CHALLENGE IN TEXTBOOK

1. What should Marcia do about this situation? _____

_____

2. Should Marcia tell the doctor about Julie's behavior? _____

_____

3. Is there any way that Marcia can suggest that Julie needs a refresher course on professionalism? _____

_____

4. What would you do in this situation? _____

_____

A. Unscramble

1. _ _ _ _ _   YETPT
2. _ _ _ _ _ _ _ _ _ _ LATNEAOIVU
3. _ _ _ _ _ _ _ _ _ _ RLXGNIPEPE
4. _ _ _ _ _   IRMTE
5. _ _ _ _ _ _ _ _ _ _ _ PDSECITRINO
6. _ _ _ _ _ _ _   ULISERE
7. _ _ _ _ _ _ _ _ _ _ VRJETENAUE

B. Brief Answer

1. What are the most important factors in the relationships among medical assistant, employers, and co-workers? _____

_____

_____

2. List positive factors of externship. _____

_____

_____

3. What are the reasons for staff meetings? _____

_____

_____

4. List some methods of intraoffice communication. _____

_____

_____

5. What is the purpose of the employee evaluation? _____

_____

_____

_____

C. Matching: MATCH the definition in column II with the correct term in column I.

COLUMN I

_____ 1. Annual evaluations
_____ 2. Positive attitude
_____ 3. Self-discipline
_____ 4. Medical assistant
_____ 5. Break-time
_____ 6. Cooperation
_____ 7. Intraoffice memo
_____ 8. Teamwork
_____ 9. Job descriptions
_____ 10. Good rapport
_____ 11. AAMA and ARMA

COLUMN II

a. Means of communicating important information to staff
b. Continuing education
c. Results in quality patient care
d. Promote efficiency
e. Necessary to accomplish objectives of physician and patient
f. Regular exercise
g. Creates pleasant work environment
h. Necessary in a professional setting
i. Essential in smooth office operation
j. Motivate employees and keep communication lines open
k. Must relate well to others
l. Essential to well-being

After your instructor has returned your work to you, make all necessary corrections and place in a three-ring notebook for future reference.

ASSIGNMENT SHEET

Chapter 5: THE OFFICE ENVIRONMENT

Review the objectives and text for each unit before completing the assignment sheet for that unit. When you have completed all sheets for the chapter, remove them from this Workbook and give them to the instructor for evaluation.

Unit 1: SAFETY, SECURITY, AND EMERGENCY PROVISIONS IN THE MEDICAL OFFICE

A. Brief Answer

1. List four things to check every morning to assure a safe environment in the medical office.

   a. _____ c. _____

   b. _____ d. _____

2. Identify four hazards to which you should be alert in the business area of an office.

   a. _____ c. _____

   b. _____ d. _____

3. Name five things in an examination room that might cause an unsafe situation.

   a. _____ d. _____

   b. _____ e. _____

   c. _____

4. What does the term *fire triangle* mean? _____

   _____

5. Name seven things that might start a fire in an office.

   a. _____ e. _____

   b. _____ f. _____

   c. _____ g. _____

   d. _____

6. What types of natural disasters require an established office policy regarding appropriate action to take?

   _____

   _____

7. Why are severe weather drills necessary? _____

8. How does knowing what to do or how to act affect a person's response to a crisis? _____

   _____

   _____

   _____

9. How would you clean up the following?

   a. Body fluids _____

   b. Glass fragments _____

10. Name the eight telephone numbers that should be posted near each office telephone.

   a. _____ e. _____

   b. _____ f. _____

   c. _____ g. _____

   d. _____ h. _____

11. Using your local phone directory, complete the "card" below listing the service and its appropriate number.

EMERGENCY NUMBERS

SERVICE	NUMBER	SERVICE	NUMBER
_____	_____	_____	_____
_____	_____	_____	_____
_____	_____	_____	_____
_____	_____	_____	_____

12. What can you do to protect yourself from skin and mucous membrane exposure to harmful organisms? List six examples of protective items. _____

13. Refer to the Role Delineation Chart in Appendix A of the textbook. Within the area of *Legal Concepts,* which three roles relate to the content of this unit? _____

_____

_____

B. Crossword Puzzle

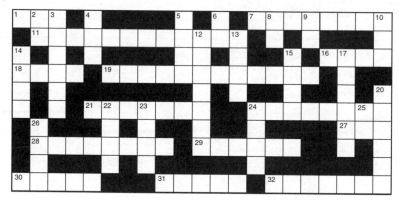

ACROSS
1. A pair
7. To leave
11. Device to put out fire
16. Entranceway
18. Floor coverings
19. Contaminated material
21. Obstruction, a guard
24. Potentially dangerous
28. Holder for soap
29. Reducing danger
30. Remains, left over
31. Covering for hand
32. A disease prevention substance

DOWN
2. Us
3. An essential element for life and combustion
4. The virus associated with AIDS
5. A federal agency
6. Myself
8. Virginia (abbreviation)
9. California (abbreviation)
10. Assists with hearing
12. Dangers
13. Unusual, not common
14. A section, place
15. Combustible material
17. Place of employment
20. Safe, protected from dange
22. The eventual result of HIV
23. Dangerous chance
24. Able to see
25. Learning disabled (abbreviation)
26. A federal agency

After your instructor has returned your work to you, make all necessary corrections and place in a three-ring notebook for future reference.

ASSIGNMENT SHEET

Chapter 5: THE OFFICE ENVIRONMENT

Unit 2: EFFICIENT OFFICE DESIGN

A. Word Puzzle: Use the clues below to spell out these terms.

1. _ _ _ I _ _
2. _ _ _ _ _ M _ _ _
3. _ _ _ _ _ _ P _ _ _ _ _
4. _ _ _ _ _ _ L _ _ _
5. _ _ _ E _ _ _ _ _ _ _
6. _ _ _ _ M _ _ _ _ _
7. _ E _ _ _ _ _ _
8. _ _ _ _ _ N _ _ _ _ _ _
9. _ _ _ T _ _ _ _ _
10. _ _ _ _ A _ _
11. _ _ _ T _ _ _ _ _ _ _ _ _ _
12. _ _ _ I _ _ _ _
13. _ _ _ O _ _ _ _
14. _ _ _ N _ _

1. Layout, arrangement
2. To act out
3. Foresight
4. Limitation, physical handicap
5. Translator
6. To serve
7. Practicable/workable
8. Infectious
9. Nurture
10. Order by law
11. To infect
12. Printing/writing system for the blind
13. Sleeplessness
14. Actions/gestures used to convey information

Name _____

B. Brief Answer

1. Explain the ADA and state when it became effective.

   _____
   _____
   _____
   _____

2. What specifically is mandated by the ADA?

   _____
   _____
   _____
   _____

3. Where in a medical facility should provisions be made for persons with disabilities?

   _____
   _____

4. Explain in your own words what is meant by "efficient office design."

   _____
   _____
   _____

5. Discuss what can make patients feel comfortable and satisfied when visiting a medical facility.

   _____
   _____

6. Discuss the reasons for separating well-visit and sick patients in the reception area.

   _____
   _____

7. Where should rest rooms, public phones, and water fountains be located for patient use in the medical facility?

   _____
   _____

8. Explain the proper way to speak to a hearing-impaired (deaf) person.

   _____
   _____
   _____

9. What may happen if the daily schedule is more often than not backed up? Why?

   _____
   _____

10. Describe how one should speak to a person in a wheelchair.

    _____
    _____

11. Where can information be obtained regarding regulations concerning persons with disabilities?

    _____
    _____

C. True or False: Place a "T" for true or "F" for false in the space provided. For false statements, explain why they are false.

_____ 1. Patients who are hearing-impaired or deaf should have a signer available to communicate their needs

_____ 2. You should talk directly to the interpreter to communicate information for the patient with disabilities.

_____ 3. Proper ventilation and moderate temperature are necessary for comfort in a public facility.

_____ 4. All patients waiting for appointments are placed at-risk for possible exposure to communicable diseases.

_____ 5. The management of the schedule is not a vital part of the medical practice.

_____ 6. All office furniture should be arranged to accommodate wheelchairs.

_____ 7. Educational programs on television for patients to view in the reception room should be very loud so that the hearing-impaired can also benefit from them.

_____ 8. It is a sensible practice when walking in hallways to keep to the right to create and maintain an orderly traffic pattern.

After your instructor has returned your work to you, make all necessary corrections and place in a three-ring notebook for future reference.

ASSIGNMENT SHEET

Chapter 5: THE OFFICE ENVIRONMENT

Unit 3: ERGONOMICS IN THE MEDICAL OFFICE

A. Multiple Choice: Place the correct letter or letters on the blank line for each question.

_____ 1. The science that applies to the physician and staff in the workplace is

     a. physics   c. ecology

     b. psychiatry   d. ergonomics

_____ 2. Considerations that should be taken when planning a medical office layout are

     a. floor plan/blueprints   c. room space

     b. environmental factors   d. all of these

_____ 3. The way to keep the medical facility free of foul odors is to

     a. remove trash as needed   c. use an air freshener

     b. clean routinely   d. all of these

_____ 4. Items that can absorb sound to keep noise at a moderate level are

     a. furniture   c. carpet

     b. reading materials   d. silk flower arrangements

_____ 5. Ergonomists recommend that computer operators

     a. wear wrist supports   c. use special keyboard

     b. vary their duties   d. all of these

B. Brief Answer

1. Why is ergonomics important?

    _____

    _____

    _____

2. What are the two most important points to consider in a medical office layout design?

    _____

    _____

    _____

3. Comment on room size in an office plan.

    _____

    _____

    _____

4. Discuss lighting and how it relates to safety.

    _____

    _____

    _____

5. What is ocular accommodation, and what can be done to prevent it?

    _____

    _____

    _____

6. How is a TV best used in a medical office reception room (if at all)?

    _____

    _____

    _____

7. Refer to Figure 5-13. Why is the work station in this picture ergonomically correct?

_____

_____

_____

C. True or False: Place a "T" for true or "F" for false in the space provided. For false statements, explain why they are false.

_____ 1. A medical office with problems in patient flow and scheduling can be helped by an ergonomist.

_____ 2. Room temperature can affect work performance.

_____ 3. Soft instrumental music can be comforting and relaxing to both staff and patients.

_____ 4. A pleasant decor in the latest color and style in the medical office is meant to impress patients with the physician's success.

_____ 5. The goal of ergonomics is to make jobs as easy and efficient as possible for optimum use of time and space.

D. Unscramble

1. _ _ _ _ _   KOVEE

2. _ _ _ _ _ _ _ _   RMETLANI

3. _ _ _ _ _   REGLA

4. _ _ _ _ _ _   MARUAT

5. _ _ _ _ _ _ _ _ _ _   SDIICEILNP

6. _ _ _ _ _ _   NUTLEN

7. _ _ _ _ _ _ _   YLASPDI

8. _ _ _ _ _ _ _ _   VANOREET

E. Fill in the Blank

1. A varied schedule of duties can help you stay _____

2. The avoidance of _____ is advised with all lighting, as it can impair vision and is uncomfortable as well.

3. _____ may signal problems such as overheating of equipment, chemical leaks, or other serious potential health hazards.

4. The proper _____ of the computer monitor will prevent glare from incoming light from windows and artificial lights in the room.

5. For those who work with computers routinely, a _____ should be used.

6. People feel more _____ in bright and colorful rooms.

7. For those who sit most of the day at work, _____ is necessary to prevent back and other work-related conditions.

8. An adjustable chair is desirable for comfort and _____ of the back.

9. Using a _____ may help in avoiding posture problems.

10. The _____ is the most critical for an ergonomically sound workplace.

After your instructor has returned your work to you, make all necessary corrections and place in a three-ring notebook for future reference.

Name _____

Date _____ Score _____

ASSIGNMENT SHEET

Chapter 5: THE OFFICE ENVIRONMENT

Unit 4: PREPARING FOR THE DAY

SUGGESTED RESPONSES TO CRITICAL THINKING CHALLENGE IN TEXTBOOK

1. Can you put yourself in Mrs. Diaz's place? _____
_____

2. How would you feel? _____
_____
_____
_____
_____
_____

3. Does a person's nationality or skin color affect how he or she are perceived? _____
_____
_____
_____

4. Do you think the office manager should mention this situation to the physician so that other people are not treated the same? _____
_____
_____
_____
_____

5. What could be done in the office to assure that this type of situation does not occur again? _____
_____

Brief Answer

1. Prepare a checklist for opening the office. (Refer to Procedure 5-1.) _____
_____
_____
_____

2. What is the role of the receptionist? _____

3. Why is the reception room atmosphere important? _____

4. Name six things to check in the reception room. _____
_____

5. List information that might be included in a practice information brochure. _____
_____
_____

6. Complete the new patient information form on the following page as if you are the patient. Then role-play being a receptionist and interview another student.

7. Why should social climate be monitored? _____
_____

Name _____

PATIENT INFORMATION   DATE:

| PATIENT'S NAME | | MARITAL STATUS | DATE OF BIRTH | SOCIAL SECURITY NO. |
| | | S | M | W | DIV | SEP | | |

| STREET ADDRESS ☐ PERMANENT ☐ TEMPORARY | CITY AND STATE | ZIP CODE | HOME PHONE NO. |

| PATIENT'S EMPLOYER | OCCUPATION (INDICATE IF STUDENT) | HOW LONG EMPLOYED? | BUSINESS PHONE NO. |

| EMPLOYER'S STREET ADDRESS | CITY AND STATE | ZIP CODE |

| IN CASE OF EMERGENCY CONTACT: | | DRIVERS LIC. NO. |

| SPOUSE'S NAME |

| SPOUSE'S EMPLOYER | OCCUPATION (INDICATE IF STUDENT) | HOW LONG EMPLOYED? | BUSINESS PHONE NO. |

| EMPLOYER'S STREET ADDRESS | CITY AND STATE | ZIP CODE |

| WHO REFERRED YOU TO THIS PRACTICE? |

IF THE PATIENT IS A MINOR OR STUDENT

MOTHER'S NAME	STREET ADDRESS, CITY, STATE AND ZIP CODE	HOME PHONE NO.
MOTHER'S EMPLOYER	OCCUPATION	HOW LONG EMPLOYED?	BUSINESS PHONE NO.
EMPLOYER'S STREET ADDRESS	CITY AND STATE	ZIP CODE
FATHER'S NAME	STREET ADDRESS, CITY, STATE AND ZIP CODE	HOME PHONE NO.
FATHER'S EMPLOYER	OCCUPATION	HOW LONG EMPLOYED?	BUSINESS PHONE NO.
EMPLOYER'S STREET ADDRESS	CITY AND STATE	ZIP CODE

INSURANCE INFORMATION

PERSON RESPONSIBLE FOR PAYMENT, IF NOT ABOVE	STREET ADDRESS, CITY, STATE AND ZIP CODE	HOME PHONE NO.
☐ COMPANY NAME & ADDRESS	NAME OF POLICYHOLDER	CERTIFICATE NO.	GROUP NO.
☐ COMPANY NAME & ADDRESS	NAME OF POLICYHOLDER	POLICY NO.
☐ COMPANY NAME & ADDRESS	NAME OF POLICYHOLDER	POLICY NO.
☐ MEDICARE	MEDICARE NO.	☐ MEDICAID	PROGRAM NO.	COUNTY NO.	ACCOUNT NO.

In order to control our cost of billing, we request that office visits be paid at the time service is rendered. We would rather control our billing costs than be forced to raise our fees.

AUTHORIZATION: I hereby authorize the physician indicated above to furnish information to insurance carriers concerning this illness/accident, and I hereby irrevocably assign to the doctor all payments for medical services rendered. I understand that I am financially responsible for all charges whether or not covered by insurance.

_____
Responsible Party Signature

New patient information form

8. List desirable characteristics for a receptionist. _____
   _____
   _____

9. Complete the charge form on page 48 to reflect the following situation. Use yourself as the patient.
   Insurance company—Health Care One
   Insurance ID—123-45-6789-A Coverage Code S—Group-II
   You have been ill for the past week: fever, chills, coughing, pain over LL chest area, expectorating, blood-tinged
        mucus
   Description Section: new patient, high complexity ($110), culture for strep ($35), therapeutic injection ($25),
   ECG ($50), respiratory function ($70), misc. drugs ($20)
   Diagnosis: acute bronchitis; pneumonia (viral), otitis media
   Doctor: use your physician's name—office visit accept assignment

10. Complete the charge form on page 49 to reflect the following situation. Use yourself as the patient, today's
    date, and the same insurance information as in question 9.
    For interview—about one week ago, you began having abdominal discomfort and occasional diarrhea. The pain
        and frequency of diarrhea have intensified.
    Diagnosis: abdominal pain; diarrhea; diverticulitis
    Description: extended exam—established patient ($85), antibiotic injection ($25)
    Procedure: high sigmoidoscopy ($90)
    Misc.: Review X-ray report ($15)
    Next appt.: one month
    Doctor: use your personal physician

11. What tasks should you do when closing the office for the day?_____
    _____
    _____
    _____

ACHIEVING SKILL COMPETENCY

Reread the performance objective for each procedure and then practice the skills listed below, following the
procedure in your textbook.
Procedure 5-1: Open the Office
Procedure 5-2: Obtain New Patient Information
Procedure 5-3: Close the Office

After your instructor has returned your work to you, make all necessary corrections and place in a three-ring
notebook for future reference.

Name _____

Patient First Name	Patient Last Name		DATE OF ONSET FOR ILLNESS OR ACCIDENT
Responsible Party Last Name	Patient Last Name (If Different)	Date	/ /

CHANGE OF: ☐ NAME ☐ ADDRESS ☐ PHONE ☐ INSURANCE ☐ EMPLOYER

DIAGNOSIS:	CODE	DIAGNOSIS:	CODE	DIAGNOSIS:	CODE	DIAGNOSIS:	CODE	DIAGNOSIS:	CODE
__ Abdominal Pain	789.0	__ Chest Pain	786.50	__ Enteritis	008.0	__ Impetigo	684	__ Pneumonia	486
__ Abrasion	959.9	__ CHF	428.0	__ Esophagitis	530.1	__ Insomnia	780.51	__ Post Menopaus. Atr. Vag.	627.3
__ Abscess	682.9	__ Cholecystitis	575.1	__ Fatigue	780.7	__ Irritable Bowel Synd.	564.1	__ Pregnancy	V22
__ Acne	706.1	__ Cirrhosis	571.5	__ Flu Syndrome	487.1	__ Keratosis	701.1	__ Prostatis Hypertrophy	600
__ Alcoholism	303.9	__ Colitis	558.9	__ FUO	780.6	__ Labyrinthitis	386.3	__ Prostatitis	601.9
__ Allergic Reaction	995.3	__ Concussion	850.9	__ Furuncle	680.9	__ Laceration	882.0	__ Pyelnophritis	590.10
__ Allergic Rhinitis	477.9	__ Conjunctivitis	372.3	__ Gastritis	535.5	__ Laryngitis	464.0	__ Radiculitis	729.2
__ Amenorrhea	626.0	__ Constipation	564.9	__ Gastroenteritis	558.9	__ Low Back Pain	847.9	__ Renal Failure	586
__ Anemia	281.9	__ Costochondritis	733.6	__ GI Bleeding	578.9	__ Lumbar Disc Dis.	847.2	__ Rheum. Arthritis	714.0
__ Angina Pectoris	413.9	__ Contusion	924.9	__ Gingivitis	523.1	__ Lumbar Strain	846.7	__ Sebaceous Cyst	706.2
__ Anxiety State	300.00	__ COPD	496	__ Gout Unspecified	274.9	__ Menopausal Syndr.	672.2	__ Seborrhea	690
__ Appendicitis	541.	__ Corneal Abrasion	918.1	__ Headache, Migraine	346.9	__ Menorrhagia	626.2	__ Seizure Disorder	345.1
__ Arrhythmia	427.9	__ Cough	786.2	__ Headache, Tension	307.81	__ Mult. Contusions	924.0	__ Sinusitis	473.9
__ ASHD	414.0	__ CVA	431	__ Hematuria	599.7	__ Myocard. Inf	429.1	__ Sprain	848.9
__ Asthma	493.9	__ Cystitis	595.9	__ Hemorrhoids	455.6	__ Myositis	729.1	__ Suture Removal	V58.3
__ Atrial Fibrillation	427.31	__ Dementia	331.0	__ Hernia Hiatal	553.3	__ Nephrosclerosis	403.9	__ Tendonitis	726.90
__ Back Pain	724.2	__ Depression	296.2	__ Hernia Ventral	553.20	__ Nose Bleed	784.7	__ Thrombophleb	451.9
__ Breast Fibrocystic Dis.	610.1	__ Derangement Knee	717.9	__ Hernia, Inguinal	550.9	__ Obesity	278	__ Tonsilitis	463
__ Breast Tumor	239.3	__ Dermatitis	692.5	__ Herpes Simplex	054.9	__ Osteoarthritis	715.9	__ Urethritis	597.80
__ Bronchitis Nos.	493.9	__ Diabetes Mellitus	250.00	__ Herpes Zoster	053.9	__ Otitis Externa	380.12	__ URI	460
__ Bursitis	727.3	__ Diarrhea	558.9	__ Hypercholesteremia	272.0	__ Otitis Media	382.9	__ Vaginitis No. 5	616.1
__ CAD	746.85	__ Diverticulitis	562.11	__ Hyperlipidemia	272.4	__ Ovarian Cyst	620.2	__ Vaginitis Trich	131.01
__ Cellulitis		__ Duodenal Ulcer	532.1	__ Hypertension	401.9	__ Pancreatitis	577	__ Vaginitis Candida	112.1
__ Cerv. Disc. Disease	722.9	__ Dysfunct. Uterus Bld.	626.8	__ Hyperventilation	786.01	__ Paronychia, Finger	681.02	__ Vertigo	780.4
__ Cervical Strain Syndr.	723.8	__ Dysmenorrhes	625.3	__ Hypoestrogenism	256.3	__ Paronychia, Toe	681.11	__ Warts, Viral	078.1
__ Cervicitis Chronic	616.0	__ Electrolyte Imb.	276.9	__ Hypothyroidism	244.9	__ Pharyngitis	462		
__ CHD	414.9	__ Endometriosis	617.9	__ Impacted Cerumen	380.4	__ PID	614.9		

DIAGNOSIS: (IF NOT CHECKED ABOVE) _____

✓	DESCRIPTION	CODE/MD	DX	FEE	✓	DESCRIPTION	CODE/MD	DX	FEE	✓	DESCRIPTION	CODE/MD	DX	FEE
	OFFICE VISIT - ESTABLISHED PATIENT					**LABORATORY**					**DIAGNOSTIC PROCEDURES (Cont'd)**			
	Minimal Exam	99211				Venipuncture-DR.	36410				Spirometry	94010YB		
	Limited Exam	99212				Venipuncture	36415				Holter Recording	93224YB		
	Intermediate Exam	99213				Handling	99000				Sigmoidoscopy	45330		
	Extended Exam	99214				Throat Culture	87060				High Sigmoidoscopy	45360		
	Comprehensive Exam	99215				Monilia Culture	87086				Sigmoidoscopy w/ Biopsy	45331		
						Urinalysis	81000							
	OFFICE VISIT - NEW PATIENT					Urine Culture	87086				**PHYSICAL THERAPY**			
	Limited Exam	99202									Hydrocollator	97010		
	Intermediate Exam	99203				**PROCEDURES**					Ultrasound	97128		
	Extended Exam	99204				Arthrocentesis Small Joint	20600				PT Unlisted	97039		
	Comprehensive Exam	99205				Arthrocentesis Interm. Joint	20605							
	Accident Work-up	90020				Arthrocentesis Major Joint	20610				**SUPPLIES**			
						Trigger Point Injection	20550				Surgical Tray A4550	99070		
	INJECTIONS					Cryosurgery Cervix	57511				Sterile Kit	84550		
	B12 J3420	90782				Face Cryosurgery	17000							
	Cortisone J0810	90782				Not Face, 1st	17100				**MISCELLANEOUS**			
	Flu	90724				Not Face, 2nd	17101				Special Reports	99080		
	Pneumovax	90732				Not Face 3 or More, Each	17102				Emergency O.V.	99058		
	Tetanus Toxoid	90703				Ear Lavage	69210				Review X-Ray Report	76140-26		
	DPT	90701												
	Polio	90712												
	MMR	90707												
	HIB	90729				**DIAGNOSTIC PROCEDURES**								
	Estrogen J0970	90782				Audiometry	92552							
	Lidocaine J2000	90782				ECG	93000YB							
	Skin Test (TB, Cocci, Histo)	86585				ECG (Medicare)	93005							
	Therapeutic Inj.	90782												
	Drug: Dose:													
	Antibiotic Inj.	90788												
	Drug: Dose:													

REC'D BY:
☐ CASH
☐ CK. # _____
☐ CO-PAY
☐ MC/VISA

TOTAL FEE	
AMT. REC'D	

Authorization/Responsibility Agreement
I hereby authorize any insurance company to pay the proceeds of any benefits due me directly to: JAY RICHARD HODES, M.D. A copy of this can be considered as an original for insurance purposes.
Signed: _____ Date: _____

I hereby agree to pay my account as services are provided. If for any reason there is a balance owing on my account, I agree to pay promptly upon receipt of the monthly statement.
Signed: _____ Date: _____

I acknowledge and understand that I am responsible for all of the charges for all of the services rendered to me or any member of my family.
Although I have requested the doctor to bill my insurance company on my behalf, I clearly understand that it is still my responsibility to make sure the bill is paid in a reasonable time. If for any reason any portion of my bill is not paid by my insurance, I further agree to make arrangements for prompt payment of the bill.
Signed: _____ Date: _____

NEXT APPOINTMENT

MON	TUES	WED	THUR	FRI	SAT
2 WKS	1 M		2 M		
3 M	6 M		12 M		

DOCTOR'S SIGNATURE & DATE

Charge form for question 9.

PATIENT INFORMATION	PATIENT'S LAST NAME	FIRST	INITIAL	BIRTHDATE		SEX ☐ MALE ☐ FEMALE	TODAY'S DATE

PATIENT INFORMATION				
ADDRESS	CITY	STATE	ZIP	RELATIONSHIP TO SUBSCRIBER	INJURY DATE

SUBSCRIBER OR POLICYHOLDER	INSURANCE CARRIER

ADDRESS	CITY	STATE	ZIP	INS. I.D.	COVERAGE CODE	GROUP

ASSIGNMENT AND RELEASE: I HEREBY AUTHORIZE MY INSURANCE BENEFITS TO BE PAID DIRECTLY TO THE UNDERSIGNED PHYSICIAN. I AM FINANCIALLY RESPONSIBLE FOR NON-COVERED SERVICES. I ALSO AUTHORIZE THE PHYSICIAN TO RELEASE ANY INFORMATION REQUIRED.

IDENTIFY
OTHER HEALTH COVERAGE ☐ YES ☐ NO
DISABILITY RELATED TO:
☐ ACCIDENT ☐ INDUSTRIAL ☐ ILLNESS ☐ OTHER

SIGNED
(PATIENT, OR PARENT, IF MINOR) _____ Date _____

DATE SYMPTOMS APPEARED, INCEPTION OF PREGNANCY, OR ACCIDENT OCCURRED:

✓	DESCRIPTION	CPT/MD	FEE	✓	DESCRIPTION	CPT/MD	FEE	✓	DESCRIPTION	CPT/MD		FEE
	OFFICE VISITS	NEW PT			LABORATORY (Cont'd.)				PROCEDURES			
	Moderate Complex	99203			Wet Mount	87210			EKG	93000	93005	
	Moderate/High Comp.	99204			Pap Smear	88150			Resp. Function Test	94010		
	High Complexity	99205			Handling	99000			Ear Lavage	69210		
	OFFICE VISITS	EST. PT			Hemoccult Stool	82270			Injection Inter. Jt.*	20605		
	Minimal	99211			Glucose	82948			Injection Major Jt.*	20610		
	Self Limited Comp.	99212			INJECTIONS				Anoscopy	46600		
	Low/Moderate Comp.	99213			Vitamin B12/B Complex	J3420			Sigmoidoscopy	45355		
	Moderate Complex	99214			ACTH	J0140			I & D*	10060		
	High Complexity	99215			Depo-Estradiol	J1000			Electrocautery*	17200		
	CONSULTATIONS	OFFICE			Depo Testosterone	J1070			Thromb Hemor.*	46320		
	Moderate Complexity	99243			Imferon	J1760			Inj. Tendon*	20550		
	Mod. to High Comp.	99244			Tetanus Toxoid	J3180						
	HOME	EST. PT			Influenza Vaccine - Flu	90724			MISCELLANEOUS			
	Moderate Complexity	99352			Pneumococcal Vaccine	90732			Drugs, Supplies, Materials	99070		
	ER				TB Tine Test	86585			Special Reports	99080		
	Moderate Severity	99283			Aminophyllin	J0280			Services After Hrs.	99050		
	High Severity	99284			Terbutaline Sulf.	J3105			Services 10pm - 8am	99052		
	LABORATORY				Demerol HCL	J0990			Services Sun. & Holidays	99054		
	Urinalysis - Complete	81000			Compazine	J0780			Counseling	99403		
	Hemoglobin	85018			Injection Therapeutic	90782						
	Culture, Strep/Monilia	87081			Estrone Susp.	J1410						

DIAGNOSIS:

☐ Allergic Rhinitis ...477.9	☐ Chronic Fatigue Synd....300.5	☐ Hemorrhoids ...455.6	☐ Peripheral Vascular Dis ...443.9
☐ Anemia ...280.9	☐ COPD ...496	☐ Hiatal Hernia ...553.3	☐ Pharyngitis ...462.0
☐ Angina Pectoris ...413	☐ Costochondritis ...733.99	☐ Hiatal Hernia & Reflux ...530.1	☐ Pneumonia, Bacterial ...482.9
☐ Anxiety ...300.00	☐ CVA ...431	☐ HVD ...402.10	☐ Pneumonia, Viral ...480.9
☐ Aortic Stenosis ...424.1	☐ Cystitis ...595.9	☐ Hyperlipidemia ...272.4	☐ Prostatitis, Chronic/Acute ...601
☐ ASCVD ...429.2	☐ Deg. Disc. Disease, CX ...722.4	☐ Hypoestrogenism ...256.3	☐ Rectal Bleeding ...569.3
☐ ASHD ...414.9	☐ Deg. Disc. Dis., Lumbar ...722.52	☐ Hypothyroidism ...244.9	☐ Renal Failure, Chronic ...585
☐ Asthma ...493.9	☐ Depression, Endogenous ...296.2	☐ Impacted Cerumen ...380.4	☐ Rheumatoid Arthritis ...714.0
☐ Atrial Fibrillation ...427.31	☐ Dermatitis ...692.9	☐ Influenza, Viral ...487.1	☐ Sinusitis ...461.9
☐ Bigeminy ...427.89	☐ Diabetes Mellitus, Adult ...250.0	☐ Irritable Bowel Syndrome ...564.1	☐ Supraventr. Tachycardia ...427.0
☐ BPH ...600	☐ Diarrhea ...558.9	☐ Laryngitis ...464.0	☐ T.I.A. ...435.9
☐ Bronchitis, Acute ...466.1	☐ Diverticulitis ...562.11	☐ Menopausal Syndrome ...627.2	☐ Tachycardia ...426.89
☐ Bronchitis, Chronic ...491.9	☐ Esophagitis ...530.1	☐ Mitral Insufficiency ...396.2	☐ Tendinitis ...726.90
☐ Bursitis ...726	☐ Fibrocystic Breast Disease ...610.11	☐ Moniliasis ...112	☐ Tonsillitis ...463
☐ Cardiomyopathy ...425.4	☐ Fissure in Ano ...565.0	☐ Myocardial Infarction ...410.9	☐ Ulcer Duodenal ...532.9
☐ Carotid Artery Disease ...433.1	☐ Gastroenteritis ...558.9	☐ Neuritis ...729.2	☐ Ulcer Gastric ...531.9
☐ Cerebral Vascular Disease ...437.9	☐ Gout ...274.9	☐ Osteoarthritis ...715.9	☐ URI ...465.9
☐ CHF ...428.0	☐ HCVD ...429.2	☐ Osteoporosis ...733.0	☐ UTI ...599.0
☐ Cholecystitis ...575.1	☐ Headache, Vascular ...784.0	☐ Otitis Media ...382.9	☐ Vaginitis ...616.10
	☐ Headache, Migraine ...346.9	☐ Parkinsonism ...332	☐ Vertigo ...780.4

DIAGNOSIS: (IF NOT CHECKED ABOVE)	REF. DR. & #

DOCTOR'S SIGNATURE / DATE	**NO SERVICES PURCHASED**	SERVICE PERFORMED	ACCEPT ASSIGNMENT	TODAY'S FEE	

INSTRUCTIONS TO PATIENT FOR FILING INSURANCE CLAIMS

1. MAIL THIS FORM DIRECTLY TO YOUR INSURANCE COMPANY. ATTACH YOUR OWN INSURANCE COMPANY'S FORM.

PLEASE REMEMBER THAT PAYMENT IS YOUR OBLIGATION, REGARDLESS OF INSURANCE OR OTHER THIRD PARTY INVOLVEMENT.

OFFICE ☐   YES ☐   AMT. REC'D TODAY
E.R. ☐   NO ☐
HOME ☐   TOTAL DUE

Charge form for question 10.

Name _____

Date _____ Score _____

ASSIGNMENT SHEET

Section 2: THE ADMINISTRATIVE ASSISTANT

Chapter 6: ORAL AND WRITTEN COMMUNICATIONS

Review the objectives and text for each unit before completing the assignment sheet for that unit. When you have completed all sheets for the chapter, remove them from this Workbook and give them to the instructor for evaluation.

Unit 1: TELEPHONE COMMUNICATIONS

A. Multiple Choice: Place the correct letter or letters on the blank line for each question.

_____ 1. Desirable skills and qualities that the medical assistant who handles phone calls should have are

    a. courtesy   c. active listening

    b. good grooming   d. great personality

_____ 2. When the phone rings in the office, it should be answered by the _____ ring.

    a. first   c. third

    b. second   d. fourth

_____ 3. When holding the phone to your ear, the receiver should be _____ inches in front of your mouth.

    a. 1–2 inches   c. 4–5 inches

    b. 2–3 inches   d. 6–8 inches

_____ 4. Patients who phone the office for an appointment should be given _____ choices.

    a. one   c. three

    b. two   d. four

_____ 5. You should _____ file a report that the physician has not seen.

    a. never   c. always

    b. sometimes   d. immediately

B. Fill in the Blank

1. Essential items that should be next to each telephone in a medical facility are a _____ _____ and a _____.

2. The _____ established by the medical assistant who answers the phone will contribute to successful communication with patients.

3. The responsibility of responding to phone calls in a medical office takes a great deal of _____ and _____.

4. It is a sensible practice to have all _____ phone numbers listed by each phone in the office.

5. All telephone messages that are urgent should be given _____ and handled as soon as possible.

6. You should be _____ about your knowledge and experience with phone systems.

7. When answering a phone call of a patient, make sure you get the caller's _____ and _____ in case the call is an emergency and it is interrupted.

8. The appointment should be _____ by reading the appointment time back to the patient after it has been recorded in the appointment book.

9. Only patient information that has been _____ by the patient in writing, with the patient's signature, may be given to another party.

10. If you have made an error on a patient's bill, be sure to _____ it, _____ and offer to send a _____ statement.

11. When placing long-distance phone calls, it is advisable to consult a telephone directory for a
_____ so you can establish the appropriate time to call.

12. Never tell anyone over the phone (or in person) that you are _____ as it may be an invitation for undesirable behavior.

13. If the physician requests that you monitor a phone call, it is important that the caller _____ to your listening and taking notes.

C. True or False: Place a "T" for true or "F" for false in the space provided. For false statements, explain why they are false.

_____ 1. A pleasant voice and good listening skills are essential in telephone communications.

_____ 2. When patients call for information about their condition or lab report results, it is not necessary to pull their chart.

_____ 3. All telephone calls, regardless of what you feel about their importance, should be documented.

_____ 4. The answering machine in the medical office should be turned on to leave a message to callers only on weekends when the physician is not in the office.

_____ 5. Telephone callers form a picture of you as they listen to your voice.

_____ 6. When you finish a conversation over the phone with a patient, you should hang up first to let the patient know you are finished talking.

_____ 7. When an attorney phones for information about a patient, you must provide the necessary information immediately.

_____ 8. Always be sure to make a copy of any correspondence mailed out so you have a copy for the patient's chart.

_____ 9. The physician usually does not wish to speak to unidentified phone callers during busy office hours.

_____ 10. When answering the medical office phone, and the physician is not there, you should always know where to reach him or her.

_____ 11. You should never leave a patient on hold for more than 10 minutes.

_____ 12. You should screen and complete as many calls as possible before adding names to the physician's call-back list.

D. Brief Answer

1. List the common types of calls that are received in a medical office. _____
_____
_____

2. Explain why a telephone triage manual should be kept by the phone to manage telephone calls in a medical facility. _____
_____
_____

3. List the important items of a telephone message. _____
_____
_____
_____

E. Crossword Puzzle

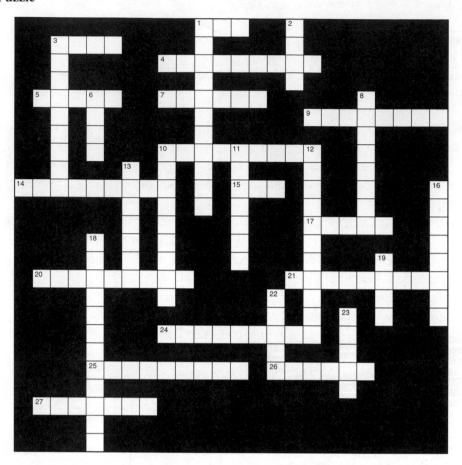

ACROSS

1. A number of sheets of paper fastened together
3. A given point of time
4. Relevant, applicable
5. To analyze by application of reagents—to prove knowledge
7. Induce to action
9. Mechanical device for recording sounds
10. An associate in an office, usually one of similar status
14. Person practicing medical profession
15. Writing instrument
17. A receptionist will answer telephone _____
20. Made known in words or actions
21. Conventional rules for correct behavior
24. A preliminary or indicating procedure
25. A helper or co-worker in a specific occupation
26. Tool or plan
27. Pertaining to medicine

DOWN

1. The personal or individual quality that makes one person different from another
2. The sound of a bell
3. A book containing lists of names and addresses
6. A chance of a life _____
8. Place for healing
10. Verified; ratified
11. Sympathetically trying to identify one's feelings with those of another
12. Pronouncing clearly
13. Sixty in each hour
16. Type of work or commerce
18. Prove to be true; supported by facts
19. Depend; trust
22. Coming next after second in a series
23. Sound produced through mouth

DIRECTIONS: Read the following situations out loud in class and role-play how you would handle them. Answers will vary. Your instructor may want to guide the situations.

TELEPHONE WORKSHEET 1: "I HAVE TO SEE THE DOCTOR—TODAY!"

Doctor's Identity: (Use names of local physicians)

Solo or Group: Two-physician partnership

Specialty: Family practice

Time: 8:30 A.M.

Situation: Both physicians are on hospital rounds and are not expected until 10:00 A.M. The appointment book is full.

Patient: (insert name of student or fictitious name), a patient since infancy

---

"I need an appointment today—right away. I'm leaving for college tomorrow, and the doctor just has to see me. Just for a minute. I need a quick physical and a form filled out. It's nothing really."

"I can't register for class unless the doctor sees me. I just have to have an appointment. I know this is last minute—but just this once, please. Certainly, you understand, you have to."

How did you handle this?

Instructor will need to evaluate each student answer. Answers will vary.

TELEPHONE WORKSHEET 2: MOTHER WHO WANTS TO MAKE AN APPOINTMENT FOR
HERSELF AND HER CHILD

Doctor's Identity: (Use name of local physician)

Solo or Group: Solo practice

Specialty: OB/GYN

Time: 10:00 A.M.

Situation: The physician is in an area where there are a number of pediatricians, and he does not
                           see pediatric patients.

Patient: (fictitious name) Mrs. _____

Mrs. _____ is new in the area and got the doctor's name from calling the county medical society. She has a
history of menstrual difficulty. She has no immediate problem, but wants to make an appointment with an
OB/GYN physician in this new location in order to establish a "regular" doctor.

She tells the medical assistant that she wants to bring (fill in name of child) with her, and wants to make an
appointment for _____ too, immediately following her appointment. _____ is her 4-year-old daughter.

Mrs. _____ does not want to accept the fact that Dr. _____ will not see _____. She argues that she has to bring
_____ with her, there is no one to take care of her, and this is not really an inconvenience to Dr. _____. It will
just take a 10-minute check for _____ , and Mrs. _____ is willing to make an appointment two or three weeks
in advance for the doctor's convenience.

How did you handle this?

Instructor will need to evaluate each student answer. Answers will vary.

TELEPHONE WORKSHEET 3: PATIENT INSISTS ON APPOINTMENT

Doctor's Identity: (Use names of local physicians)

Solo or Group: Two-physician partnership

Specialty: Internal medicine

Time: 3:30 P.M.

Situation: Dr. _____ is out of the office today.
          Dr. _____ is in the examining room with a patient. The office is already behind schedule because Dr. _____ has had to work in a couple of emergency patients of Dr. _____.

Patient: (fictitious name) Mrs. _____ is a regular patient (she has been to the office two or three times a year). The medical assistant knows her well enough to recognize the name and identify it with a 64-year-old widow living alone. Mrs. _____ has always been very nice, but is a little bit on the "dramatic" side.

Mrs. _____ calls and says she is very ill and would like to see (Dr. who is out of the office) right away. She says she has had a headache since mid-morning and it is getting worse. She has had these headaches before, and Dr. _____ has always given her something to stop them. She doesn't have any more of the little pills and she feels just awful. She knows she will be sick all night if something isn't done right away. Although she feels real bad, she will get in a cab and come to the office right now.

She will see (Dr. in office) if necessary, but she prefers to see (Dr. who is out of the office) since he is her regular doctor. She thinks the doctor should see her now when she feels so bad. There is no use for the doctor to see her two or three days from now, when she may be feeling all right—if she lives through the night.

She doesn't threaten or get abusive, but is persistent and keeps repeating that she must see the doctor right now.

How did you handle this?
Instructor will need to evaluate each student answer. Answers will vary.

TELEPHONE WORKSHEET 4: "WE'RE ON VACATION"

Doctor's Identity: (Use name of local physician)

Solo or Group: Solo practice

Specialty: Internist

Time: Late afternoon in July

Situation: The doctor is in and he is seeing his last scheduled patient for the day.

Patient: (fictitious name)

The caller simply identifies herself as Mrs. _____. She has a thick southern accent. The medical assistant does not know her.

The woman is sniffling and is saying, "My baby, my baby, _____ is so sick. Is the doctor there? I just know my baby needs help. Is the doctor there? I'm just visiting here, my husband left me in the hotel here and has been out fishing and camping for two days. The baby has a high fever and just keeps crying. I'm all alone, I don't know what to do."

How did you handle this?

Instructor will need to evaluate each student answer. Answers will vary.

TELEPHONE WORKSHEET 5: THE ANGRY AND ABUSIVE PATIENT

Doctor's Identity: (Use name of local physician)

Solo or Group: Solo practice

Specialty: Family practice

Time: 1:30 P.M.

Situation: The appointment book is completely filled and the only time for a regular office visit is 2½ weeks ahead, on Thursday at 2:00 P.M.

Patient: (fictitious name) Mrs. _____ has been in the office two or three times during the past year, and has always been rather quiet and reserved. Mrs. _____ has high blood pressure, which is being handled very well with medication, but she is supposed to come into the office every three or four months for a checkup. This office does not schedule appointments that far in advance. The doctor has simply said, "Come back every two or three months." Mrs. _____ has never seemed unreasonable before, but today she is in a very bad mood.

Mrs. _____ calls for an appointment and the medical assistant advises her that the first opening is 2½ weeks ahead. When the medical assistant gives her this information, her immediate response is that this is not at all convenient. She says that she planned to see the doctor in the next several days and that she has no idea where she will be in 2½ weeks. She thinks she might be taking a vacation trip somewhere, and she simply does not want to wait this long for an appointment.

As the conversation continues, Mrs. _____ gets more and more argumentative and points out that all she wants is a checkup, which will take the doctor only a few minutes, and that if it was anything more than that she would probably be dead before the doctor could get around to seeing her. She argues that she isn't demanding to see the doctor immediately, that an appointment in the next three or four days will be satisfactory, but that waiting 2½ weeks for a simple checkup is not reasonable.

Finally, Mrs. _____ gets nasty. She says she wants to talk to the doctor. She wants to know just who is running the medical practice. She doesn't think the doctor really knows what is going on. She mentions that she is running low on her pills and doesn't think that her medication will last for 2½ weeks more.

How did you handle this?
Instructor will need to evaluate each student answer. Answers will vary.

Name _____

TELEPHONE WORKSHEET 6: INSISTS ON TALKING TO THE DOCTOR

Doctor's Identity: (Use name of local physician)

Solo or Group: Solo practice

Specialty: Family practice

Time: Early Monday morning

Situation: The doctor is in the examining room with a patient. The appointment schedule is already overbooked, and this is going to be another day when all of the patients have a long wait in the reception room, and both the doctor and the medical assistant will be working overtime.

Patient: (fictitious name) An elderly widower, a regular patient who makes an appointment to see the doctor almost every month most of the time for imagined ills.

Mr. _____ calls and says, "I need to talk with Dr. _____. I've had a splitting headache all weekend. I knew he would be out on the golf course or some such thing—so I waited until now to call. I just can't wait any longer. Put me through to him. I'll only take a minute."

The medical assistant replies that Dr. _____ is seeing a patient in the examining room and that he will call back.

"That's what you always say," Mr. _____ replies. "If I was dying I would have to wait for a convenient time? All I want to do is talk to the doctor for just a minute."

The medical assistant repeats that the doctor is in the examining room and suggests a call-back.

Mr. _____, "I had to get out of bed to come to the phone, so I'll just hang on. That certainly isn't going to inconvenience him. You just tell him that I'm holding the phone. I don't like waiting—I waited all weekend and I don't want to be put off a moment longer than necessary. I pay my bills and I deserve to talk to the doctor when I need him."

How did you handle this?
Instructor will need to evaluate each student answer. Answers will vary.

59

TELEPHONE WORKSHEET 7: CALL TO NOTIFY PATIENT

Doctor's Identity: (Use names of local physicians)

Solo or Group: Partnership

Specialty: OB/GYN

Time: 1:00 P.M.

Situation: Both physicians have called in to say that they will be late in returning to the office.
It seems all of the babies in town decided to be born today. Dr. _____ , anticipating
a caesarean section, says he may not be in at all. Dr. _____ says that he will be at
least one hour late, and maybe longer. Here office protocol is to notify patients, who
have not as yet arrived, of the delay.

Patient: (fictitious name)

You call Mrs. _____ and tell her of the delay. She has an appointment for 3:00 P.M., which she made about three
weeks ago. She is upset—you can tell this from the tone of her voice.
The medical assistant knows from past experience that the best thing to do would be to cancel Mrs. _____'s
appointment and reschedule her. This can't be done. About the earliest time that Dr. _____ can see Mrs. _____
will be 5:00 to 5:30 P.M.
Mrs. _____ is not enthusiastic about either alternative.

How did you handle this?
Instructor will need to evaluate each student answer. Answers will vary.

Name _____

TELEPHONE WORKSHEET 8: THE CASE OF THE HOLD BUTTON

Doctor's Identity: (Use name of local physician, female)

Solo or Group: Solo practice

Specialty: General surgery

Time: 10:00 A.M.

Situation: Dr. _____ has advised the patient that if her incision continues to ooze, she is to call the doctor. The doctor has advised the medical assistant that if the patient calls, she will want to talk with her.

Patient: (fictitious name)

Mrs. _____ calls; the doctor is in her consulting office and the medical assistant plans to transfer the call immediately to Dr. _____. Mrs. _____ is not upset, or doesn't seem to be, on the telephone. Dr. _____ is upset after talking with Mrs. _____ because she was having no trouble with her incision. All she needed was an appointment.

What did the medical assistant fail to do?
Instructor will need to evaluate each student answer. Answers will vary.

Name _____

TELEPHONE WORKSHEET 9: THE PATIENT WHO HAS BEEN A NO-SHOW

Doctor's Identity: (Use name of local physician)

Solo or Group: Solo practice

Specialty: Family practice

Time: 11:30 A.M.

Situation: The patient calls for an appointment. The patient had an appointment the previous week, but didn't show or call in. The patient simply says she was busy last Thursday and just couldn't make it. The appointment was only for a checkup, but she wants to make another appointment for now.

Patient: (fictitious name)

The medical assistant can make an appointment for approximately two weeks from today. Mrs. _____ is willing to accept that.

What should the medical assistant say in regard to the previous "no-show"?
Instructor will need to evaluate each student answer. Answers will vary.

TELEPHONE WORKSHEET 10: "I *MUST* SPEAK TO THE DOCTOR!"

Doctor's Identity: (Use names of local physicians)

Solo or Group: Two-physician partnership

Specialty: OB/GYN

Time: 3:00 P.M.

Situation: Both physicians are in the office, and are busy seeing patients. They have a well-established practice and haven't been taking new patients unless they have been referred by associates.

Patient: (fictitious name)

A woman calls and identifies herself as _____. Mrs. _____ is obviously very upset. She says, "I need to talk with a doctor right away. My friend _____ told me that Dr. _____ was the best doctor in town." The medical assistant explains the doctor's policy.

Breathlessly, Mrs. _____ continues. "I need to talk to the doctor, really. I'm new in town. I don't know what to do. My sister in Omaha just called to say that she has found a lump on her breast and it has been identified as cancer. We lost our mother from cancer last year. I'm scared. I need to talk to the doctor. Please—can't you make an exception just this once?" Mrs. _____ then begins sobbing on the telephone.

How did you handle this?
Instructor will need to evaluate each student answer. Answers will vary.

ASSIGNMENT SHEET

Chapter 6: ORAL AND WRITTEN COMMUNICATIONS

Unit 2: SCHEDULE APPOINTMENTS

A. Brief Answer

1. What are the most important points in scheduling when a patient calls the office for an appointment?

_____

_____

2. Describe the best way to schedule a patient who is always late. _____

_____

3. List the advantages of a computer scheduling system. _____

_____

_____

4. What information should be in the office procedure manual that would be helpful in making appointments outside the office? _____

_____

_____

B. Multiple Choice: Place the correct letter or letters on the blank line for each question.

_____ 1. Time blocked off in the schedule book that is not for patient appointments is called the
    a. schedule   c. manual
    b. matrix   d. cancelation

_____ 2. When patients cancel appointments, you should
    a. cross them off the schedule with one line through their name
    b. note C & C on the chart and the reason for canceling
    c. notify the physician
    d. a and b only

_____ 3. How long should medical office appointment books be kept in a secured area away from patient access and any unauthorized persons?
    a. indefinitely   c. five years
    b. three years   d. seven years

_____ 4. The preferred method of payment for services provided by the physician is/are
    a. cash   c. credit card
    b. check/money order   d. a and b

_____ 5. To keep medical records updated, how often should you ask patients about any changes in their personal data (insurance, phone number, address, etc,)?
    a. at each visit   c. once a year
    b. every six months   d. not necessary, patient will tell you

_____ 6. When do patients have to precertify services with their insurance company to ensure coverage?
    a. mental health counseling   c. emergency services where they live
    b. all office visits   d. substance abuse counseling

C. Matching: MATCH the definition in column II with the correct term in column I.

COLUMN I

_____ 1. Wave
_____ 2. Open hours
_____ 3. Streaming
_____ 4. Clustering
_____ 5. Single-booking
_____ 6. Modified wave
_____ 7. Double-booking

COLUMN II

a. Appointments are made to accommodate specific needs of patients according to the amount of time that is generally adequate (for continuous patient flow)

b. This method is used for patients who will take a considerable amount of time-45 minutes to an hour

c. Appointment times are given to two or more patients for the same time

d. No appointments made; patients sign, in noting time of arrival

e. Appointments are made in the first 30 minutes of each hour—second half hour is for work-ins

f. A group of patients with the same complaint, diagnosis, or other commonality are scheduled sequentially every 10 minutes

g. Same as wave with additional scheduling of the second half of the hour in 10- to 20-minute intervals, according to the medical problem

D. True or False: Place a "T" for true or "F" for false in the space provided. For false statements, explain why they are false.

_____ 1. Information regarding office hours should be placed in phone directories and wherever applicable.

_____ 2. Downtime refers to the time when the computer is not functional.

_____ 3. You should place an OUTguide in place of every chart that is pulled for the daily schedule.

_____ 4. The process of rescheduling involves calling each scheduled patient and offering an alternative appointment time as close to the original one as possible.

_____ 5. When scheduling an appointment for a patient, you should offer several choices of times for the appointment.

_____ 6. The term *precertification* means that certain procedures and treatments must be approved with the patient's insurance company for guaranteed payment of services before the patient receives the service.

_____ 7. Leaving the appointment book open for unauthorized persons to view breaks the laws of confidentiality.

_____ 8. Delays in the appointment schedule do not have to be made known to patients because it will upset them.

_____ 9. Appropriate printed information and instructions should be given to a patient for a referral appointment.

E. Word Search: Find the following words hidden in the puzzle.

SERVICE	RAPPORT	WAVE
SEVERE	CODES	STAFF
TRIAGE	DOWNTIME	STYLE
GATEKEEPER	ROUTINE	FLEX
PERIODIC	CRITERION	PHONE
PRECERTIFICATION	PATIENT	REMOTE
APPOINTMENT	SCHEDULE	GUARANTOR
STREAMING	COMPLICATIONS	INFORMATION
SEQUENTIALLY	DELAY	STRESS
GOALS		

```
P E R I O D I C S O M R I S S
G O A L S C L O S W A A N E E
A P P O I N T M E N T P F Q V V
T R I A G E D P R S R P O U E C
E C O D E S H L T T I O R E R R
K D A I L Y J I S A X R M N E I
E M S E R V I C E F I T A T R T
E W S T Y L E A Z F L P T I O E
P A I D O W N T I M E H I A U R
E V E A P A T I E N T O O L T I
R E M O T E D O U B F N N L I O
S T R E A M I N G T L E K Y N N
D E L A Y F E S C H E D U L E Z
G U A R A N T O R A X P B C V O
P R E C E R T I F I C A T I O N
```

F. Completion

Use the appointment schedule provided. Establish the matrix. Office hours are:

Mondays: 8–5 P.M. (Lunch break 12:00–1:15 P.M.)
Tuesdays: 8:30 A.M.–2:30 P.M. (Lunch break 12–12:30 P.M.)
Wednesdays: 12:30–6:00 P.M.

Use the list of patients and list of abbreviations in Figure 6-14 of the textbook to fill in the appointment schedule. You should be able to find room for all on the schedule.

INFORMATION SHEET FOR APPOINTMENTS

NAME	PHONE	COMPLAINT OR PROCEDURE	MINUTES	BEST TIME
1. Koch, Curtis	555-0123	Stepped on rusty nail	15	emergency
2. Harris, Dezzie	555-1234	Shortness of breath, dizziness	14	early p.m.
3. Hall, Pauline	555-2345	Smallpox vaccination for travel	15	any time
4. Graves, Connie	555-3456	Headache and sinus trouble	15	after work
5. Ford, Kenneth	555-4567	Cough and cold	15	any time
6. Edwards, Melvin	555-5678	Rectal examination and consultation	15	late p.m.
7. Dennis, Mrs. P.A.	555-6789	Annual physical exam; Pap test	30	a.m.
8. Daniels, Dave	555-8910	New patient	30	Monday
9. Carr, Bruce	555-9102	Company examination, new employee	30	Monday
10. Booth, Vivian	555-1023	Injury to ankle	15	Monday, p.m.
11. Block, Jimmy	555-3457	Check leg cast	15	a.m.
12. Bergstrom, Stephen	555-4680	Examination; complaint of pain in hands and knees	15	late Wednesday
13. Applegate, Elmo	555-1357	Follow-up exam and ECG	15	Monday, late p.m.
14. Anders, L.K.	555-0987	Treatment of leg ulcer	15	early a.m.
15. Appleby, Nathan	555-1193	Injection and consultation	15	Monday, late p.m.
16. Jefferson, Thomas	555-7890	Remove sutures and dressing, following hernia operation	15	any time
17. Benson, Mrs. C.L.	555-5789	Exam and consult regarding gallbladder surgery	30	Wednesday, after 4
18. Hanning, Dianne	555-6890	Remove small growth by eye under local	30	a.m.
19. Blair, Robert	555-7901	Chest congestion	15	receive complaint today
20. Frost, Theresa	555-8012	IUD insertion	30	late p.m.
21. Booth, Earl	555-9123	Injury to ankle	15	Monday, p.m.
22. Ford, Anna	555-0985	Dressing to injured finger	15	Wednesday
23. Callahan, Barbara	555-0984	Remove wood splinter in leg	30	emergency
24. Dyer, Sandra	555-0983	Excise lesion on back	30	early p.m.
25. Carter, Gertrude	555-0982	Infection on face	15	Wednesday
26. Davis, Charles L.	555-0981	Examination, possible hernia	15	Tuesday
27. Guthrie, Mrs. June	555-0980	Desires weight reduction	15	a.m.
28. Underwood, Edgar	555-0979	Dog bite; left hand	15	emergency
29. Landers, Hubert	555-0978	Consultation regarding plastic surgery for facial scars from auto accident	10	near noon
30. Meyer, Thomas	555-0977	College examination, urinalysis, drug screen	30	any time
31. Thornton, Helen	555-0976	Weakness; patient thinks she is anemic	15	any time
32. Ochs, Glenn	555-0975	Preschool exam, booster injection	15	a.m.
33. Saunders, Mrs. G.	555-0974	Post-op dressing, breast surgery	15	early p.m.
34. Poff, Richard	555-0973	Crushed finger in car door	15	emergency
35. Rambo, Clyde	555-0963	Complete physical exam	30	early p.m.
36. Quinn, Mrs. Mary J.	555-0953	Influenza vaccine injection	5	any time
37. Owens, Russell	555-0954	Aspirate left elbow	15	late a.m.
38. Stone, Ann	555-0843	Prolonged menstrual periods	15	after work
39. Lee, Felix	555-0732	Dressing to toe injury	15	noon
40. Nye, Peter	555-0132	Check blood pressure, weight, urine	15	a.m.

Name _____

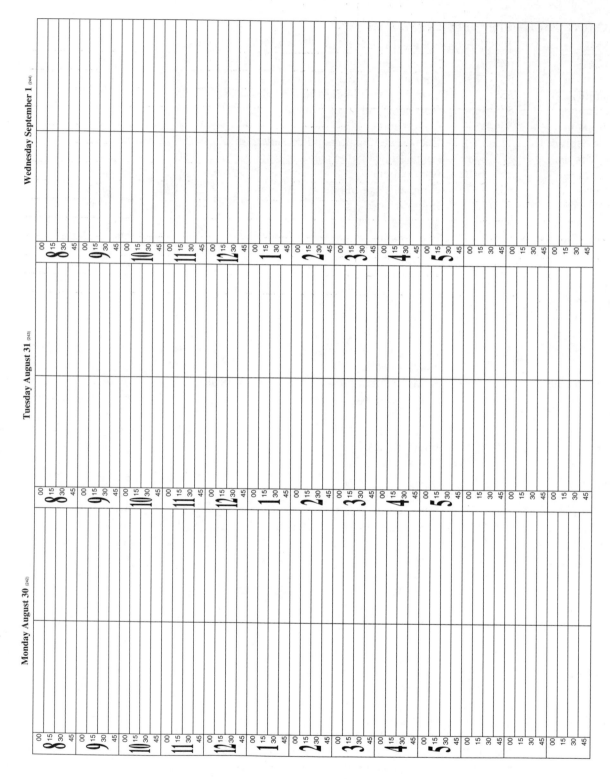

Monday August 30 (242)	Tuesday August 31 (243)	Wednesday September 1 (244)

Appointment Schedule

G. Brief Answer: Spell out the following abbreviations.

1. NP _____
2. CPE or CPX _____
3. FU _____
4. NS _____
5. RS _____
6. C & C _____
7. Ref _____
8. Re _____
9. PT _____
10. Cons _____
11. Inj _____
12. ECG _____
13. Sig _____
14. Surg _____

After your instructor has returned your work to you, make all necessary corrections and place in a three-ring notebook for future reference.

ASSIGNMENT SHEET

Chapter 6: ORAL AND WRITTEN COMMUNICATIONS

Unit 3: WRITTEN COMMUNICATIONS

A. Brief Answer

1. List seven types of communication medical assistants may need to compose. _____

_____

_____

2. Prepare an IOC to inform six persons in your class about the following: Field trip to your local Health Department, one month from today at 9:00 A.M., returning by noon. Request verification of reading.

_____

_____

_____

_____

_____

_____

_____

_____

_____

3. List six instances when form letters are appropriate. _____

_____

_____

_____

4. Fill in the Blank: Using the following abbreviations, determine which type of correspondence is appropriate to the stated situation.

Types: IOC, IN (informal note), Per Let (personal letter), Pro Let (professional letter), BL (business letter), IS (information sheet)

_____ a. Sending information to a referred patient

_____ b. Correspondence to colleagues on hospital board

_____ c. Congratulations to a friend

_____ d. Instructions for a diagnostic procedure

_____ e. Request for membership information at a golf club

_____ f. Request to accountant for mid-year status

_____ g. Employee memo regarding change in office insurance benefits

_____ h. Request for medical practice reciprocity in another state

5. Spelling: Each line contains three different spellings of a word. Underline the correctly spelled word.

apostrophy	apostrofe	apostrophe
communication	comunication	communikation
congratulations	congradulations	congratulashuns
contraction	contrackion	contracshun
coresspondence	correspondence	correspondance
hiphen	hyfen	hyphen
mispelled	misspeled	misspelled
modafies	modifies	modifyes
stationery	stationairy	stationare

6. Following information in the textbook on punctuation, capitalization, and mailable standards, type Letters 1, 2, and 3 following the instruction for each letter; letterheads are provided. Final copy should meet mailable standards. _____

7. List the problem areas to watch when proofreading. _____

_____

8. Prepare corrected Letter 4 by interpreting proofreader's marks.

9. Given a dictating machine tape, produce a mailable letter according to Procedure 6-7, Compare a Business Letter. _____

10. Refer to the CAAHEP Standards in Appendix B of the textbook. Within the area of *Communication,* which three curriculum standards are discussed in this unit? _____

_____

LETTER 1

The first letter is to Robert Jones, M.D., 5000 N. High Street, Yourtown, US 43200. The name of the patient is Juan Gomez. Use full block style seen in Figure 6-20(B) and proper capitalization, punctuation, and placement on the paper.

Dear dr jones

your patient juan gomez was first seen October 7, complaining of severe tinnitus in both ears.

On physical examination his hearing was 15/20 right ear 13/20 left ear audiogram was made which showed considerable loss of high tones Mr. gomez's complaints of tinnitus and decreased hearing are in accordance with the audiometric and clinical findings of beginning degeneration of his nerve of hearing. In all probability this condition has been caused by loud noises which he has encountered in his work.

despite treatment his hearing has not increased and tinnitus persists.

thank you for referring mr gomez.

very truly yours

LETTER 2

Type the second letter using modified block style seen in Figure 6-20(C). Use current date for the letter. Address the letter to John Jones, M.D., 3530 Main Street, Cold Springs, KY 41076. The name of the patient is Mrs. Patty Segal. The dictating physician is Samuel E. Matthews, M.D.

I saw _____ on _____ for X-ray examination.

AP and lateral roentgenograms of the cervical spine show an aberration of the normal cervical curve. The curve is convexed posteriorly at the level of the fifth, sixth, and seventh cervical vertebrae. Normally, the posterior curve should be concave. There are no significant hypertrophic changes, but there are minimal true arthritic changes involving the articular facets in the lower cervical region.

A roentgenogram of the right shoulder shows no evidence of intrinsic bone disease. There is no periarticular soft tissue calcification in the region of the bruise.

Thank you for your referral

Very truly yours,

LETTER 3

Type the following letter using modified block with indented paragraphs as seen in Figure 6-20(D). The letter is to Robert Jones, M.D., 5000 N. High Street, Yourtown, US 98765. The patient is Patricia Moriarty. The letter is from Kerry Smith, M.D.

Dear Dr. Jones:

I saw _____ in the office today. You will recall that she has suffered from menstrual discomfort and intermenstrual pain for the past 6 months.

On examination, the breasts are well developed and free of masses. On pelvic examination, the hymen is intact; and vaginal examination was not performed. On rectal examination, the uterus was anterior and freely movable. The right adnexa were normal. The left ovary was enlarged to the size of a walnut or slightly larger and was cystic. Compression of this ovary reproduced the patient's pain.

Patricia was asked to return in three weeks for re-examination to determine the need for treatment of ovarian enlargement.

Thank you for referring this patient.

Sincerely,

LETTERHEAD 1

SAMUEL E. MATTHEWS, M.D.

SUITE 120 100 E. MAIN STREET

YOURTOWN, US 98765-4321

LETTERHEAD 2

SAMUEL E. MATTHEWS, M.D.

SUITE 120 100 E. MAIN STREET

YOURTOWN, US 98765-4321

Name _____

LETTERHEAD 3

KERRY SMITH, M.D.

101 LANE AVENUE

YOURTOWN, US 12345

LETTER 4: Letter to Be Corrected

Kerry Smith, M.D.
101 Lane Avenue
Yourtown, US 12345

Rob*e*rt Jones, M.D.
5000 N. High Street
Yourtown, US 98765

Dear Dr. Jones:

I saw Patricia Moriarty in the office today. You will recall that she has
suffered from menstrual discomfort and intermenstrual pain since July.

On examination, the breasts are well developed and free of masses. on
pelvic examination, the hymen is intact; and vaginal examination was not

lc performed. On Rectal examination, the uterus was anterior and freely
movable. The right adnexa were normal. The left ovary was enlarged to
the size of a walnut or slightly larger and was cystic. Compression of this
ovary reproduced the patient's pain. Patricia was asked to return in three
weeks for re-examination to determine the need for treatment of ovarian
enlargement.

Thank you for referring this patient.

Sincerely,

Kerry Smith, M.D.

LETTER 4

KERRY SMITH, M.D.

101 LANE AVENUE

YOURTOWN, US 12345

B. Word Puzzle: Use the definitions below to spell out these terms.

```
 1.        _ _ _ T _ _ _
 2.       _ _ _ _ R _ _ _ _ _ _
 3.          _ _ A _ _ _ _
 4.         _ _ _ N _ _ _
 5.   _ _ _ _ _ S _ _
 6.             C _ _ _ _ _ _ _
 7            _ R _ _ _ _ _ _ _
 8.          _ _ I _ _ _ _ _
 9.            P _ _ _ _ _ _ _ _ _ _
10.         _ _ T _ _ _ _ _
11.          _ I _ _ _ _ _ _
12.          _ O _ _ _ _ _ _
13.         _ _ N _ _ _
14.    _ _ _ _ I _ _ _ _ _
15. _ _ _ _ _ S _
16.             T _ _ _ _ _ _ _
```

1. The part of a written or spoken statement that surrounds a particular word or passage and can clarify its meaning
2. A shortened word or words formed by omitting or combining some of the letters or sounds
3. A section of a sentence
4. A noun substitute
5. A mark or series of marks used in writing or printing to indicate an omission, especially of letters or words
6. A critical examination of a thing or situation
7. Carefully read material for errors
8. An item suitable for mailing
9. An addition to a letter written after the writer's name
10. A mark imprinted on paper that is visible when it is held up to the light, usually a sign of quality
11. The name of a person as written by himself or herself
12. To qualify or limit the meaning
13. To indicate, to mean
14. Paper used for letters
15. To write, to form by combination of units or parts
16. A reference book containing words and their synonyms

ASSIGNMENT SHEET

Chapter 6: ORAL AND WRITTEN COMMUNICATIONS

Unit 4: RECEIVING AND SENDING OFFICE COMMUNICATIONS

A. Brief Answer

1. What supplies and equipment are needed to open the mail? _____

_____

2. What information may be different on the envelope than on the contents of the letter? _____

_____

3. The U.S. Postal Service has identified certain features of a letter that might be suspicious. List the three that would be the most inappropriate for a physician's office. _____

_____

4. What should you do with a suspicious letter or package? _____

_____

5. What incoming mail may be handled by the medical assistant alone? _____

_____

6. How should unwanted drug samples be disposed of? _____

7. Using the following information, address the envelope below so it can be read by the OCR and sorted by the BCS. Send to: Medical Records, University Hospital, 100 E. First Street, Ourtown, US 12345-6789 (You may print your answer in lieu of typing.) Use Elizabeth R. Evans, M.D., Suite 205, 100 E. Main St., Yourtown, US 98765-4321 as the return address.

_____

Fill in the Blank:

8. Below are some abbreviations pertaining to mail; spell out the words they stand for.

    A. USPS _____

    B. OCR _____

    C. BCS _____

    D. APT _____

E. ATTN _____

F. AVE _____

G. BLVD _____

H. HTS _____

I. HOSP _____

J. INST _____

K. LN _____

L. PKY _____

M. PL _____

N. PO _____

O. RR _____

9. What do the numbers in the following zip code 43221-4940 stand for?

  4- _____

  32- _____

  21- _____

  49- _____

  40- _____

10. Name four things to remember in processing metered mail. _____

_____

11. Where can current postal information be obtained? _____

12. List the six classifications of mail. _____

_____

13. What special sending or receiving features are associated with the following types of mailings?

A. Express— _____

B. Certificate of mailing— _____

C. Certified mail— _____

D. Registered— _____

E. Restricted delivery— _____

14. Refer to the Role Delineation Chart in Appendix A of the textbook. Within the area of *Operational Functions,* what role relates to the content of this unit? _____

B. Matching: MATCH the definition in column II with the correct term in column I.

COLUMN I

_____ 1. Fax

_____ 2. Pager

_____ 3. Voice mail

_____ 4. Cellular

_____ 5. Conference call

_____ 6. Teleconference

_____ 7. Telemedicine

_____ 8. E-mail

_____ 9. Internet

COLUMN II

a. Involves phones, cameras, and television

b. Portable telephone

c. Needs computer, electronic address, and phone to receive messages

d. Requires appropriate software, a modem, a service provider, and a search engine

e. Sends written material electronically over phone lines

f. Long-distance physical assessment

g. Small receiver of electronic messages by phone signal

h. Multi-phone call

i. Receives messages in a "mailbox"

C. Word Puzzle: Use the clues below to spell out these terms.

1. _ _ C _ _ _ _ _
2. O _ _ _ _ _
3. _ _ _ _ M _ _ _
4. _ _ M _ _ _ _
5. _ U _ _ _ _ _ _ _ _
6. _ _ N _ _ _ _ _ _
7. _ _ _ _ I _ _ _ _
8. _ _ C _ _ _ _ _ _
9. _ _ _ _ _ A _ _ _
10. _ _ _ _ T
11. _ _ I _ _ _ _ _
12. _ O _ _ _ _ _
13. _ N _ _ _ _ _ _
14. _ _ _ _ S _ _ _ _ _ _

1. A copy
2. Where one works
3. Placed on mail by post office
4. At home mail
5. Assures
6. To note
7. Provide written proof
8. Receiver
9. Uses heat
10. Number one
11. Overweight first-class mail
12. Not domestic
13. Holds letter
14. Sent

ASSIGNMENT SHEET

Chapter 6: ORAL AND WRITTEN COMMUNICATIONS

Unit 5: OFFICE MANAGEMENT EQUIPMENT

SUGGESTED RESPONSES TO CRITICAL THINKING CHALLENGE IN TEXTBOOK

1. Should Ruth be required to make the payment in order to continue her relationship with the doctor? _____

_____

_____

_____

_____

_____

_____

2. Do you think a patient might say she or he canceled an appointment to avoid the charge? _____

_____

_____

_____

_____

3. Is a physician's time so valuable that a charge should be made for a missed appointment? _____

_____

_____

_____

_____

4. Why do you think Miss Chan is no longer there? _____

_____

_____

ANSWERS TO WORKBOOK ASSIGNMENT

A. Brief Answer

1. Demonstrate the use of a calculator, with emphasis on accuracy in determining the total of each column of figures:

	a.	b.	c.
	85.00	40.00	70.00
	10.00	16.00	25.00
	10.00	−12.00	65.00
	−15.00	100.00	−125.00
	4.00	18.00	37.00
	10.00	−35.00	−54.00
Total	_____	_____	_____

2. Use a calculator to determine the balance due o\n the following patient account. Total each appointment and payment, list monthly balances and final balance due. (Insurance filing charge not reimbursable.)

		Charges	Receipts	Balance
6/1/97	Office consult—extensive	105.00		
	Diagnostic X-ray testing	67.00		
	Laboratory	35.00		_____
6/10/97	Office, follow-up, extensive	85.00		
	ECG	65.00		
	Culture	40.00		
	Injection, antibiotic	30.00		_____
7/1/97	Office, intermediate	65.00		_____
7/21/97	Office intermediate	65.00		_____
8/1/97	Insurance filed (Medicare, Travelers)	10.00		_____
9/15/97	Medicare payment		272.16	
	Medicare write off		226.80	_____
9/25/97	Travelers payment		58.04	_____

B. Brief Answer

1. List the nine examples of items frequently copied. _____

_____

2. What is microfilming? _____

_____

3. How can microfilmed material be read? _____

_____

4. You are having difficulty transcribing dictation due to the following possible reasons. What could you say to the physician to improve the quality of the content?
   a. You are not sure what type of dictation is to be transcribed or when it was recorded. _____

   _____

   b. The message is clear, but you do not know to whom it goes or where to send it. _____

   _____

   c. You can't tell if a pause is the end of the sentence or a break in dictation. _____

   _____

   d. The dictation seems to be muffled and slurred at times and often barely audible because of background noise. _____

   _____

   e. You are never sure if the dictation is finished or if it's a break in the message. _____

   _____

5. List four features of a word processor. _____

_____

_____

6. What is a computer? _____

_____

_____

7. Name three types of printers _____

_____

8. Give 10 examples of medical management software uses. _____

_____

_____

9. Refer to the ABHES Course Content Requirements in Appendix C of the textbook. Within the area of *Basic Keyboarding*, which content requirement relates to the content in this unit? _____

_____

C. Matching: MATCH the definition in column II with the correct term in column I.

COLUMN I

_____ 1. Batch
_____ 2. Bug
_____ 3. Cursor
_____ 4. Data
_____ 5. Disk
_____ 6. File
_____ 7. Font
_____ 8. Hard copy
_____ 9. Initialize
_____ 10. Memory
_____ 11. Modem
_____ 12. Monitor
_____ 13. Peripheral
_____ 14. Program
_____ 15. Scroll
_____ 16. Write-protect

COLUMN II

a. A readable paper copy or printout
b. Information that can be processed or produced by a computer
c. A single stored unit of information that is named
d. Formatting
e. Video display unit with a screen
f. To move the cursor up, down, right, or left
g. An error in a program
h. Anything plugged into a computer
i. A set of instructions written in computer language
j. An accumulation of data to be processed
k. Data held in storage
l. Process or code that prevents overwriting data or a program on a disk
m. A marker on the screen showing where the next character will be placed
n. An assortment of characters of a given size and style
o. A magnetic storage device made of plastic
p. A peripheral device that enables a computer to communicate over phone lines

D. Word Search: Find the following words hidden in the puzzle.

ACRONYM   MICROFILM
CALCULATOR   PAYEE
COMPUTER   PROCESSOR
DICTATION   PROGRAM
ELECTRONIC   SOFTWARE
HARDWARE   TECHNOLOGY
MENU   TRANSCRIPTION
MICROFICHE

```
E C P G T O U R A D W Y C M I B
X T R A C Q S P R O G R A M C T
U D O D B W C M I C R O F I L M
H R C D I C T A T I O N L C G E
A V E T O M E N U R P C S R Q Y
R X S A D L C U Z F G O O O H K
D J S L M Z H T S P C M F F W F
W B O T R A N S C R I P T I O N
A K R A C R O N Y M G U W C H J
R C A L C U L A T O R T A H K L
E L E C T R O N I C M E R E N P
S V A D C O G G H F C R E T R O
D G V K P A Y E E R H P Z W C A
```

ACHIEVING SKILL COMPETENCY

Reread the performance objective for each procedure and then practice the skills listed below, following the procedure in your textbook.

Procedure 6-1:   Answer the Office Phone
Procedure 6-2:   Process Phone Message
Procedure 6-3:   Record Telephone Mesage on Recording Device
Procedure 6-4:   Obtain Telephone Message from Phone Recording Device
Procedure 6-5:   Schedule Appointments
Procedure 6-6:   Arrange Referral Appointment
Procedure 6-7:   Compose a Business Letter
Procedure 6-8:   Total Charges on Calculator
Procedure 6-9:   Operate Copy Machine
Procedure 6-10: Operate Transcriber
Procedure 6-11: Operate Office Computer

When you feel you have mastered performance of a skill, sign your name on the appropriate evaluation sheet and give it to your instructor to indicate you are prepared to perform the procedure for evaluation.

After your instructor has returned your work to you, make all necessary corrections and place in a three-ring notebook for future reference.

ASSIGNMENT SHEET

Chapter 7: RECORDS MANAGEMENT

Review the objectives and text for each unit before completing the assignment sheet for that unit. When you have completed all sheets for the chapter, remove them from this Workbook and give them to the instructor for evaluation.

Unit 1: THE PATIENT'S MEDICAL RECORD

A. Brief Answer

1. Define *subjective information.* _____

_____

2. Define *objective information.* _____

_____

_____

3. What is a progress note? _____

_____

4. Describe methods of recording progress notes. _____

_____

5. Describe the correct procedure for making corrections on progress notes. _____

_____

_____

_____

6. List the differences between a traditional record and the Problem Oriented Medical Record (POMR).

_____

_____

_____

_____

_____

_____

7. What is a procrastinator? In terms of the medical office, what effect would this have on patients' records?

_____

_____

_____

B. Word Scramble

1. _ _ _ _ _ _ _ _   DIFIGNSN
2. _ _ _ _ _ _ _ _   PSEFICCI
3. _ _ _ _ _ _   RDOCRE
4. _ _ _ _ _ _ _ _ _ _   CEJEVTIBSU
5. _ _ _ _ _ _ _ _ _   SPGESRRO
6. _ _ _ _ _ _ _   ACEDITT
7. _ _ _ _ _ _ _ _ _ _ _ _ _ _ _   NFOICTTYLIDAEIN
8. _ _ _ _ _ _ _ _ _ _ _ _ _   TANECIVOONNL
9. _ _ _ _ _ _ _ _ _   CEBTJIOVE
10. _ _ _ _ _ _ _ _ _   MDDCEUONTE
11. _ _ _ _ _ _ _   RTSHYIO
12. _ _ _ _ _ _ _ _ _   ENIOMRIPSS

B. Write a sentence with each unscrambled word regarding the patient's medical record.

1. _____
2. _____
3. _____
4. _____
5. _____
6. _____
7. _____
8. _____
9. _____
10. _____
11. _____
12. _____

C. Multiple Choice: Place the correct letter or letters on the blank line for each question.

_____ 1. What information in a medical record makes it a useful legal document?

a. progress notes   c. dates of injuries
b. dates of treatments   d. all of these

_____ 2. Which of the symptoms listed below are objective?

a. headache   c. swelling
b. rash   d. bleeding

_____ 3. Which of the symptoms listed below are subjective?

a. red throat   c. bruise
b. nausea   d. abdominal pain

_____ 4. Besides the clinical visit findings, what additional information is recorded on progress notes?

a. phone messages   c. phone/fax refills
b. marital status   d. cancelations

_____ 5. What color of ink should be used in recording patient information?

a. blue   c. red
b. black   d. any color

C. True or False: **Place a "T" for true or "F" for false in the space provided. For false statements, explain why they are false.**

_____ 1. The confidentiality of the patient's medical record must be maintained by careful management as it is used.

_____ 2. Only parts of the patient's record are necessary when the patient wishes the physician to testify in an injury case.

_____ 3. The patient must always sign an authorization form before any information can be released.

_____ 4. All patient information contained in the medical record is considered subjective information.

_____ 5. Progress notes should be arranged in chronological order with the most recent date on top.

_____ 6. The date and time should be recorded on the page for progress notes each time the patient is seen.

_____ 7. Using correction fluid is recommended to completely eliminate an error made on a patient's record.

_____ 8. Using black ink on the patient's record is important for making good copies.

_____ 9. The POMR record begins with the standard database.

After your instructor has returned your work to you, make all necessary corrections and place it in a three-ring notebook for future reference.

ASSIGNMENT SHEET

Chapter 7: RECORDS MANAGEMENT

Unit 2: FILING

SUGGESTED RESPONSES TO CRITICAL THINKING CHALLENGE IN TEXTBOOK

1. What did Judy's apparent haste cause to happen? _____

_____

2. Do you think Judy had good intentions? _____

3. What do you think needs to be done to Mr. Jeffries' chart? _____

_____

4. What do you think Francene said to Judy about this error? _____

_____

5. Who should record the data on Mr. Stephens' chart? _____

_____

6. What would you have done in this situation? _____

_____

_____

7. Would you call the temporary service to report Judy's error? _____

_____

8. What do you think of the temporary service? _____

_____

9. Would you call the temporary service again? _____

A. Brief Answer

1. What is meant by *indexing*? _____

_____

2. Name and define the four basic filing methods.

    a. _____
    b. _____
    c. _____
    d. _____

3. Name and define the five steps in filing.

    a. _____

    _____
    b. _____
    c. _____
    d. _____
    e. _____

4. Describe the proper method of placing material in a file folder. _____

_____

5. Describe the most efficient method of removing and replacing patient files. _____

_____

_____

6. List the storage media used for "paperless" filing systems. _____

_____

7. Describe ways to help find a missing chart. _____

_____

_____

_____

_____

B. Indexing Practice

1. Index each name below on a 3 × 5 card or paper cut to that size. Start each name ½ inch from the top and ½ inch from the left margin. Arrange the cards in alphabetical order.

   a. Curtis Koch
   b. Dianne Hanning
   c. Dezzie Harris
   d. Connie Graves
   e. Anna Epstein
   f. Melvin Edwards
   g. Charles L. Davis
   h. Gertrude Carter
   i. Barbara Cahill
   j. Earl Block

   k. Robert Blair
   l. C.L. Benson
   m. L.K. Ander
   n. Elmo Applegate
   o. Nathan Appleby
   p. Bruce Carr
   q. Sandra Dyer
   r. Pauline Hall
   s. P.A. Dennis
   t. Dave Daniels

2. Index each name below on a 3 × 5 card or paper cut to that size. Start each name ½ inch from the top and ½ inch in from the left margin. Arrange the cards in alphabetical order.

   a. Edgar Underwood
   b. Richard Poff
   c. Thomas Meyer
   d. Felix Lee
   e. Helen Thornton
   f. Hubert Landers
   g. Ann Stone
   h. Mary June Quinn
   i. Peter Nye
   j. G. Saunders

   k. Glen Ochs
   l. Clyde Rambo
   m. Russel Owens
   n. Thomas Jefferson
   o. June Guthrie
   p. Theresa Frost
   q. Kenneth Ford
   r. Vivian Booth
   s. Jimmy Block
   t. Stephen Bergstrom

3. Code the names listed below by underlining the first unit and place 2, 3, 4 above other units in correct filing order. Then arrange the names in correct alphabetic and indexing order on the form provided.

Ex: L$\overset{2}{\text{i}}$sa / $\overset{3}{\text{A}}$nn / Hale

a. Steve Van Meter
b. Victor Li-Lelaez
c. Min Kwang-Shik
d. Joan Vanmatre
e. Judy Kavang
f. Esther Corbie-Bender
g. Marila Corbitt
h. Asad Al-Alowi
i. Louise Gage
j. Frances Buntyn
k. Letticia Galindo
l. Don Durflinger
m. Anna Gunton

n. Louie Gage
o. Alfred D'Ambrosio
p. A./M. FitzHugh
q. Kelly LaBarba
r. Sylvia D'Ambrogi
s. Bill Fitz
t. Bryan LaBeff
u. C. W. McBrayer
v. Dr. Larry Mathis
• w. Mrs. M.W. Smith (Mary)
x. Rev. Joan Sanders
y. Mrs. Carol Long (Mrs. William)
   Carol Long (Mrs.) William

WORKSHEET FOR FILING ASSIGNMENTS

1st Unit	2nd Unit	3rd Unit	4th Unit
a.			
b.			
c.			
d.			
e.			
f.			
g.			
h.			
i.			
j.			
k.			
l.			
m.			
n.			
o.			
p.			
q.			
r.			
s.			
t.			
u.			
v.			
w.			
x.			
y.			

4. Code the names listed below by underlining the first unit and place 2, 3, 4 above other units in correct filing order. Then arrange the names in correct alphabetic and indexing order on the form provided.

Ex: Abbott-Coltman. / Inc.

a. Neu-Mor/Corp.
b. Mt./Vernon/Mobile/Homes
c. Richard's/Antiques
d. Robt./Moriconi, (Jr.)
e. Japan/Air Lines
f. Aus-/Tex/Garden/Supply
g. A./Ingram
h. Northwest/Airlines
i. Bill/New/Law/Office
j. San/Antonio/Tours,/Inc.
k. So-Lo/Diet/Center
l. M/N/Insurance/Agency
m. McFarland/Down Town/Motor/Co.
n. Vivian/Richards, (M.D.)
o. St./Paul/Printing/Co.

WORKSHEET FOR FILING ASSIGNMENTS

1st Unit	2nd Unit	3rd Unit	4th Unit
a.			
b.			
c.			
d.			
e.			
f.			
g.			
h.			
i.			
j.			
k.			
l.			
m.			
n.			
o.			

5. Use the 25 cards prepared in question 3. Write the following registry numbers in the upper-right-hand corner of the cards. Arrange the cards in numerical order and list the 25 names in the order in which they now appear.

a. _____   j. _____   r. _____
b. _____   k. _____   s. _____
c. _____   l. _____   t. _____
d. _____   m. _____   u. _____
e. _____   n. _____   v. _____
f. _____   o. _____   w. _____
g. _____   p. _____   x. _____
h. _____   q. _____   y. _____
i. _____

Van Meter 19-2-10   Kavang 10-11-65   Gage, Louise 12-70-45
Li-Lelaez 22-12-65   Corbie-Bender 50-30-25   Buntyn 60-20-15
Kwang-Shik 13-11-65   Corbitt 13-30-25   Galindo 12-70-45
Vanmatre 10-22-10   Al-Alowi 10-10-15   Durflinger 40-40-25
Gunton 10-70-45   D'Ambrogi 19-40-25   Mathis 40-12-75
Gage, Louise 12-70-45   Fitz 20-60-35   Smith 13-23-95
D'Ambrosio 10-10-25   LaBeff 20-12-65   Sanders 18-10-95
FitzHugh 10-13-35   McBrayer 30-23-75   Long 13-30-65
LaBarba 11-12-65

C. Word Search: Find the following words hidden in the puzzle.

ACCUMULATED	NUMERICAL
ALPHABETICAL	SEQUENCE
CODING	SORT
DATA	STORE
EXPEDITE	SUBSEQUENT
FILING	SUPPLEMENTED
GEOGRAPHIC	SYSTEMATICALLY
ILLUMINATING	UNIT
INDEXING	UNPRODUCTIVE
INSPECT	

```
P O I U L K J H M N B V O I U Y L L A C I T A M E T S Y S
Q W E R F D S A Z X C V K J H N B U N P R O D U C T I V E
H J K F G H D F H S T O R E S D A W Q E T R E F O C N M Q
B V C X Z G F D S O M D E T A L U M U C C A I U D O S N U
L K J M N B T Y U R I O T M N B H G F A P O I U I K P L E
S U B S E Q U E N T X P I W A B M Y I P O U J H N B E M N
L O J Y F E D S W G Z Q D B Y N T M I T T R E W G D C X C
O P U I T Y T R E N A S E W E R I P F I L I N G Y N T G E
L K J M N B H G F I P L P D E X N V B O M I Y R E D D L K
A S D W E Q R T B X N H X I L L U M I N A T I N G C A B N
P O K I J M N B F E D T E H G F D S A Q W E R T Y O T L K
F D S A E R T W C D B N M J H L A C I T E B A H P L A K J
L O I K J M N H Y N P O M N U M E R I C A L J N B M L O P
E R W D S F B V C I M J H K I U O C I H P A R G O E G I N
P O I N T S U P P L E M E N T E D P O K E R D C S Q N T L
```

D. Multiple Choice: Place the correct letter on the blank line for each question.

_____ 1. Bar code files eliminate the need for

     a. data entry   c. progress notes

     b. OUTguides   d. all of these

_____ 2. Placing all documents in a patient's chart in _____ order makes it easier to obtain information.

     a. color-coded   c. chronological

     b. alphabetical   d. categorical

_____ 3. The method of filing that provides the most patient privacy is

     a. alphabetical   c. categorical

     b. numeric   d. chronological

_____ 4. In a miscellaneous file, when there are more than ____ papers on one subject or person, you should remove them and make a separate folder.

     a. two   c. four

     b. three   d. five

_____ 5. _____ make it easy to obtain phone numbers and addresses.

     a. bar code files   c. tickler files

     b. desktop files   d. numeric files

_____ 6. Removing the files of patients who are no longer being seen by the physician is called
   a. processing   c. sorting
   b. indexing   d. purging

_____ 7. When there is a signature on a patient's chart, J. Williams (CL), whose initials are in the parentheses?
   a. patient's   c. medical assistant's
   b. physician's   d. office manager's

ACHIEVING SKILL COMPETENCY

Reread the performance objective for each procedure and then practice the skills listed below, following the procedure in your textbook.

Procedure 7-1: File Item(s) Alphabetically

Procedure 7-2: Pull File Folder from Alphabetic files

Procedure 7-3: File Item(s) Numerically

Procedure 7-4: Pull file Folder from Numeric Files

When you have mastered the performances of a skill, sign your name on the appropriate evaluation sheet and give it to your instructor to indicate you are prepared to perform the procedure for evaluation.

After your instructor has returned your work to you, make all necessary corrections and place in a three-ring notebook for future reference.

Name _____

Date _____ Score _____

ASSIGNMENT SHEET

Chapter 8: COLLECTING FEES

Review the objectives and text for each unit before completing the assignment sheet for that unit. When you have completed all sheets for the chapter, remove them from this Workbook and give them to the instructor for evaluation.

Unit 1: MEDICAL CARE EXPENSES

A. Brief Answers

1. What are the factors to consider in determining fees for patient care?

_____
_____

2. When insurance companies and government agencies establish a fee profile for physicians, how does it affect payment for patients?

_____
_____

3. Explain what you should do if an indigent patient wants an appointment in your facility and your physician cannot accept another indigent patient at this time.

_____
_____
_____
_____

4. List the information that should be obtained on the personal data sheet of each patient.

a. _____
b. _____
c. _____
d. _____
e. _____
f. _____
g. _____
h. _____
i. _____
j. _____

B. True or False: Place a "T" for true or "F" for false in the space provided. For false statements, explain why they are false.

_____ 1. Physicians are the ones who discuss fees with patients.

_____ 2. Insurance companies and government agencies establish a fee profile for physicians based on charges averaged over a period of time.

_____ 3. Physicians should never be told when a patient is unhappy with the cost of treatment.

_____ 4. Indigent patients should receive the same care as paying patients.

_____ 5. Two copies of the reduced fee agreement, with the words "without prejudice" stated, should be witnessed as they are signed for those with limited income.

_____ 6. Each time the patient comes in for an appointment, you should verify the personal data sheet information.

_____ 7. The personal data sheet should ask for additional insurance coverage.

_____ 8. It is not necessary for the records release form to have a witness sign it.

_____ 9. On the third-party liability statement, the name of the patient and the name of the responsible party are always one and the same person.

C. Word Puzzle: **For each word listed below, provide another word that has the same meaning (or is similar in meaning) to fill in the blank spaces.**

1. Complicated   1. __ __ __ __ __ __ __ __ __ __

2. Poor   2. __ __ __ __ __ __ __ __

3. Inexpensive   3. __ __ __ __ __ __ __

4. Succeeding   4. __ __ __ __ __ __ __ __ __

5. Confirm   5. __ __ __ __ __ __

D. Multiple Choice: **Place the correct letter on the blank line for each question.**

_____ 1. Completed annually, this form provides a "signature on file" for your records.

     a. personal/patient data sheet   c. medication list

     b. medical history form   d. charges statement

_____ 2. Fees should be discussed with patients

     a. in the reception area   c. in a private area

     b. in the exam room   d. in groups

_____ 3. At each office visit you should ask patients for their insurance card so that you can

     a. read it   c. release information

     b. copy it   d. check their birth date

_____ 4. If a third party is responsible for a patient's charges, that person should sign a

     a. liability statement   c. records release form

     b. data sheet   d. estimate form

_____ 5. You should obtain a release of information form

     a. as needed   c. at the first visit

     b. when patients are moving   d. at each visit

After your instructor has returned your work to you, make all necessary corrections and place in a three-ring notebook for future reference.

ASSIGNMENT SHEET

Chapter 8: COLLECTING FEES

Unit 2: CREDIT ARRANGEMENTS

A. Brief Answers

1. Explain when you should discuss payment planning and health insurance coverage with patients and give examples.

   _____

   _____

   _____

   _____

2. What is specified in the Truth in Lending Act?

   _____

   _____

3. How are physicians required under the AMA Code of Ethics to allow patients to use credit cards for services?

   _____

   _____

4. Why are credit card payments advantageous if there is a 1% to 3% assessment charged to the physician?

   _____

   _____

   _____

5. What is the purpose of the Bureau of Medical Economics?

   _____

6. If a request is received from a credit bureau regarding a patient, what information are you to disclose in your answer?

   _____

   _____

B. Multiple Choice: Place the correct letter or letters on the blank line for each question.

_____ 1. Assisting patients with a plan for payment of costly medical expenses is the responsibility of the
   a. physician   c. medical assistant
   b. interpreter   d. physician assistant

_____ 2. How long must the (signed) Truth in Lending form be kept on file?
   a. two years   c. 10 years
   b. six years   d. indefinitely

_____ 3. Patients should be reminded to check with their ____ for the amount that they are responsible for (co-pay), if their insurance does not pay the total cost.
   a. bank   c. insurance company
   b. financial planner   d. loan company

_____ 4. In large cities it is wise to check _____ before extending credit for a large medical expense.
    a. marital status   c. credit references
    b. medical history   d. insurance

_____ 5. It is a violation of the law if you disclose _____ in requests from creditors regarding patients.
    a. opening date of account   c. character of patient
    b. paying habits   d. largest amount of account

C. Word Search: Find the following words hidden in the puzzle.

```
I A D V A N C E A C T
A D D I S C L O S E H
D E L I N Q U E N T C
V C L O E T H I C S O
T R U T H   C A R D S
I N S T A L L M E N T
C P A Y M E N T D E S
I A F I N A N C I N G
L T E S T I M A T E F
O I N C H A R G E S A
S U B S T A N T I A L
```

CARDS
INSTALLMENT
CHARGES
FINANCING
ETHICS
COSTS
DISCLOSE
PAYMENT
TRUTH
ESTIMATE
DELINQUENT
ADVANCE
ACT
CREDIT
SOLICIT
SUBSTANTIAL

D. True or False: Place a "T" for true or "F" for false in the space provided. For false statements, explain why they are false.

_____ 1. A cost estimate sheet for surgery should include cost of the surgery and the approximate cost of the anesthesia, consultants, and hospital costs.

_____ 2. The Truth in Lending Act is enforced by the International Trade Commission.

_____ 3. Physicians may increase charges for services to patients who wish to use credit cards for medical services.

_____ 4. It is not only lawful but good practice to disclose information to referring offices regarding paying habits of patients.

_____ 5. The Truth in Lending form must be signed by the patient in your presence.

    After your instructor has returned your work to you, make all necessary corrections and place in a three-ring notebook for future reference.

ASSIGNMENT SHEET

Chapter 8: COLLECTING FEES

Unit 3: BOOKKEEPING PROCEDURES

A. Multiple Choice: Place the correct letter or letters on the blank line for each question.

_____ 1. A patient account shows the
    a. balance due   c. payments
    b. charges   d. a and b only

_____ 2. Besides the appointment schedule, the ___ will reflect the names of all patients seen each day.
    a. patient's ledger   c. itemized statement
    b. daily log sheet   d. all receipts

_____ 3. Patients should be ____ from sending cash payments through the mail.
    a. encouraged   c. discouraged
    b. stopped   d. restrained

_____ 4. Dividing account cards into groups to correspond to the number of times billing is done is called
    a. bookkeeping   c. business transactions
    b. cycle billing   d. balancing

_____ 5. Patients who have filed bankruptcy may continue to see the physician, but must pay with
    a. cash   c. insurance
    b. credit card   d. check

B. Matching: Match the definition in column II with the correct term in column I.

COLUMN I

_____ 1. Posted
_____ 2. Trial balance
_____ 3. Cash payment
_____ 4. Petition
_____ 5. Proprietorship
_____ 6. Bankruptcy
_____ 7. Bookkeeper
_____ 8. Journalizing

COLUMN II

a. Owner-manager of a business
b. Formal written application seeking specific judicial action
c. Legal petition to the courts if one is unable to pay creditors
d. One who records transactions/accounts of a business
e. To record bookkeeping transactions in a journal
f. Total owed/record of accounts receivable
g. Transfer of information from one record to another
h. Write-it-once bookkeeping system
i. Must be given a receipt

C. Brief Answer

1. Use half sheets of paper and type the invoice shown in Figure 8-7. Type itemized statements from the five families who still owe money. _____

_____

2. Describe the exceptions to the usual billing procedures. _____

_____

_____

_____

_____

_____

3. Describe the advantages of a write-it-once bookkeeping system. _____

_____

_____

_____

_____

D. 1. Use the following information to fill in a daily log for each of the three days indicated. Be careful to calculate charges when more than one is listed and put only the total in the charge column. Be sure to itemize in column listing description. Be careful to list payments in payment column and break down each in either cash or check payment column.

December 27, XX____

    Juan Gomez - paid $17.00 ck

    Sue Schmidt - O.C. limited $27.00; Inj. B 12 $15.00

    Susan Segal - O.C. New intermediate $48.00

    Sue Schmidt - paid $62.00 ck

    Carol Sue Kostrevski - O.C. Comprehensive $70.00; paid $50.00 cash

    LaChar Holley - (NP) Comprehensive $85.00

January 5, XX____

    Geoff Segal - paid $48.00 cash for Susan

    Juan Gomez - Extended exam $46.00

    June Kostrevski - Allergy testing $100.00

    Carol Sue Kostrevski - Inj. Penicillin $12.00

    Joan Moriarty - O.C. Intermediate $30.00; x-ray left knee $76.00; paid $50.00 ck

    Carol Schmidt - O.C. Extended $46.00

    Boris Kostrevski - Paid $150.00 ck

January 8, XX____

    Boris Kostrevski - CPE comprehensive New $85.00; chest x-ray $79.00;

      ECG $50.00; Lab Physical Profile $113.00;

      Draw blood $5.00; Urinalysis $10.00

    Patrick Moriarty - O.C. Intermediate $30.00; paid $38.00 ck

    Tina Schmidt - cast removal $35.00

    Juan Gomez- O.C. Limited $27.00

    Geoff Segal - N.C.

    June Kostrevski - Ck. Aetna Ins. $100.00

    LaChar Holley - Hospital 12/29 thru 1/6

      Initial visit $85.00

      6 days at $25.00

      Total charges $235.00

    Boris Kostrevski - Medicare pd. ck $40.00

    Juan Gomez - Medical pd. ck $12.50

    After your instructor has returned your work to you, make all necessary corrections and place in a three-ring notebook for future reference.

Name _____

DATE	NAME	DESCRIPTION	CHARGES	CREDITS		CASH	CHK
				PAYMENTS	ADJ.		

Name _____

DATE	NAME	DESCRIPTION	CHARGES	√	CREDITS		CASH	CHK
					PAYMENTS	ADJ.		

DATE	NAME	DESCRIPTION	CHARGES	√	CREDITS PAYMENTS	ADJ.	CASH	CHK

2. Prepare ledger cards for the patients listed below. The additional names are of family members who would be listed on the separate account cards. After the account cards are prepared, post the three daily log days to the account cards. Be sure to itemize all charges under description column. Your instructor may provide you with account cards, or you may use the blank cards printed in this Workbook for completion of this assignment. If you use separate cards, they should always be in alphabetical order. _____

Boris Kostrevski - Mrs. June; Carol Sue
1493 S. James Road
(Your city and ZIP code)
$55.00 Balance brought forward

Patrick Moriarty - Mrs. Joan
397 North Tony Road
(Your city and ZIP code)
$38.00 Balance brought forward

George Schmidt - Mrs. Sue; Tina; Carol Susan
2349 E. Remington Road
(Your city and ZIP code)
$75.00 Balance brought forward

Juan Gomez
293 West High Street
(Your city and ZIP code)
$25.00 Balance brought forward

Patty and Geoff Segal - Susan
410 North Tony Road
(Your city and ZIP code)

LaChar Holley
4567 Charcoal Lane
(Your city and ZIP code)

If you would like more practice experience in completion of day sheets and account cards, your instructor has additional assignments in the Instructor's Manual.

Samuel E Matthews, M D
Suite 120
100 E Main Street
Yourtown US 98765-4321
(654) 789-0123

Segal, Patty
410 North Tony Road
Anywhere, USA 00000

| DATE | DESCRIPTION | CHARGE | CREDITS | | CURRENT |
			PAYMENTS	ADL.	BALANCE
	BALANCE FORWARD ➔				

PLEASE PAY LAST AMOUNT IN THIS COLUMN ◀

276L

Samuel E Matthews, M D
Suite 120
100 E Main Street
Yourtown US 98765-4321
(654) 789-0123

Gomez, Juan
293 West High Street
Anywhere, USA 00000

| DATE | DESCRIPTION | CHARGE | CREDITS | | CURRENT |
			PAYMENTS	ADL.	BALANCE
	BALANCE FORWARD ➔				

PLEASE PAY LAST AMOUNT IN THIS COLUMN ◀

276L

Statement 1

Samuel E Matthews, M D
Suite 120
100 E Main Street
Yourtown US 98765-4321
(654) 789-0123

Holley, LaChar
4567 Charcoal Lane
Anywhere, USA 00000

DATE	DESCRIPTION	CHARGE	CREDITS PAYMENTS	ADL.	CURRENT BALANCE
	BALANCE FORWARD →				

PLEASE PAY LAST AMOUNT IN THIS COLUMN ←

276L

Statement 2

Samuel E Matthews, M D
Suite 120
100 E Main Street
Yourtown US 98765-4321
(654) 789-0123

Moriarty, Ioan
397 Tony Road
Anywhere, USA 00000

DATE	DESCRIPTION	CHARGE	CREDITS PAYMENTS	ADL.	CURRENT BALANCE
	BALANCE FORWARD →				

PLEASE PAY LAST AMOUNT IN THIS COLUMN ←

276L

Name _____

Samuel E Matthews, M D
Suite 120
100 E Main Street
Yourtown US 98765-4321
(654) 789-0123

Moriarty, Patrick
397 North Tony Road
Anywhere, USA 00000

DATE	DESCRIPTION	CHARGE	CREDITS PAYMENTS	ADL.	CURRENT BALANCE
	BALANCE FORWARD				

PLEASE PAY LAST AMOUNT IN THIS COLUMN

276L

Samuel E Matthews, M D
Suite 120
100 E Main Street
Yourtown US 98765-4321
(654) 789-0123

Kostrevski, Carol Sue
1493 S. James Road
Anywhere, USA 00000

DATE	DESCRIPTION	CHARGE	CREDITS PAYMENTS	ADL.	CURRENT BALANCE
	BALANCE FORWARD				

PLEASE PAY LAST AMOUNT IN THIS COLUMN

276L

Statement 1

Samuel E Matthews, M D
Suite 120
100 E Main Street
Yourtown US 98765-4321
(654) 789-0123

Kostrevski, June
1493 S. James Road
Anywhere, USA 00000

DATE	DESCRIPTION	CHARGE	CREDITS PAYMENTS	ADL	CURRENT BALANCE
	BALANCE FORWARD →				

PLEASE PAY LAST AMOUNT IN THIS COLUMN

276L

Statement 2

Samuel E Matthews, M D
Suite 120
100 E Main Street
Yourtown US 98765-4321
(654) 789-0123

Kostrevski, Boris
1493 S. James Road
Anywhere, USA 00000

DATE	DESCRIPTION	CHARGE	CREDITS PAYMENTS	ADL	CURRENT BALANCE
	BALANCE FORWARD →				

PLEASE PAY LAST AMOUNT IN THIS COLUMN

276L

Form 1 (top right)

Samuel E Matthews, M D
Suite 120
100 E Main Street
Yourtown US 98765-4321
(654) 789-0123

Schmidt, Sue
2349 E. Remington Road
Anywhere, USA 00000

| DATE | DESCRIPTION | CHARGE | CREDITS | | CURRENT |
			PAYMENTS	ADL.	BALANCE
	BALANCE FORWARD				

PLEASE PAY LAST AMOUNT IN THIS COLUMN

276L.

Form 2 (bottom left)

Samuel E Matthews, M D
Suite 120
100 E Main Street
Yourtown US 98765-4321
(654) 789-0123

Schmidt, George
2349 E. Remington Road
Anywhere, USA 00000

| DATE | DESCRIPTION | CHARGE | CREDITS | | CURRENT |
			PAYMENTS	ADL.	BALANCE
	BALANCE FORWARD				

PLEASE PAY LAST AMOUNT IN THIS COLUMN

276L.

111

Statement 1

Samuel E Matthews, M D
Suite 120
100 E Main Street
Yourtown US 98765-4321
(654) 789-0123

Schmidt, Carol Susan
2349 E. Remington Road
Anywhere, USA 00000

DATE	DESCRIPTION	CHARGE	CREDITS PAYMENTS	ADJ.	CURRENT BALANCE
	BALANCE FORWARD				

PLEASE PAY LAST AMOUNT IN THIS COLUMN

276L

Statement 2

Samuel E Matthews, M D
Suite 120
100 E Main Street
Yourtown US 98765-4321
(654) 789-0123

Schmidt, Tina
2349 E. Remington Road
Anywhere, USA 00000

DATE	DESCRIPTION	CHARGE	CREDITS PAYMENTS	ADJ.	CURRENT BALANCE
	BALANCE FORWARD				

PLEASE PAY LAST AMOUNT IN THIS COLUMN

276L

Samuel E Matthews, M D
Suite 120
100 E Main Street
Yourtown US 98765-4321
(654) 789-0123

Segal, Susan
410 North Tony Road
Anywhere, USA 00000

DATE	DESCRIPTION	CHARGE	CREDITS PAYMENTS	ADL.	CURRENT BALANCE
		BALANCE FORWARD →			

PLEASE PAY LAST AMOUNT IN THIS COLUMN ←

276L.

Samuel E Matthews, M D
Suite 120
100 E Main Street
Yourtown US 98765-4321
(654) 789-0123

Segal, Geoff
410 North Tony Road
Anywhere, USA 00000

DATE	DESCRIPTION	CHARGE	CREDITS PAYMENTS	ADL.	CURRENT BALANCE
		BALANCE FORWARD →			

PLEASE PAY LAST AMOUNT IN THIS COLUMN ←

276L.

ASSIGNMENT SHEET

Chapter 8: COLLECTING FEES

Unit 4: COMPUTER BILLING

A. Brief Answer

1. Describe the advantages of computerized billing. _____

_____

_____

_____

_____

2. Describe different ways to locate an account in a computer system. _____

_____

3. List reasons why billing statements would/should be withheld. _____

_____

_____

4. Define *alpha search.* _____

_____

_____

B. Multiple Choice: Place the correct letter on the blank line for each question.

_____ 1. A patient's account history is also referred to as a
       a. family history   c. fee statement
       b. monthly summary   d. patient ledger

_____ 2. A back-up file disk of all transactions ___ is necessary to keep billing records secure.
       a. often   c. weekly
       b. daily   d. monthly

_____ 3. In computer terminology, a record of the information obtained for every patient is a(n)
       a. account history   c. charge slip
       b. insurance form   d. journal report

_____ 4. _____ should be programmed into the computer along with their descriptions and the fees to be charged for each.
       a. ICD codes   c. CPT codes
       b. account numbers   d. insurance numbers

_____ 5. A computer statement should show the portion of the amount due that is current,
       a. over 30 days   c. over 90 days
       b. over 60 days   d. all of these

B. True or False: **Place a "T" for true or "F" for false in the space provided. For false statements, explain why they are false.**

_____ 1. So that you don't have to ask patients to sign insurance forms each time they are seen, you can have them sign a form initially and keep it as a "signature on file."

_____ 2. When the computer system accepts a number only, you must maintain a cross-reference file of an alphabetical listing of patients along with their account numbers.

_____ 3. For an alpha search, the account number is entered in the computer to find the patient's ledger card.

After your instructor has returned your work to you, make all necessary corrections and place in a three-ring notebook for future reference.

ASSIGNMENT SHEET

Chapter 8: COLLECTING FEES

Unit 5: COLLECTING OVERDUE PAYMENTS

SUGGESTED RESPONSES TO CRITICAL THINKING CHALLENGE IN TEXTBOOK

1. Does there seem to be a lack of continuity and communication among the office personnel? _____

2. What should have been done about this? Whose fault was it? _____
   . _____

3. What should Clara have done when she realized the patient couldn't understand her? _____
   _____

4. Should the person who took care of the cash payment have alerted someone about having very little information about this lady? _____
   _____

5. What happens if the patient has a reaction to the medication? _____
   _____

6. Do you think this is a critical issue that should be discussed at a staff meeting? _____

7. What would you have done in this situation? _____
   _____

A. Brief Answer

1. Define *aging of accounts.* _____
   _____

2. How long are accounts ordinarily carried before being referred to a collection agency? _____
   _____

3. Should accounts automatically be referred to collection after the prescribed period of time? Why? _____
   _____

4. List the advantages of the use of telephone calls for account collection. _____
   _____

5. List conditions necessary when using the telephone for account collection.
   a. _____
   b. _____
   c. _____
   d. _____
   e. _____
   f. _____
   g. _____
   h. _____
   i. _____
   j. _____

6. Compose and type collection letters for the accounts of LaChar Holley, Juan Gomez, George Schmidt, and Boris Kostrevski. Use the examples in Figure 8-11 as a guide. If you use dates, be sure they compatible with the account cards you are using for a reference. Use a different form for each letter. Read typed letters.

7. Define *statute of limitations.* _____
   _____
   _____

B. True or False: **Place a "T" for true or "F" for false in the space provided. For false statements, explain why they are false.**

_____ 1. Making idle threats can encourage patients to pay their bill.

_____ 2. The process of computer analysis of accounts receivable is known as aging of accounts.

_____ 3. If you make collection calls early in the morning or late at night, you can be held liable for harassment.

_____ 4. You should have a reminder file to help you follow up on promises to pay.

SAMUEL E. MATTHEWS, MD
SUITE 120
100 E. MAIN STREET
YOURTOWN, US 98765-4321
(654) 789-0123

SAMUEL E. MATTHEWS, MD
SUITE 120
100 E. MAIN STREET
YOURTOWN, US 98765-4321
(654) 789-0123

Name _____

SAMUEL E. MATTHEWS, MD
SUITE 120
100 E. MAIN STREET
YOURTOWN, US 98765-4321
(654) 789-0123

SAMUEL E. MATTHEWS, MD
SUITE 120
100 E. MAIN STREET
YOURTOWN, US 98765-4321
(654) 789-0123

ACHIEVING SKILL COMPETENCY

Reread the performance objective for each procedure and then practice the skills listed below, following the procedure in your textbook.

        Procedure 8-1: Prepare Patient Ledger Card

        Procedure 8-2: Record Charges and Credits

        Procedure 8-3: Generate Itemized Statement

        Procedure 8-4: Compose Collection Letter

When you feel you have mastered the performance of the skill, sign your name on the appropriate evaluation sheet and give it to your instructor to indicate you are prepared to perform the procedure for evaluation.

After your instructor has returned your work to you, make all necessary corrections and place in a three-ring notebook for future reference.

ASSIGNMENT SHEET

Chapter 9: HEALTH CARE COVERAGE

Review the objectives and text for each unit before completing the assignment sheet for that unit. When you have completed all sheets for the chapter, remove them from this Workbook and give them to the instructor for evaluation.

Unit 1: FUNDAMENTALS OF MANAGED CARE

A. Brief Answer

1. What type of medical insurance has created competition in the insurance industry? _____
   _____

2. Why are HMOs so popular? _____
   _____

3. How did the phrase *managed care* originate? _____
   _____

4. What is generally the cost of health care to employees whose employer offers an HMO as part of their benefit package? _____
   _____

5. Describe managed care today. _____
   _____
   _____

6. What is the initial purpose of the HMO? _____
   _____

7. What are the two major types of health insurance? _____
   _____

8. In regard to health insurance coverage, how can the medical assistant be helpful to patients? _____
   _____
   _____

9. Where can patients find the names of physicians who participate in their HMO? _____
   _____

10. Describe a helpful practice that should be performed at the beginning of each office visit regarding the patient's insurance card. _____
    _____

11. List the four conditions of the birthday rule in regard to insurance coverage. _____
    _____
    _____

12. What is critical to ensure successful reimbursement for medical services rendered to patients? _____
    _____
    _____

13. List the subject areas the medical assistant must be knowledgeable about to process medical claims forms and explain why they are important. _____

_____

14. Refer to the CAAHEP Standards in Appendix B of the textbook. Within the area of *Medical Assisting Administrative Procedures,* which curriculum standard is discussed in this unit? _____

_____

B. Matching: Match the definition in column II with the correct term in column I.

COLUMN I

_____ 1. Attending physician
_____ 2. Signed authorization
_____ 3. Advance directives
_____ 4. Admitting physician
_____ 5. Capitation
_____ 6. Balance billing
_____ 7. Assignment of benefits
_____ 8. Accounts receivable
_____ 9. Claim

COLUMN II

a. Fixed amount paid to physician per month
b. Physician who admits patient to hospital
c. Total charges that have not been paid
d. Patient authorizes payment directly to the physician
e. Physician who cares for patient in hospital
f. Authorization to release medical information
g. Also known as a living will
h. Charges insurance did not pay
i. Request for insurance company payment

C. Fill in the Blank

1. _____ was established to aid personnel and dependents of the armed services with medical expenses.

2. _____ was established for disabled veterans, their spouses, and their dependents to aid with medical expenses.

3. A predetermined amount that the insured must pay before the insurance company pays is called the

_____.

4. A printed description of the benefits provided by the insurer to the beneficiary is known as the _____

_____

5. _____ is the term given to the primary care physician for coordinating the patient's care to specialists, hospital admissions, and so on.

6. A specific amount that the insured must pay toward the charge for professional services rendered is called

_____

7. The _____ is the one who writes his or her signature on the back of a check that is made out to him or her.

8. A list of approved professional services for which the insurance company will pay along with the maximum fee is called a _____

9. A _____ is a printed form that has patient information and a listing of the services and code numbers with the total charges.

10. A program that provides complete health care for children and encourages early detection of health problems is known as _____

11. _____ is a system of medical team members organized into groups to provide quality and cost-effective care that encompasses both the delivery of health care and the payment of services

Name _____

D. Word Search: Provide the term for each definition below. Then find the terms and the words in italics hidden in the puzzle. (Abbreviations may be used.)

1. Standard claims *form* of the *Health* Care Finance Administration to submit for third-*party* payment.

   _____

2. A joint funding program by the federal and by state governments (but not Arizona) for those on public assistance for medical *care.* _____

3. Private *insurance* to supplement Medicare benefits for non-covered services. _____

4. A *group* of physicians who continue to practice independently in their own offices. _____

5. Coding system used to *document* diseases, injuries, illnesses, and modalities. _____

6. Non-profit organization created to improve patient care *quality* and health plan performance. _____

7. Another name for *encounter* form. _____

8. Transferring words into numbers to facilitate use of *computers* in claims processing. _____

9. Moneys paid for an insurance *contract.* _____

10. *Fee* schedule based on relative *value* of resources that physicians spend to provide services to Medicare patients. _____

11. The person who has been insured; insurance *policy* holder. _____

12. Prior authorization must be obtained before the patient is admitted to the hospital or receives some specified outpatient or in-office *procedures.* _____

```
V A L U E R M I N S U R A N C E
E R A C I D E M N C Z A U C O D
R A M I F I D A C O A T I E N T
B O C A R E I D Q D H E A L T H
R W O R A H C F A I 5 0 0 L R D
V S M M C H A J P N S W X L A T
S U P E R B I L L G Y B P F C J
P B U D I C D 9 C M F O R M T Q
O S T I F E N C O U N T E R E U
L C E F E E G P R T F A M I P A
I R R I P A R T Y S X D I K U L
C I S L N C O G J X K O U Z M I
Y B M L B T U X D O C U M E N T
M E D I G A P R O C E D U R E Y
P R E C E R T I F I C A T I O N
```

125

E. True or False: **Place a "T" for true or "F" for false in the space provided. For false statements, explain why they are false.**

_____ 1. An indemnity plan is a company that bills the physician for medical services.

_____ 2. The Medicare fee schedule is a list of approved professional services that includes the maximum fee that Medicare will pay for each service.

_____ 3. A preexisting condition is a condition that existed before the insured's policy was issued.

_____ 4. A contract is an agreement between two or more parties for certain services or obligations to be discussed.

_____ 5. For patients who are minors or who are incompetent, a guardian must sign for any release of information and for any services to be completed.

_____ 6. Utilization management refers to a panel that keeps track of what services were ordered and checks if medical care was completed.

_____ 7. The usual fee is the charge that physicians make for services for their private patients.

_____ 8. A skilled nursing facility is a medical facility licensed primarily to provide skilled nursing care to patients ordered by workers' compensation.

After your instructor has returned your work to you, make all necessary corrections and place in a three-ring notebook for future reference.

ASSIGNMENT SHEET

Chapter 9: HEALTH CARE COVERAGE

Unit 2: HEALTH CARE PLANS

A. Brief Answer

1. What is significant regarding premiums and benefits of private commercial insurance companies?

   _____

2. Why was Blue Cross health insurance originally set up?

   _____

3. What coverage does Blue Cross now include besides hospital expenses?

   _____

4. Name the additional plans Blue Cross Blue Shield offer today.

   _____

5. What do indemnity plans require of the patient regarding payments?

   _____

6. What is the usual co-payment required of patients who have an HMO plan?

   _____

7. List the available types of HMOs and briefly describe each of them.

   a. _____

   b. _____

   c. _____

   d. _____

8. What are the responsibilities of the NCQA?

   _____

9. Refer to the CAAHEP Standards in Appendix B of the textbook. Within the area of *Medical Assisting Administrative Procedures,* which role relates to the content of this unit? _____

10. In October 2001, what four changes were made to help inform Medicare recipients? _____

   _____

   _____

B. Fill in the Blank: For each plan below, identify if it is considered private or government by placing a "P" or "G" in the space provided.

_____ 1. Foundations for medical care

_____ 2. Medicare

_____ 3. Blue Shield

_____ 4. TRICARE (CHAMPUS)

_____ 5. Workers' compensation

_____ 6. Blue Cross

_____ 7. Easter Seal Rehabilitation Centers

_____ 8. Medicaid

_____ 9. Commercial health insurance

_____ 10. Health maintenance organizations

C. Fill in the Blank

1. To qualify as a(n) _____ an organization must present proof of its ability to provide comprehensive health care.

2. One of the four levels of NCQA accreditation is full accreditation given for _____ indicating excellent performance.

3. The primary care physician is also referred to as _____

4. HMOs mail _____ to the provider's office to keep the office apprised of policy changes between representatives' visits.

5. Besides the four principal types of state benefits, workers' compensation also includes _____ _____ for severely disabled employees.

6. Patients who have had an industrial injury should have a _____ and a separate account card for that injury.

7. One common reason for delay in payment of claims is that they are _____

8. Medicare B is the coverage that pays for _____

9. Physicians who choose not to be participating providers must collect _____ _____ for the services rendered.

10. If the physician provides a non-covered service for a Medicare patient, an _____ must be signed by the patient.

11. There is a special _____ on the HCFA-1500 form that allows the claims processor to assign a unique identification number to the claim during microfilming.

12. In processing Medicare forms, use ICDA codes for _____ CPT codes for _____ and HCPCS codes for _____

D. True or False: Place a "T" for true or "F" for false in the space provided. For false statements, explain why they are false.

_____ 1. TRICARE (CHAMPUS) covers all military personnel.

_____ 2. Medicare encourages all providers to file claims electronically.

_____ 3. The NPI (National Provider Identification) is used in blocks 24k and 33 of the HCFA-1500 to identify the location of the service.

_____ 4. Ideally, all insurance forms should be signed and dated by the patient.

_____ 5. The only time a patient's signature is not necessary is when you have been given verbal permission from that patient to release information.

_____ 6. Claims will be returned to the provider if the NPI number is missing from the HCFA form.

_____ 7. Medicare Part B patients usually are responsible for the first $100 of covered services.

_____ 8. For Medicaid patients, a general rule is that prior authorization is necessary to provide medical treatment except in an emergency.

_____ 9. Workers' compensation requires that a patient have reevaluations at intervals with her or his physician, who must promptly give a supplemental report regarding the patient's condition.

After your instructor has returned your work to you, make all necessary corrections and place in a three-ring notebook for future reference.

ASSIGNMENT SHEET

Chapter 9: HEALTH CARE COVERAGE

Unit 3: PREPARING CLAIMS

SUGGESTED RESPONSES TO CRITICAL THINKING CHALLENGE IN TEXTBOOK

1. What should Maria do? _____
_____
_____
_____

2. Is she liable for filing fraudulent insurance claims when in reality she just enters what the physician has indicated? _____

3. There is a phone number to report Medicare fraud (800-447-8477). Should she call and report her suspicion? _____
_____

4. What do you think would be the ramifications if she approaches the physician with her observations? _____
_____
_____

5. Because this position is so perfect for her and she is paid well, should she just overlook the occasional irregularities? After all, physicians are only allowed to charge so much for services, and they need to add a little to help make up the difference. _____

6. Do you think it is possible that the physician realizes her personal situation and might take advantage of her loyalty? _____
_____
_____

ANSWERS TO WORKBOOK ASSIGNMENT

Mixed Quiz

1. What does the phrase *third-party reimbursement* mean? _____
_____

2. Why were claim forms developed? _____

3. When did the first attempt at classifying the causes of deaths occur? _____
4. What significant event occurred in 1938? _____
_____

5. Fill in the blank

Coding is, in reality, the _____ of _____ or _____ of _____ or _____ into _____ to _____ _____ which can be _____ into _____ and _____

6. List three reasons why coding is beneficial.

   a. _____

   _____

   b. _____

   c. _____

   _____

7. What change occurred with the Catastrophic Coverage Act of 1988? _____

8. What does *sequencing* mean? _____

9. What is the main rule to remember when coding, and what does it mean? _____

10. Look at a copy of an approved HCFA-1500 insurance form. Where would you enter the following information?

   _____ A. Health care coverage being billed
   _____ B. Patient's name
   _____ C. Insured's name
   _____ D. Patient's condition is result of employment
   _____ E. Name of insured's employer
   _____ F. Indicate there is another health plan
   _____ G. Have patient sign
   _____ H. Dates patient unable to work
   _____ I. Diagnosis codes
   _____ J. Procedure codes
   _____ K. Physician's tax ID number
   _____ L. Assignment acceptance
   _____ M. Physician's signature

11. Complete the five insurance forms provided using the following information: Code 11, office, for places of service: (24B) The physician is Samuel E. Matthews, MD, Suite 120, 100 E. Main Street, Yourtown, US 98765-4321. His SS# is 987654321. Phone 654-789-0123. PIN 7654321. The patients all live in Yourtown, US.

   a. Juan Gomez, 293 West High Street 98765

   Medicare. Phone 263-5538. BD 2/17/21. Male. SS# 291166966-A. Patient is insured person. Other insurance BC, BS #2911669660; signature on file. Abdominal pain and diabetes mellitus. (Consult this unit for code numbers. Consult code book for code numbers needed for procedures.) Seen in office.

   5/18/__ Office visit, intermediate 30.00
   Test feces for blood   15.00
   Automated hemogram   10.00
   Blood drawing   5.00

   b. LaChar Holley, 4567 Charcoal Lane 98765

   Travelers Insurance. Phone 122-7768. BD 10/7/60. Female. SS# 505209821. Patient is insured person. No other insurance. Not related to employment or accident. Signature on file. Arthritis, acute back pain. Seen in office.

   6/15/__ Office visit, intermediate 30.00
   X ray lumbar spine, AP & lateral 118.00
   Blood drawing   5.00
   Automated hemogram   10.00

c. Tina Schmidt, daughter. BD 12/27/90. Phone 891-7145. Insured George Schmidt, 1249 E. Remington Road 98769. Self-employed. BC and BS Insurance. SS# of insured 888207777. BD 10/6/49. No other insurance. Phone 441-0050. Signature on file. Impetigo. Seen in office.

6/20/__   Office visit, limited   27.00

d. Joan Moriarty, wife. BD 12/19/62. Insured Patrick Moriarty, 397-½ North Tony Road 98768. Self-employed. Metropolitan-Insurance. SS# of insured 887105566. BD 11/14/60. Phone 431-6943. No other insurance. Signature on file. Cervicitis, cystitis, acute edema. Patient seen in office.

9/20/__   Office visit, extended   46.00

             Catheterization, urethra   20.00

             Endometrial biopsy   125.00

             Urinalysis   10.00

e. Boris Kostrevski, 1493 S. James Road 98765. Medicare and Aetna Insurance. SS# of insured 505208800-A. BD 7/14/22. Phone 298-6483. Signature on file. Diabetes mellitus, coronary atherosclerosis. Seen in office.

6/20/__   Office visit, intermediate 30.00

             Assay blood fluid, glucose   10.00

             Blood drawing   5.00

12. Refer to ABHES Course Content Requirements in Appendix C of the textbook. Within the area of *Medical Office Business Procedures/Management,* which content requirement is discussed in this unit?

_____

Name _____

PLEASE
DO NOT
STAPLE
IN THIS
AREA

APPROVED OMB-0938-0008

PICA

HEALTH INSURANCE CLAIM FORM

PICA

1. MEDICARE ☐ (Medicare #)   MEDICAID ☐ (Medicaid #)   CHAMPUS ☐ (Sponsor's SSN)   CHAMPVA ☐ (VA File #)   GROUP HEALTH PLAN ☐ (SSN or ID)   FECA BLK LUNG ☐ (SSN)   OTHER ☐ (ID)

1a. INSURED'S I.D. NUMBER   (FOR PROGRAM IN ITEM 1)

2. PATIENT'S NAME (Last Name, First Name, Middle Initial)

3. PATIENT'S BIRTH DATE   MM   DD   YY   SEX   M ☐   F ☐

4. INSURED'S NAME (Last Name, Firts Name, Middle Initial)

5. PATIENT'S ADDRESS (No., Street)

6. PATIENT RELATIONSHIP TO INSURED   Self ☐   Spouse ☐   Child ☐   Other ☐

7. INSURED'S ADDRESS (No., Street)

CITY   STATE

8. PATIENT STATUS   Single ☐   Married ☐   Other ☐

CITY   STATE

ZIP CODE   TELEPHONE (Include Area Code)   ( )

Employed ☐   Full-Time Student ☐   Part-Time Student ☐

ZIP CODE   TELEPHONE (Include Area Code)   ( )

9. OTHER INSURED'S NAME (Last Name, First Name, Middle Initial)

10. IS PATIENT'S CONDITION RELATED TO:

11. INSURED'S POLICY GROUP OR FECA NUMBER

a. OTHER INSURED'S POLICY OR GROUP NUMBER

a. EMPLOYMENT? (CURRENT OR PREVIOUS)   YES ☐   NO ☐

a. INSURED'S DATE OF BIRTH   MM   DD   YY   SEX   M ☐   F ☐

b. OTHER INSURED'S DATE OF BIRTH   MM   DD   YY   SEX   M ☐   F ☐

b. AUTO ACCIDENT?   PLACE (State)   YES ☐   NO ☐

b. EMPLOYER'S NAME OR SCHOOL NAME

c. EMPLOYER'S NAME OR SCHOOL NAME

c. OTHER ACCIDENT?   YES ☐   NO ☐

c. INSURANCE PLAN NAME OR PROGRAM NAME

d. INSURANCE PLAN NAME OR PROGRAM NAME

d. RESERVED FOR LOCAL USE

d. IS THERE ANOTHER HEALTH BENEFIT PLAN?   YES ☐   NO ☐   If yes, return to and complete item 9 a-d.

READ BACK OF FORM BEFORE COMPLETING & SIGNING THIS FORM.

12. PATIENT'S OR AUTHORIZED PERSON'S SIGNATURE I authorize the release of any medical or other information necessary to process this claim. I also request payment of government benefits either to myself or to the party who accepts assignments below.

SIGNED_____ DATE_____

13. INSURED'S OR AUTHORIZED PERSON'S SIGNATURE I authorize payment of medical benefits to the undersigned physician or supplier for services described below.

SIGNED_____

14. DATE OF CURRENT: MM   DD   YY   ILLNESS (First sympton) OR INJURY (Accident)OR PREGNANCY (LMP)

15. IF PATIENT HAS HAD SAME OR SIMILAR ILLNESS. GIVE FIRST DATE   MM   DD   YY

16. DATES PATIENT UNABLE TO WORK IN CURRENT OCCUPATION   MM   DD   YY   MM   DD   YY   FROM   TO

17. NAME OR REFERRING PHYSICIAN OR OTHER SOURCE

17a. I.D. NUMBER OF REFERRING PHYSICIAN

18. HOSPITALIZATION DATES RELATED TO CURRENT SERVICES   MM   DD   YY   MM   DD   YY   FROM   TO

19. RESERVED FOR LOCAL USE

20. OUTSIDE LAB?   YES ☐   NO ☐ $ CHARGES

21. DIAGNOSIS OR NATURE OF ILLNESS OR INJURY. (RELATE ITEMS 1,2,3 OR 4 TO ITEM 24E BY LINE)

1.I_____._____   3. I_____._____

2.I_____._____   4. I_____._____

22. MEDICAID RESUBMISSION CODE   ORIGINAL REF. NO.

23. PRIOR AUTHORIZATION NUMBER

24.	A		B	C	D		E	F	G	H	I	J	K
	DATE(S) OF SERVICE		Place of Service	Type of Service	PROCEDURES, SERVICES, OR SUPPLIES (Explain Unusual Circumstances)		DIAGNOSIS CODE	$ CHARGES	DAYS OR UNITS	EPSDT Family Plan	EMG	COB	RESERVED FOR LOCAL USE
	From MM DD YY	To MM DD YY			CPT/HCPCS	MODIFIER							
1													
2													
3													
4													
5													
6													

25. FEDERAL TAX I.D. NUMBER   SSN ☐ EIN ☐

26. PATIENT'S ACCOUNT NO.

27. ACCEPT ASSIGNMENT? (For govt. claims, see back)   YES ☐   NO ☐

28. TOTAL CHARGE $

29. AMOUNT PAID $

30. BALANCE DUE $

31. SIGNATURE OF PHYSICIAN OR SUPPLIER INCLUDING DEGREES OR CREDENTIALS (I certify that the statements on the reverse apply to this bill and are made a part thereof.)

SIGNED _____ DATE _____

32. NAME AND ADDRESS OF FACULTY WHERE SERVICES WERE RENDERED (If other than home or office)

33. PHYSICIAN'S, SUPPLIER'S BILLING NAME, ADDRESS, ZIP CODE & PHONE#

PIN #   GRP #

(APPROVED BY AMA COUNCIL ON MEDICAL SERVICE 8/88)   **PLEASE PRINT OR TYPE**

FORM HCFA-1500 (U2) (12-90)
FORM OWCP -1500   FORM RRB-1500

CARRIER →   PATIENT AND INSURED INFORMATION   PHYSICIAN OR SUPPLIER INFORMATION

HEALTH INSURANCE CLAIM FORM

PLEASE
DO NOT
STAPLE
IN THIS
AREA

APPROVED OMB-0938-0008

PICA   PICA

1. MEDICARE   MEDICAID   CHAMPUS   CHAMPVA   GROUP   FECA   OTHER   1a. INSURED'S I.D. NUMBER   (FOR PROGRAM IN ITEM 1)
                                                        HEALTH PLAN BLK LUNG
☐(Medicare #) ☐(Medicaid #) ☐(Sponsor's SSN) ☐(VA File #) ☐(SSN or ID) ☐(SSN) ☐(ID)

2. PATIENT'S NAME (Last Name, First Name, Middle Initial)   3. PATIENT'S BIRTH DATE   SEX   4. INSURED'S NAME (Last Name, Firts Name, Middle Initial)
                                                              MM   DD   YY
                                                                              M☐ F☐

5. PATIENT'S ADDRESS (No., Street)   6. PATIENT RELATIONSHIP TO INSURED   7. INSURED'S ADDRESS (No., Street)
                                                   ☐Self ☐Spouse ☐Child ☐Other

CITY   STATE   8. PATIENT STATUS   CITY   STATE
                                                   ☐Single ☐Married ☐Other

ZIP CODE   TELEPHONE (Include Area Code)   ZIP CODE   TELEPHONE (Include Area Code)
                    (   )   Employed ☐ Full-Time ☐ Part-Time   (   )
                                                            Student   Student

9. OTHER INSURED'S NAME (Last Name, First Name, Middle Initial)   10. IS PATIENT'S CONDITION RELATED TO: 11. INSURED'S POLICY GROUP OR FECA NUMBER

a. OTHER INSURED'S POLICY OR GROUP NUMBER   a. EMPLOYMENT? (CURRENT OR PREVIOUS)   a. INSURED'S DATE OF BIRTH   SEX
                                                    ☐ YES   ☐ NO   MM   DD   YY
                                                                                                         M☐ F☐

b. OTHER INSURED'S DATE OF BIRTH   SEX   b. AUTO ACCIDENT?   PLACE (State)   b. EMPLOYER'S NAME OR SCHOOL NAME
   MM   DD   YY
                        M☐ F☐   ☐ YES   ☐ NO

c. EMPLOYER'S NAME OR SCHOOL NAME   c. OTHER ACCIDENT?   c. INSURANCE PLAN NAME OR PROGRAM NAME
                                                    ☐ YES   ☐ NO

d. INSURANCE PLAN NAME OR PROGRAM NAME   d. RESERVED FOR LOCAL USE   d. IS THERE ANOTHER HEALTH BENEFIT PLAN?
                                                                                          ☐ YES   ☐ NO If yes, return to and complete item 9 a-d.

READ BACK OF FORM BEFORE COMPLETING & SIGNING THIS FORM.   13. INSURED'S OR AUTHORIZED PERSON'S SIGNATURE I authorize
12. PATIENT'S OR AUTHORIZED PERSON'S SIGNATURE I authorize the release of any medical or other information necessary   payment of medical benefits to the undersigned physician or supplier for
to process this claim. I also request payment of government benefits either to myself or to the party who accepts assignments below.   services described below.

SIGNED_____   DATE_____   SIGNED_____

14. DATE OF CURRENT: ◄ILLNESS (First sympton) OR   15. IF PATIENT HAS HAD SAME OR SIMILAR ILLNESS.   16. DATES PATIENT UNABLE TO WORK IN CURRENT OCCUPATION
    MM   DD   YY   INJURY (Accident)OR   GIVE FIRST DATE   MM   DD   YY   MM   DD   YY   MM   DD   YY
                        PREGNANCY (LMP)   FROM   TO

17. NAME OR REFERRING PHYSICIAN OR OTHER SOURCE   17a. I.D. NUMBER OF REFERRING PHYSICIAN   18. HOSPITALIZATION DATES RELATED TO CURRENT SERVICES
                                                                                          MM   DD   YY   MM   DD   YY
                                                                                      FROM   TO

19. RESERVED FOR LOCAL USE   20. OUTSIDE LAB? $ CHARGES
                                                                                          ☐YES ☐NO

21. DIAGNOSIS OR NATURE OF ILLNESS OR INJURY. (RELATE ITEMS 1,2,3 OR 4 TO ITEM 24E BY LINE)   22. MEDICAID RESUBMISSION
                                                                                          CODE   ORIGINAL REF. NO.
  1.I_____.___   3. I_____.___
                                                                                        23. PRIOR AUTHORIZATION NUMBER
  2.I_____.___   4. I_____.___

24.	A		B	C	D		E	F	G	H	I	J	K
	DATE(S) OF SERVICE		Place of Service	Type of Service	PROCEDURES, SERVICES, OR SUPPLIES (Explain Unusual Circumstances)		DIAGNOSIS CODE	$ CHARGES	DAYS OR UNITS	EPSDT Family Plan	EMG	COB	RESERVED FOR LOCAL USE
	From MM DD YY	To MM DD YY			CPT/HCPCS	MODIFIER							
1													
2													
3													
4													
5													
6													

25. FEDERAL TAX I.D. NUMBER   SSN EIN   26. PATIENT'S ACCOUNT NO.   27. ACCEPT ASSIGNMENT?   28. TOTAL CHARGE   29. AMOUNT PAID   30. BALANCE DUE
                              ☐   ☐   (For govt. claims, see back) $ $ $
                                                                        ☐YES ☐NO

31. SIGNATURE OF PHYSICIAN OR SUPPLIER   32. NAME AND ADDRESS OF FACULTY WHERE SERVICES WERE   33. PHYSICIAN'S, SUPPLIER'S BILLING NAME, ADDRESS, ZIP CODE
INCLUDING DEGREES OR CREDENTIALS   RENDERED (If other than home or office)   & PHONE#
(I certify that the statements on the reverse
apply to this bill and are made a part thereof.)

SIGNED _____ DATE _____   PIN #   GRP #

(APPROVED BY AMA COUNCIL ON MEDICAL SERVICE 8/88)   **PLEASE PRINT OR TYPE**   FORM HCFA-1500 (U2) (12-90)
                                                                                    FORM OWCP -1500   FORM RRB-1500

Name _____

APPROVED OMB-0938-0008

PICA

HEALTH INSURANCE CLAIM FORM

PICA

1. MEDICARE MEDICAID CHAMPUS CHAMPVA GROUP HEALTH PLAN FECA BLK LUNG OTHER

☐ (Medicare #) ☐ (Medicaid #) ☐ (Sponsor's SSN) ☐ (VA File #) ☐ (SSN or ID) ☐ (SSN) ☐ (ID)

1a. INSURED'S I.D. NUMBER   (FOR PROGRAM IN ITEM 1)

2. PATIENT'S NAME (Last Name, First Name, Middle Initial)

3. PATIENT'S BIRTH DATE   SEX
MM   DD   YY
M ☐   F ☐

4. INSURED'S NAME (Last Name, Firts Name, Middle Initial)

5. PATIENT'S ADDRESS (No., Street)

6. PATIENT RELATIONSHIP TO INSURED
☐ Self ☐ Spouse ☐ Child ☐ Other

7. INSURED'S ADDRESS (No., Street)

CITY   STATE

8. PATIENT STATUS
☐ Single   ☐ Married   ☐ Other

CITY   STATE

ZIP CODE   TELEPHONE (Include Area Code)
(   )

Employed ☐ Full-Time ☐ Part-Time ☐
Student   Student

ZIP CODE   TELEPHONE (Include Area Code)
(   )

9. OTHER INSURED'S NAME (Last Name, First Name, Middle Initial)

10. IS PATIENT'S CONDITION RELATED TO:

11. INSURED'S POLICY GROUP OR FECA NUMBER

a. OTHER INSURED'S POLICY OR GROUP NUMBER

a. EMPLOYMENT? (CURRENT OR PREVIOUS)
☐ YES   ☐ NO

a. INSURED'S DATE OF BIRTH   SEX
MM   DD   YY
M ☐   F ☐

b. OTHER INSURED'S DATE OF BIRTH   SEX
MM   DD   YY
M ☐   F ☐

b. AUTO ACCIDENT?   PLACE (State)
☐ YES   ☐ NO

b. EMPLOYER'S NAME OR SCHOOL NAME

c. EMPLOYER'S NAME OR SCHOOL NAME

c. OTHER ACCIDENT?
☐ YES   ☐ NO

c. INSURANCE PLAN NAME OR PROGRAM NAME

d. INSURANCE PLAN NAME OR PROGRAM NAME

d. RESERVED FOR LOCAL USE

d. IS THERE ANOTHER HEALTH BENEFIT PLAN?
☐ YES   ☐ NO If yes, return to and complete item 9 a-d.

READ BACK OF FORM BEFORE COMPLETING & SIGNING THIS FORM.
12. PATIENT'S OR AUTHORIZED PERSON'S SIGNATURE I authorize the release of any medical or other information necessary to process this claim. I also request payment of government benefits either to myself or to the party who accepts assignments below.

SIGNED_____ DATE_____

13. INSURED'S OR AUTHORIZED PERSON'S SIGNATURE I authorize payment of medical benefits to the undersigned physician or supplier for services described below.

SIGNED_____

14. DATE OF CURRENT: ILLNESS (First sympton) OR
MM   DD   YY   INJURY (Accident) OR
                      PREGNANCY (LMP)

15. IF PATIENT HAS HAD SAME OR SIMILAR ILLNESS. GIVE FIRST DATE   MM   DD   YY

16. DATES PATIENT UNABLE TO WORK IN CURRENT OCCUPATION
MM   DD   YY   MM   DD   YY
FROM   TO

17. NAME OR REFERRING PHYSICIAN OR OTHER SOURCE

17a. I.D. NUMBER OF REFERRING PHYSICIAN

18. HOSPITALIZATION DATES RELATED TO CURRENT SERVICES
MM   DD   YY   MM   DD   YY
FROM   TO

19. RESERVED FOR LOCAL USE

20. OUTSIDE LAB? $ CHARGES
☐ YES   ☐ NO

21. DIAGNOSIS OR NATURE OF ILLNESS OR INJURY. (RELATE ITEMS 1,2,3 OR 4 TO ITEM 24E BY LINE)

1. I_____.___   3. I_____.___

2. I_____.___   4. I_____.___

22. MEDICAID RESUBMISSION
CODE   ORIGINAL REF. NO.

23. PRIOR AUTHORIZATION NUMBER

24.	A		B	C	D		E	F	G	H	I	J	K
	DATE(S) OF SERVICE		Place of Service	Type of Service	PROCEDURES, SERVICES, OR SUPPLIES (Explain Unusual Circumstances)		DIAGNOSIS CODE	$ CHARGES	DAYS OR UNITS	EPSDT Family Plan	EMG	COB	RESERVED FOR LOCAL USE
	From MM DD YY	To MM DD YY			CPT/HCPCS	MODIFIER							
1													
2													
3													
4													
5													
6													

25. FEDERAL TAX I.D. NUMBER   SSN EIN
☐ ☐

26. PATIENT'S ACCOUNT NO.

27. ACCEPT ASSIGNMENT? (For govt. claims, see back)
☐ YES   ☐ NO

28. TOTAL CHARGE
$

29. AMOUNT PAID
$

30. BALANCE DUE
$

31. SIGNATURE OF PHYSICIAN OR SUPPLIER INCLUDING DEGREES OR CREDENTIALS (I certify that the statements on the reverse apply to this bill and are made a part thereof.)

SIGNED _____ DATE _____

32. NAME AND ADDRESS OF FACULTY WHERE SERVICES WERE RENDERED (If other than home or office)

33. PHYSICIAN'S, SUPPLIER'S BILLING NAME, ADDRESS, ZIP CODE & PHONE#

PIN #   GRP #

(APPROVED BY AMA COUNCIL ON MEDICAL SERVICE 8/88)   **PLEASE PRINT OR TYPE**

FORM HCFA-1500 (U2) (12-90)
FORM OWCP -1500   FORM RRB-1500

CARRIER

PATIENT AND INSURED INFORMATION

PHYSICIAN OR SUPPLIER INFORMATION

PLEASE
DO NOT
STAPLE
IN THIS
AREA

APPROVED OMB-0938-0008

← CARRIER →

PICA

HEALTH INSURANCE CLAIM FORM

PICA

1. MEDICARE   MEDICAID   CHAMPUS   CHAMPVA   GROUP HEALTH PLAN   FECA BLK LUNG   OTHER
☐ (Medicare #) ☐ (Medicaid #) ☐ (Sponsor's SSN) ☐ (VA File #) ☐ (SSN or ID) ☐ (SSN) ☐ (ID)

1a. INSURED'S I.D. NUMBER   (FOR PROGRAM IN ITEM 1)

2. PATIENT'S NAME (Last Name, First Name, Middle Initial)

3. PATIENT'S BIRTH DATE   SEX
   MM ¦ DD ¦ YY   M ☐   F ☐

4. INSURED'S NAME (Last Name, Firts Name, Middle Initial)

5. PATIENT'S ADDRESS (No., Street)

6. PATIENT RELATIONSHIP TO INSURED
   ☐ Self ☐ Spouse ☐ Child ☐ Other

7. INSURED'S ADDRESS (No., Street)

CITY   STATE

8. PATIENT STATUS
   ☐ Single ☐ Married ☐ Other

CITY   STATE

ZIP CODE   TELEPHONE (Include Area Code)
(   )

Employed ☐ Full-Time Student ☐ Part-Time Student ☐

ZIP CODE   TELEPHONE (Include Area Code)
(   )

9. OTHER INSURED'S NAME (Last Name, First Name, Middle Initial)

10. IS PATIENT'S CONDITION RELATED TO:

11. INSURED'S POLICY GROUP OR FECA NUMBER

a. OTHER INSURED'S POLICY OR GROUP NUMBER

a. EMPLOYMENT? (CURRENT OR PREVIOUS)
   ☐ YES ☐ NO

a. INSURED'S DATE OF BIRTH   SEX
   MM ¦ DD ¦ YY   M ☐ F ☐

b. OTHER INSURED'S DATE OF BIRTH   SEX
   MM ¦ DD ¦ YY   M ☐ F ☐

b. AUTO ACCIDENT?   PLACE (State)
   ☐ YES ☐ NO

b. EMPLOYER'S NAME OR SCHOOL NAME

c. EMPLOYER'S NAME OR SCHOOL NAME

c. OTHER ACCIDENT?
   ☐ YES ☐ NO

c. INSURANCE PLAN NAME OR PROGRAM NAME

d. INSURANCE PLAN NAME OR PROGRAM NAME

d. RESERVED FOR LOCAL USE

d. IS THERE ANOTHER HEALTH BENEFIT PLAN?
   ☐ YES ☐ NO If yes, return to and complete item 9 a-d.

READ BACK OF FORM BEFORE COMPLETING & SIGNING THIS FORM.

12. PATIENT'S OR AUTHORIZED PERSON'S SIGNATURE I authorize the release of any medical or other information necessary to process this claim. I also request payment of government benefits either to myself or to the party who accepts assignments below.

SIGNED_____ DATE_____

13. INSURED'S OR AUTHORIZED PERSON'S SIGNATURE I authorize payment of medical benefits to the undersigned physician or supplier for services described below.

SIGNED_____

14. DATE OF CURRENT: ILLNESS (First symptom) OR INJURY (Accident) OR PREGNANCY (LMP)
    MM ¦ DD ¦ YY

15. IF PATIENT HAS HAD SAME OR SIMILAR ILLNESS. GIVE FIRST DATE   MM ¦ DD ¦ YY

16. DATES PATIENT UNABLE TO WORK IN CURRENT OCCUPATION
    MM ¦ DD ¦ YY   MM ¦ DD ¦ YY
    FROM   TO

17. NAME OR REFERRING PHYSICIAN OR OTHER SOURCE

17a. I.D. NUMBER OF REFERRING PHYSICIAN

18. HOSPITALIZATION DATES RELATED TO CURRENT SERVICES
    MM ¦ DD ¦ YY   MM ¦ DD ¦ YY
    FROM   TO

19. RESERVED FOR LOCAL USE

20. OUTSIDE LAB? $ CHARGES
    ☐ YES ☐ NO

21. DIAGNOSIS OR NATURE OF ILLNESS OR INJURY. (RELATE ITEMS 1,2,3 OR 4 TO ITEM 24E BY LINE)

1.I_____.___   3.I_____.___

2.I_____.___   4.I_____.___

22. MEDICAID RESUBMISSION CODE   ORIGINAL REF. NO.

23. PRIOR AUTHORIZATION NUMBER

24.	A				B	C	D		E	F	G	H	I	J	K
	DATE(S) OF SERVICE				Place of Service	Type of Service	PROCEDURES, SERVICES, OR SUPPLIES (Explain Unusual Circumstances)		DIAGNOSIS CODE	$ CHARGES	DAYS OR UNITS	EPSDT Family Plan	EMG	COB	RESERVED FOR LOCAL USE
	From		To				CPT/HCPCS	MODIFIER							
	MM	DD	YY	MM	DD	YY										
1																
2																
3																
4																
5																
6																

25. FEDERAL TAX I.D. NUMBER   SSN EIN
    ☐ ☐

26. PATIENT'S ACCOUNT NO.

27. ACCEPT ASSIGNMENT? (For govt. claims, see back)
    ☐ YES ☐ NO

28. TOTAL CHARGE
    $

29. AMOUNT PAID
    $

30. BALANCE DUE
    $

31. SIGNATURE OF PHYSICIAN OR SUPPLIER INCLUDING DEGREES OR CREDENTIALS (I certify that the statements on the reverse apply to this bill and are made a part thereof.)

SIGNED _____ DATE _____

32. NAME AND ADDRESS OF FACULTY WHERE SERVICES WERE RENDERED (If other than home or office)

33. PHYSICIAN'S, SUPPLIER'S BILLING NAME, ADDRESS, ZIP CODE & PHONE#

PIN #   GRP #

(APPROVED BY AMA COUNCIL ON MEDICAL SERVICE 8/88)

PLEASE PRINT OR TYPE

FORM HCFA-1500 (U2) (12-90)
FORM OWCP -1500   FORM RRB-1500

← PATIENT AND INSURED INFORMATION →

← PHYSICIAN OR SUPPLIER INFORMATION →

Name _____

APPROVED OMB-0938-0008

HEALTH INSURANCE CLAIM FORM

PICA   PICA

1. MEDICARE MEDICAID CHAMPUS CHAMPVA GROUP HEALTH PLAN FECA BLK LUNG OTHER   1a. INSURED'S I.D. NUMBER   (FOR PROGRAM IN ITEM 1)
   ☐ (Medicare #) ☐ (Medicaid #) ☐ (Sponsor's SSN) ☐ (VA File #) ☐ (SSN or ID) ☐ (SSN) ☐ (ID)

2. PATIENT'S NAME (Last Name, First Name, Middle Initial)   3. PATIENT'S BIRTH DATE SEX   4. INSURED'S NAME (Last Name, Firts Name, Middle Initial)
                                                               MM DD YY   M☐ F☐

5. PATIENT'S ADDRESS (No., Street)   6. PATIENT RELATIONSHIP TO INSURED   7. INSURED'S ADDRESS (No., Street)
                                        ☐ Self ☐ Spouse ☐ Child ☐ Other

CITY   STATE   8. PATIENT STATUS   CITY   STATE
                                        ☐ Single ☐ Married ☐ Other

ZIP CODE   TELEPHONE (Include Area Code)   Employed ☐ Full-Time Student ☐ Part-Time Student ☐   ZIP CODE   TELEPHONE (Include Area Code)
           (   )   (   )

9. OTHER INSURED'S NAME (Last Name, First Name, Middle Initial)   10. IS PATIENT'S CONDITION RELATED TO: 11. INSURED'S POLICY GROUP OR FECA NUMBER

a. OTHER INSURED'S POLICY OR GROUP NUMBER   a. EMPLOYMENT? (CURRENT OR PREVIOUS) ☐ YES ☐ NO   a. INSURED'S DATE OF BIRTH SEX
                                                                                                 MM DD YY   M☐ F☐

b. OTHER INSURED'S DATE OF BIRTH SEX   b. AUTO ACCIDENT? PLACE (State) ☐ YES ☐ NO   b. EMPLOYER'S NAME OR SCHOOL NAME
   MM DD YY   M☐ F☐

c. EMPLOYER'S NAME OR SCHOOL NAME   c. OTHER ACCIDENT? ☐ YES ☐ NO   c. INSURANCE PLAN NAME OR PROGRAM NAME

d. INSURANCE PLAN NAME OR PROGRAM NAME   d. RESERVED FOR LOCAL USE   d. IS THERE ANOTHER HEALTH BENEFIT PLAN?
                                                                        ☐ YES ☐ NO If yes, return to and complete item 9 a-d.

READ BACK OF FORM BEFORE COMPLETING & SIGNING THIS FORM.
12. PATIENT'S OR AUTHORIZED PERSON'S SIGNATURE I authorize the release of any medical or other information necessary to process this claim. I also request payment of government benefits either to myself or to the party who accepts assignments below.   13. INSURED'S OR AUTHORIZED PERSON'S SIGNATURE I authorize payment of medical benefits to the undersigned physician or supplier for services described below.

SIGNED_____ DATE_____   SIGNED_____

14. DATE OF CURRENT: MM DD YY ILLNESS (First sympton) OR INJURY (Accident)OR PREGNANCY (LMP)   15. IF PATIENT HAS HAD SAME OR SIMILAR ILLNESS. GIVE FIRST DATE MM DD YY   16. DATES PATIENT UNABLE TO WORK IN CURRENT OCCUPATION MM DD YY FROM TO MM DD YY

17. NAME OR REFERRING PHYSICIAN OR OTHER SOURCE   17a. I.D. NUMBER OF REFERRING PHYSICIAN   18. HOSPITALIZATION DATES RELATED TO CURRENT SERVICES MM DD YY FROM TO MM DD YY

19. RESERVED FOR LOCAL USE   20. OUTSIDE LAB? ☐ YES ☐ NO $ CHARGES

21. DIAGNOSIS OR NATURE OF ILLNESS OR INJURY. (RELATE ITEMS 1,2,3 OR 4 TO ITEM 24E BY LINE)
   1.I____.___   3.I____.___
   2.I____.___   4.I____.___

22. MEDICAID RESUBMISSION CODE   ORIGINAL REF. NO.
23. PRIOR AUTHORIZATION NUMBER

24.	A DATE(S) OF SERVICE			B Place of Service	C Type of Service	D PROCEDURES, SERVICES, OR SUPPLIES (Explain Unusual Circumstances) CPT/HCPCS MODIFIER	E DIAGNOSIS CODE	F $ CHARGES	G DAYS OR UNITS	H EPSDT Family Plan	I EMG	J COB	K RESERVED FOR LOCAL USE
	From MM DD YY	To MM DD YY											
1													
2													
3													
4													
5													
6													

25. FEDERAL TAX I.D. NUMBER SSN ☐ EIN ☐   26. PATIENT'S ACCOUNT NO.   27. ACCEPT ASSIGNMENT? (For govt. claims, see back) ☐ YES ☐ NO   28. TOTAL CHARGE $ 29. AMOUNT PAID $ 30. BALANCE DUE $

31. SIGNATURE OF PHYSICIAN OR SUPPLIER INCLUDING DEGREES OR CREDENTIALS (I certify that the statements on the reverse apply to this bill and are made a part thereof.)   32. NAME AND ADDRESS OF FACULTY WHERE SERVICES WERE RENDERED (If other than home or office)   33. PHYSICIAN'S, SUPPLIER'S BILLING NAME, ADDRESS, ZIP CODE & PHONE#

SIGNED_____ DATE_____   PIN #   GRP #

(APPROVED BY AMA COUNCIL ON MEDICAL SERVICE 8/88)   **PLEASE PRINT OR TYPE**   FORM HCFA-1500 (U2) (12-90) FORM OWCP -1500 FORM RRB-1500

136

ACHIEVING SKILL COMPETENCY

Reread the performance objective for the procedure and then practice the skill listed below, following the procedure in your textbook.

Procedure 9-1: Complete a Claim Form

When you have mastered the performance of the skill, sign your name on the appropriate evaluation sheet and give it to your instructor to indicate you are prepared to perform the procedure for evaluation.

After your instructor has returned your work to you, make all necessary corrections and place in a three-ring notebook for future reference.

ASSIGNMENT SHEET

Chapter 10: MEDICAL OFFICE MANAGEMENT

Review the objectives and text for each unit before completing the assignment sheet for that unit. When you have completed all sheets for the chapter, remove them from this Workbook and give them to the instructor for evaluation.

Unit 1: THE LANGUAGE OF BANKING

Mixed Quiz

1. Matching: Match the definition in column II with the correct term in column I.

COLUMN I

_____ 1. Agent
_____ 2. Bankbook
_____ 3. Bank statement
_____ 4. Cashier's check
_____ 5. Check register
_____ 6. Certified check
_____ 7. Checking account
_____ 8. Currency
_____ 9. Deposit
_____ 10. Debit
_____ 11. Deposit record
_____ 12. Deposit slip

COLUMN II

a. Record of deposit given to customer by bank
b. A person authorized to act for another
c. A bank account against which checks are written
d. Record of deposits, withdrawals, and interest earned
e. An itemized list of cash and checks deposited
f. Check stub
g. Purchaser pays full amount of check issued by bank
h. Paper money issued by government
i. A record sent to customer showing all banking activity for a set period of time
j. Money being placed in a bank account
k. Bank stamps customer's own check and holds funds aside to cover check
l. An entry of an amount owed that has been charged to the account

2. Matching: Match the definition in column II with the correct term in column I.

COLUMN I

_____ 1. Endorsement
_____ 2. Endorser
_____ 3. Insufficient funds
_____ 4. Limited check
_____ 5. Maker
_____ 6. Money order
_____ 7. Note
_____ 8. Payee
_____ 9. Payer
_____ 10. Postdated check
_____ 11. Direct deposit

COLUMN II

a. Negotiable instrument purchased for a fee to be used instead of a check
b. Check made out for a future date
c. Person to whom check is written
d. Payee's signature on back of check
e. A bank term used to indicate that writer of check did not have enough money in account to cover check
f. Person who signs check
g. An amount sent electronically to a savings or checking account
h. Legal evidence of debt
i. Same as payee on check
j. Check that will be void if written over designated amount or kept beyond time limit of when it should be cashed
k. Individual who signs a check

3. Matching: Match the definition in column II with the correct term in column I.

COLUMN I

_____ 1. Power of attorney

_____ 2. Savings account

_____ 3. Service charge

_____ 4. Stale check

_____ 5. Negotiable

_____ 6. Stop payment

_____ 7. Teller

_____ 8. Traveler's check

_____ 9. Voucher check

_____ 10. Warrant

_____ 11. Withdrawal

COLUMN II

a. Bank employee who is main contact between customer and bank

b. Fees charged by bank for services rendered

c. Removal of funds from depositor's account

d. Method by which maker of check may change his mind about making payment

e. Check with detachable form used to state purpose for which check was written

f. A bank account upon which depositor earns interest

g. Evidence of a debt due but is not negotiable

h. Special check issued by bank in exchange for cash that must be signed when purchased and again when used

i. A check presented for payment after date specified when would be honored

j. A legal procedure that authorizes one person to act as agent for another

k. Something that is able to be transferred or exchanged

4. Explain the bank code on a check.

   a. What is an ABA number? _____

   b. Who originated the number concept? _____

   c. What is its purpose? _____

   _____

5. Spell out the acronym MICR. _____

   a. Explain what each series of numbers means.

      1. _____

      2. _____

      3. _____

   b. What does a bank add to the check? _____

   c. Why is MICR used? _____

   _____

Name _____

6. Label the ABA and MICR codes on the check. Refer to Figure 10-1 in the textbook.

Labeling:

JAMES C. MORRISON
1765 SHERIDAN DRIVE
YOUR CITY, STATE, 12345

_____, 19____   00–6789/0000   ] A

101

PAY TO THE ORDER OF _____ | $ _____

_____ DOLLARS

DELUXE CHECK PRINTERS
YOUR CITY, U.S.A. 12345

MEMO _____

|:00006 7894|: 12345678;' 0101 ;0000039158;

B   C   D   E

a. _____
b. _____
c. _____
d. _____
e. _____

7. Explain the difference between overdraft and overdrawn. _____
_____
_____

8. a. List five pieces of information the bank requires to stop payment on a check.
1. _____
2. _____
3. _____
4. _____
5. _____

b. For what reasons may payment be stopped?
1. _____
2. _____

9. Define the term *postdated check* and explain what you must do with such a check. _____
_____
_____

10. What is an electronic fund transfer system? _____
_____

11. Describe the one-write check writing system. _____
_____

12. What would you do in the event a bank deposit is not credited? _____
_____
_____

13. Refer to the Role Delineation Chart in Appendix A of the textbook. Within the area of *Practice Finances,* which two roles relate to the content of this unit?

    a. _____

    b. _____

       After your instructor has returned your work to you, make all necessary corrections and place in a 3-ring notebook for future reference.

ASSIGNMENT SHEET

Chapter 10: MEDICAL OFFICE MANAGEMENT

Unit 2: CURRENCY, CHECKS, AND PETTY CASH

Mixed Quiz

1. Explain why comparing shipments to packing lists or invoices is important. _____
   _____
   _____
   _____

2. Using the following information, write four checks to suppliers of goods and services. Use the current date and sign the checks with the physician's name with your name below the line. Complete the stub end, subtracting each subsequent check. (Two extra checks are provided in case you make an error.)
   a. Physician's Supply, Inc. $125.50
   b. Clinical Laboratory Services $987.45
   c. Brown Office Equipment $535.99
   d. Jones Building Maintenance $1,248.75

3. Fill in the Blanks
   Currency is the name given to _____ It can be made up of _____ and
   _____ When receiving cash from a patient, always _____ the money while the patient is
   watching. When the amount is entered on the ledger card or other form, always indicate the payment is in
   _____ All cash in an offfice should be kept _____ Daily proceeds are usually
   _____ or _____ at the close of the day.

4. List the seven features you must examine to be sure the check is valid. _____
   _____
   _____

5. Why should you refuse a third-party check? _____

6. Why should you not accept a check for more than the amount due? _____
   _____

7. Why may a check marked "payment in full" be a problem? _____
   _____

8. Name the two kinds of endorsements, explaining the meaning of each one.
   a. _____
   _____
   b. _____

9. How do you process a check when the name of the payee is misspelled? _____
   _____

10. Where should a check be endorsed? _____

Check 1490

1490

BAL. BRO'T FOR'D		
_____ 19 ___		
TO _____	DEPOSITS	
FOR _____		
TOTAL		
THIS CHECK		
BALANCE		

ELIZABETH R. EVANS, M.D.
SUITE 205 100 E. MAIN ST.
YOURTOWN, US 98765-4321

1490

_____ 19 ___   25-64/440

PAY
TO THE
ORDER OF _____ $ _____

_____ DOLLARS

THE NEVER FAIL BANK
ANYWHERE, U.S.A 00000

7-88-25

FOR _____

|:00006 7894|: 12345678;' 01490 ;0000039158;

Check 1491

1491

BAL. BRO'T FOR'D		
_____ 19 ___		
TO _____	DEPOSITS	
FOR _____		
TOTAL		
THIS CHECK		
BALANCE		

ELIZABETH R. EVANS, M.D.
SUITE 205 100 E. MAIN ST.
YOURTOWN, US 98765-4321

1491

_____ 19 ___   25-64/440

PAY
TO THE
ORDER OF _____ $ _____

_____ DOLLARS

THE NEVER FAIL BANK
ANYWHERE, U.S.A 00000

7-88-25

FOR _____

|:00006 7894|: 12345678;' 01491 ;0000039158;

Check 1492

1492

BAL. BRO'T FOR'D		
_____ 19 ___		
TO _____	DEPOSITS	
FOR _____		
TOTAL		
THIS CHECK		
BALANCE		

ELIZABETH R. EVANS, M.D.
SUITE 205 100 E. MAIN ST.
YOURTOWN, US 98765-4321

1492

_____ 19 ___   25-64/440

PAY
TO THE
ORDER OF _____ $ _____

_____ DOLLARS

THE NEVER FAIL BANK
ANYWHERE, U.S.A 00000

7-88-25

FOR _____

|:00006 7894|: 12345678;' 01492 ;0000039158;

Check 1493

1493

BAL. BRO'T FOR'D		
_____ 19 ___		
TO _____	DEPOSITS	
FOR _____		
TOTAL		
THIS CHECK		
BALANCE		

ELIZABETH R. EVANS, M.D.
SUITE 205 100 E. MAIN ST.
YOURTOWN, US 98765-4321

1493

_____ 19 ___   25-64/440

PAY
TO THE
ORDER OF _____ $ _____

_____ DOLLARS

THE NEVER FAIL BANK
ANYWHERE, U.S.A 00000

7-88-25

FOR _____

|:00006 7894|: 12345678;' 01493 ;0000039158;

Check 1494

1494

BAL. BRO'T FOR'D		
_____ 19 ___		
TO _____	DEPOSITS	
FOR _____		
TOTAL		
THIS CHECK		
BALANCE		

ELIZABETH R. EVANS, M.D.
SUITE 205 100 E. MAIN ST.
YOURTOWN, US 98765-4321

1494

_____ 19 ___   25-64/440

PAY
TO THE
ORDER OF _____ $ _____

_____ DOLLARS

THE NEVER FAIL BANK
ANYWHERE, U.S.A 00000

7-88-25

FOR _____

|:00006 7894|: 12345678;' 01494 ;0000039158;

Check 1495

1495

BAL. BRO'T FOR'D		
_____ 19 ___		
TO _____	DEPOSITS	
FOR _____		
TOTAL		
THIS CHECK		
BALANCE		

ELIZABETH R. EVANS, M.D.
SUITE 205 100 E. MAIN ST.
YOURTOWN, US 98765-4321

1495

_____ 19 ___   25-64/440

PAY
TO THE
ORDER OF _____ $ _____

_____ DOLLARS

THE NEVER FAIL BANK
ANYWHERE, U.S.A 00000

7-88-25

FOR _____

|:00006 7894|: 12345678;' 01495 ;0000039158;

11. Prepare a bank deposit using the following list of cash and check payments.

Currency/coin: $35.50, $40.00, $50.75, $25.00, $15.75

Checks: Holley, check #134—$40.00

Segal, check #285—$25.00

Gomez, check #596—$55.00

Schmidt, check #436—$32.00

Moriarty, check #1073—$38.00

Kostrevski, check #735—$47.00

Kendrix, check #489—$150.00

Cartloano, check #634—$45.00

Money orders: Chin, $45.00; Jackson, $55.00

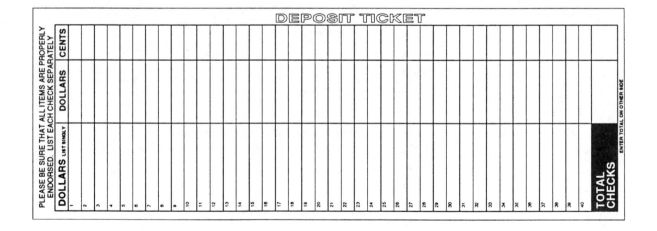

12. What must you do if a mail deposit is lost? _____

_____

13. Use the following figures to reconcile the bank account on the form provided. You may assume the opening balance agrees with the previous statement.

STATEMENT OF ACCOUNT

THE NEVER FAIL BANK • ANYWHERE, USA 00000

For the month of _____, _____(year)

Checks written during the month

#101	25.00	111	500.00	122	35.00		
102	600.00	112	18.22	123	95.94		
103	75.00	113	133.28	124	19.00		
104	37.54	114	57.50	125	75.00		
105	30.00	115	38.60	126	400.00		
106	95.94	116	500.00	127	78.37		
107	73.87	117	785.00	128	95.94		
108	44.00	118	28.37	129	200.00		
109	130.00	119	60.00	130	33.60		
110	95.94	120	36.30	131	1200.00		
		121	115.45	132	100.00		

Checkbook balance end of last month $3173.71

Deposit mailed but not appearing on statement $191.00

Checks Paid Out		Deposits	Balance
Balance Brought Forward			1840.57
25.00	95.94	500.00	1815.57
600.00	44.00	750.00	1715.57
30.00	500.00	350.00	2339.63
73.87	38.60	700.00	2441.76
95.94	115.45	335.00	2394.32
57.50	95.94	500.00	2133.22
28.37	75.00	440.50	2604.85
60.00	78.37	180.00	2985.35
36.30	33.60	175.00	3013.60
35.00	130.00	520.00	3057.66
19.00	18.22	522.50	3483.66
400.00	500.00	720.00	3431.85
200.00	95.94	600.00	3918.25
100.00	133.28	662.00	4414.98
	3.27 SC		5076.98

No. checks 28

No. deposits 14

Service charge 3.27

Ending balance 5076.98

RECONCILE THE BANK STATEMENT

Bank statement balance   _____

Outstanding checks

_____

_____

_____

_____

_____

Subtract total outstanding checks   _____

Adjusted balance   _____

Add deposits not credited   _____

Corrected bank statement balance   _____

Checkbook balance   _____

Subtract bank charges   _____

Corrected checkbook balance   _____

14. For what purpose is a petty cash fund used? _____

_____

15. Word Puzzle: Use the clues below to spell out these terms.

```
 1.              _ E _ _ _ _ _ _
 2.              _ _ _ _ N _ _ _ _
 3.              _ _ _ _ D _ _ _ _ _
 4.              _ O _ _
 5.              _ _ _ R _ _ _ _
 6.              _ _ _ S _ _ _
 7              _ E _ _ _ _ _
 8.              _ _ _ M _ _ _
 9.              _ _ _ _ _ E _
10.              _ _ _ N _ _ _ _ _ _ _
11. _ _ _ _ _ _ _ _ _ T _ _ _
```

1. All consumed, none left
2. Make agree
3. Payee other than patient
4. Cancel, make invalid
5. Cash
6. A record
7. To place in an account
8. A sum paid toward a balance
9. A paper designating payment
10. Action occurring
11. Power given, permission granted

16. Refer to the Role Delineation Chart in Appendix A of the textbook. Within the area of *Practice Finances,* which three roles relate to the content of this unit? _____

_____

After your instructor has returned your work to you, make all necessary corrections and place in a three-ring notebook for future reference.

ASSIGNMENT SHEET

Chapter 10: MEDICAL OFFICE MANAGEMENT

Unit 3: SALARY, BENEFITS, AND TAX RECORDS

Mixed Quiz

1. Fill in the Blanks

    All employees in a physician's office must have a _____ Forms to apply for the number can be obtained from local _____ and _____ Each employee must also complete an _____ indicating the number of exemptions claimed. In addition, recent federal legislation requires the completion of an _____ This form is issued by the _____ _____ Its purpose is to ensure all persons employed are either _____ or _____ In addition to these federal requirements, forms must also be processed for _____ and _____ tax records.

2. What information should be listed on payroll record keeping forms?

    a. _____

    b. _____

    c. _____

    d. _____

    e. _____

    f. _____

    g. _____

    h. _____

    i. _____

    j. _____

    k. _____

    l. _____

    m. _____

3. a. What determines the amount of federal tax withheld?

    1. _____

    2. _____

    3. _____

    4. _____

   b. How are state and local taxes determined? _____

   c. What is net pay? _____

4. What is the physician's responsibility in relation to state and federal regulations?

    a. _____

    b. _____

    c. _____

    d. _____

5. List twelve examples of fringe benefits.

a. _____ g. _____
b. _____ h. _____
c. _____ i. _____
d. _____ j. _____
e. _____ k. _____
f. _____ l. _____

6. What does the term *vested* mean? _____

7. Spelling: Each line contains three different spellings of a word. Underline the correctly spelled word.

accountent   accontant   accountant
disability   disibility   disebility
longevity   lonjevity   longitevy
egemption   exeption   exemption
deducktions   deductions   deductshuns

8. Refer to the Role Delineation Chart in Appendix A of the textbook. Within the area of *Practice Finances*, which role relates specifically to the content of this unit? _____

9. Word Puzzle: Use the clues below to spell out these terms.

1. ___ ___ ___   ___ ___ ___ ___ ___ ___
2. ___ ___ ___ ___ ___   ___ ___ ___ ___
3. ___   ___ ___ ___ ___ ___ ___
4. ___ ___ ___   ___ ___ ___ ___ ___ ___ ___ ___
5. ___ ___ ___ ___   ___ ___ ___ ___
6. ___ ___ ___ ___ ___ ___   ___ ___ ___
7. ___ ___   ___ ___
8. ___ ___ ___ ___ ___ ___ ___ ___
9. ___   ___ ___ ___ ___ ___ ___
10. ___   ___ ___ ___ ___
11. ___ ___
12. ___ ___ ___ ___   ___ ___ ___ ___ ___ ___

1. Eligible credits to reduce tax
2. One who examines fiscal matters
3. Additional to salary
4. Without work
5. To excuse
6. Lack of ability
7. Total earnings
8. Length of time
9. One hired for a job
10. Eligible to receive
11. Remaining
12. Participation in distribution of earnings

After your instructor has returned your work to you, make all necessary corrections and place in a three-ring notebook for future reference.

ASSIGNMENT SHEET

Chapter 10: MEDICAL OFFICE MANAGEMENT

Unit 4: GENERAL MANAGEMENT DUTIES

SUGGESTED RESPONSES TO CRITICAL THINKING CHALLENGE IN TEXTBOOK

1. What are some options open to Michelle? _____
_____

2. What do you think about establishing a different job description with perhaps a little more responsibility in order to justify a salary increase? _____
_____
_____
_____

3. Could additional fringe benefits be established for employees such as Rosie, who have been employed for five years? _____
_____
_____

4. Is there any guarantee that Rosie would stay even if Michelle did manage to arrange a salary increase? _____
_____
_____
_____
_____

5. What really is important for job satisfaction? _____
_____
_____
_____

6. How would being given more responsibility, a *title,* and a sense of control over some portion of the operation provide any incentive? _____
_____
_____
_____
_____
_____
_____
_____

A. Mixed Quiz

1. Why is it necessary to maintain a sense of fiscal status? _____
_____

2. What kinds of information are supplied to the practice monthly by an accountant?
   a. _____
   b. _____
   c. _____

3. What are three consequences of a missed appointment?

   a. _____

   b. _____

   c. _____

4. List eight topics that should be covered by the office policy manual: _____

   _____

   _____

5. What is the purpose of an office procedure manual? _____

   _____

6. What kind of information should be indicated on an inventory card?

   a. _____

   b. _____

   c. _____

   d. _____

7. When might a patient's account be overpaid? _____

   What must you check before refunding any amount? _____

8. All items must be stored properly. Identify the following correct storage places.

   a. Medications in _____

   b. Narcotics in _____

   c. Some laboratory supplies in _____

   d. Supplies _____

9. List an office manager's responsibility to the support staff.

   a. _____

   b. _____

   c. _____

   d. _____

   e. _____

   f. _____

   g. _____

10. List an office manager's responsibilities to physicians.

   a. _____

   b. _____

   c. _____

   d. _____

   e. _____

11. List six organizations that might conduct an on-site visit. _____

   _____

12. Refer to the ABHES Course Content Requirements in Appendix C of the textbook. Within the area of *Medical Office Business Procedures/Management,* which **three** content requirements are discussed in this unit?

   _____

   _____

13. Unscramble

```
A P R E M I U M S D B C D
M E E S F G E D H E MA I
A C I T F I X R J L A C N
N A MA I N T E N A N C E
A L B T S C E C K G U O G
G I U U C O N O L A A U L
E B R S A M S R M T L N I
M R S N L E I D O I P T G
E A E Q R S V S T O U V E
N T M W X R E F U N D Y N
T I E X P E D I T U R E T
Z O N I N V E N T O R Y A
B N T C P O L I C Y D E F
```

ACCOUNT	MANAGEMENT
CALIBRATION	MANUAL
DELEGATION	NEGLIGENT
EXPENDITURE	POLICY
EXTENSIVE	PREMIUMS
FISCAL	RECORDS
INCOME	REFUND
INVENTORY	REIMBURSEMENT
MAINTENANCE	STATUS

ACHIEVING SKILL COMPETENCY

Reread the performance objective for each procedure and practice the skills listed below, following the procedures in your textbook.

Procedure 10-1: Prepare a Check

Procedure 10-2: Prepare a Deposit Slip

Procedure 10-3: Reconcile a Bank Statement

When you feel you have mastered the performance of the skill, sign your name on the appropriate evaluation sheet and give it to your instructor to indicate you are prepared to perform the procedure for evaluation.

After your instructor has returned your work to you, make all necessary corrections and place in a three-ring notebook for future reference.

ASSIGNMENT SHEET

Section 3: THE CLINICAL MEDICAL ASSISTANT

Chapter 11: PREPARING FOR CLINICAL DUTIES

Review the objectives and text for each unit before completing the assignment sheet for that unit. When you have completed all sheets for the chapter, remove them from this Workbook and give them to the instructor for evaluation.

Unit 1: GUIDELINES FOR THE PERSONAL SAFETY AND WELL-BEING OF STAFF AND PATIENTS

A. Brief Answer

1. How can the medical assistant be considerate of patients when assisting with procedures? _____
_____

2. Besides being apprehensive about procedures, what else might a patient be afraid of? _____
_____

3. List the types of patients who will need the undivided attention of the medical assistant. _____
_____
_____

4. How should you speak to patients, and why? _____
_____

5. What special instructions should you give to a patient who is blind? deaf? _____
_____
_____

B. Multiple Choice: Place the correct letter or letters on the blank line for each question.

_____ 1. Assistance dogs (or other assistance animals) should be left alone because the animal
    a. might bite   c. is protecting its owner
    b. is working   d. may feel threatened or distracted

_____ 2. The state of being free of all pathogenic microorganisms is
    a. sanitization   c. disinfection
    b. asepsis   d. esthetic

_____ 3. The ideal temperature setting in a medical office is
    a. 72°F   c. 76°F
    b. 74°F   d. 78°F

_____ 4. After a tissue has been used to catch a sneeze, it should be
    a. put in your pocket   c. placed in a waste receptacle
    b. placed in a sharps container

_____ 5. In the medical facility a foamed alcohol preparation is used to ____ hands.
    a. disinfect   c. sterilize
    b. clean   d. soothe

_____ 6. To turn water faucets on and off for handwashing you should use a
    a. tissue   c. paper towel
    b. gauze square   d. glove

_____ 7. Disposable gloves are available with or without
    a. cuffs   c. lotion
    b. powder   d. disinfectant

8. Areas of the skin that should be covered with a bandage after handwashing and drying and before gloving are
   a. moles and scars
   c. burns
   b. breaks, scratches, cuts
   d. all of these

9. Disposable instruments and _____ should be deposited in the sharps container after use.
   a. lancets
   c. bandages
   b. syringes
   d. needles

10. Electrical wiring and appliances should be checked periodically and tagged for ___ as necessary.
    a. repair
    c. expiration date
    b. cleaning
    d. date of purchase

11. Phone numbers that should be posted near the phone are
    a. personal
    c. patients'
    b. retailers
    d. emergency

12. One who wears loose-fitting clothing and jewelry when working with machines or equipment can contribute to
    a. attractiveness
    c. asepsis
    b. accuracy
    d. accidents

C. True or False: Place a "T" for true or "F" for false in the space provided. For false statements, explain why they are false.

1. There should be a scheduled time weekly for inspection of the entire medical facility.
2. Medical facilities are prime targets of pathogenic organisms.
3. Periodic remodeling of a medical facility should be done only after furniture and carpets become a safety hazard.
4. A disinfectant spray should be kept in a convenient place to disinfect small areas and to help eliminate unpleasant odors.
5. Small toys are not recommended in the pediatric area of the reception room because babies might swallow them.
6. Soap and water should be used every time you wash your hands.
7. If you wear gloves for assisting with invasive procedures, you will not need to wash your hands as often.
8. Emergency exits should be clearly posted with easy-to-follow paths for evacuation in each room of the medical facility.

D. Brief Answer

1. List the reasons for wearing latex gloves.
   a. _____
   _____
   b. _____
   c. _____

2. What information should be documented in case of an accident at a medical facility? _____
   _____

3. What should you do (and what should you tell patients to do) if stricken with a case of the flu/bad cold?
   _____

4. Why should hand lotion be available to the medical assistant in a medical facility? _____
   _____

E. Fill in the Blank

1. A _____ eliminates the possibility of dropping a bar of soap in the sink or on the floor when performing the handwashing procedure.

2. When performing the handwashing procedure, a _____ should be used to dislodge microorganisms around cuticles and under the fingernails.

3. Spills should be cleaned up immediately to prevent _____

4. Lab test results should be recorded _____ on charts and in logs to ensure accuracy.

5. _____ chemicals should be kept away from flames and gas lines.

After your instructor has returned your work to you, make all necessary corrections and place in a three-ring notebook for future reference.

ASSIGNMENT SHEET

Chapter 11: PREPARING FOR CLINICAL DUTIES

Unit 2: INFECTION CONTROL

SUGGESTED RESPONSES TO CRITICAL THINKING CHALLENGE IN TEXTBOOK

1. What is being jeopardized here? _____
_____

2. What gain is there in rushing through your work? _____
_____

3. Is Ella likely to contract what the patient has? _____
_____

4. Who else is being subjected to becoming sick? _____
_____

5. What should she have done? _____
_____

6. Should Ella be reprimanded? _____
_____

7. How do you think the patient felt? _____
_____

8. Would you like to have Ella be your medical assistant if you get sick? Why or why not? _____
_____
_____
_____
_____

ANSWERS TO WORKBOOK ASSIGNMENT

A. Unscramble

1. _ _ _ _ _ _ _ _ _ _ _ _ _   HRDBUZISAOAO

2. _ _ _ _ _ _ _ _   TICAREAB

3. _ _ _ _ _ _ _   SELAMIA

4. _ _ _ _ _ _ _ _ _ _   YORMPGOOHL

5. _ _ _ _ _ _ _ _ _ _ _   UCTESPBSELI

6. _ _ _ _ _ _   ORPSSE

7   _ _ _ _ _ _ _ _ _ _   TNESISAERC

8. _ _ _ _ _ _ _   PSSASIE

9. _ _ _ _ _ _ _ _   EOPHAGTN

10. _ _ _ _ _ _ _ _ _ _ _   EFNCONINTME

11. _ _ _ _ _ _ _   RLEDTPO

B. Matching: Match the definition in column II with the correct term in column I.

COLUMN I

_____ 1. Cholera
_____ 2. Autotrophs
_____ 3. Obligate parasite
_____ 4. Tinea pedis
_____ 5. Viruses
_____ 6. *Escherichia coli*
_____ 7. Dysentery
_____ 8. Facultative parasites
_____ 9. Ticks and fleas
_____ 10. Heterotrophs
_____ 11. Pathogens
_____ 12. Anaerobes

COLUMN II

a. Fungus condition
b. Can live independently
c. Feed on organic matter
d. External parasites
e. From contaminated food/water
f. Disease-producing microorganisms
g. Feed on inorganic matter
h. Grow best in the absence of oxygen
i. Non-pathogen
j. Smallest of microorganisms
k. Completely dependent on host
l. Common cause of urinary tract infections
m. Protozoa

C. Brief Answer

1. Name the common pathogens known to man. _____

2. What are the growth requirements for microorganisms? _____

_____

3. Explain the infection cycle.

   a. _____

   b. _____

   c. _____

   d. _____

   e. _____

4. Name a disinfectant and an antiseptic that are commonly used in the medical office. _____

_____

5. What is most commonly used in preparing a patient's skin for injection or surgery procedures? _____

_____

6. Describe the proper method of cleaning instruments. _____

_____

7. Why should precautions be taken in the storage of instruments? _____

8. Explain the precautions to be taken when you are exposed to all blood and body fluids. (These precautions are known as the "blood and body fluid standard precautions.") Why is it vitally important to follow these precautions carefully? _____

_____

_____

_____

_____

9. How are used needles, scalpels, and other sharp instruments to be handled? Why? _____

_____

_____

_____

10. How should waste be treated before it is disposed of from a medical office or clinic? _____

_____

11. Name the two most feared communicable diseases that health care facilities must strive to prevent
transmitting to the public. _____

D. Matching: Match the disease in column I with the common name in column II.

COLUMN I	COLUMN II
_____ 1. Varicella	a. Pinworms
_____ 2. URI	b. Scabies
_____ 3. Conjunctivitis	c. Chickenpox
_____ 4. Pediculosis	d. Scarlet fever
_____ 5. Herpes simplex	e. Hepatitis B
_____ 6. *Enterobius vermicularis*	f. Common cold
_____ 7. Scarlatina	g. Fever blister
	h. Head lice
	i. Pinkeye

E. Fill in the Blank

1. Antibacterial agents, antibiotics, or corticosteroids, depending on the causative agent, is the treatment for

   _____

2. Cleansing of areas with antibacterial soap and water and topical and/or oral antibiotics is the treatment for

   _____

3. Topical application of drying medications and antibiotics for secondary infections is the treatment for

   _____

4. 2–3 weeks, usually 13–17 days, is the incubation period for _____

5. In one week nits (eggs) hatch; in two weeks they mature. This describes the incubation period for

   _____

6. Bed rest, antipyretics, and topical antipruritics is the treatment for _____

7. 14–50 days is the incubation period for both _____ and _____

8. Blister-like lesions, which later become crusted and itchy, are symptoms of _____

9. Antibiotics, analgesics, antipyretics, increase in fluid intake, and bed rest is the treatment for _____

10. Strawberry tongue, rash of skin and inside of mouth, high fever, nausea, and vomiting are symptoms of

    _____

F. Brief Answer

1. How is impetigo transmitted? _____

2. What is the treatment for hepatitis A and hepatitis B? _____

   _____

3. How long is the incubation period for aseptic meningitis? for bacterial meningitis? _____

   _____

4. Explain the treatment for pediculosis and why it is important to follow it carefully. _____

   _____

   _____

   _____

   _____

   _____

5. What is the incubation period of pinworms and how are they transmitted? _____
_____

6. What are the symptoms of *Enterobius vermicularis* and how is it treated? _____
_____
_____

7. List the symptoms of aseptic meningitis and bacterial meningitis. _____
_____
_____

8. How is aseptic meningitis transmitted? bacterial meningitis? _____
_____

9. What is the treatment of aseptic meningitis? bacterial meningitis? _____
_____
_____

10. What are the symptoms of influenza? _____
_____

11. What is the means of transmission of the common cold? _____
_____

12. How is conjunctivitis transmitted? _____
_____

13. What are the symptoms of hepatitis A? of hepatitis B? _____
_____

14. How is hepatitis A transmitted? hepatitis B? _____
_____

15. What are symptoms of pediculosis and how is it transmitted? _____
_____

16. List the symptoms of scabies. _____
_____

17. How is scabies transmitted? _____
18. How are strep throat and scarlet fever transmitted, and how long are the incubation periods? _____
_____

19. List the symptoms of strep throat and scarlet fever and the treatment for each. _____
_____
_____
_____

20. List the symptoms of AIDS. _____
_____
_____

21. What is the incubation period for AIDS? _____

_____

22. What are the symptoms of *Haemophilus influenzae* type B? _____

_____

23. How is *Haemophilus influenzae* type B transmitted? _____

_____

G. Multiple Choice: Place the correct letter or letters on the blank line for each question.

_____ 1. Red, itching, burning eyes with matted eyelashes are symptoms of
   a. impetigo   c. varicella
   b. scarlatina   d. conjunctivitis

_____ 2. Crops of pruritic vesicular eruptions on the skin, slight fever, headache, and malaise are symptoms of
   a. cholera   c. pediculosis
   b. varicella   d. scabies

_____ 3. This disease is transmitted by direct contact with an infected person who has painful blisters on her lips (pustular/then crusted scabs) and small ulcerated oral lesions.
   a. bacterial meningitis   c. herpes simplex
   b. tinea pedis   d. cholera

_____ 4. Bed rest, increased intake of fluids, and antipyretics is the treatment for
   a. Hepatitis B   c. dysentery
   b. influenza   d. bacterial meningitis

_____ 5. The treatment listed in #4, plus a decongestant and mild analgesics. is the treatment for
   a. common cold   c. cholera
   b. measles   d. scarlatina

_____ 6. The incubation period for scabies is
   a. 2–6 months   c. 2–3 days
   b. 2–6 weeks   d. none of these

_____ 7. The incubation period for the common cold is
   a. 12–72 hours   c. 12–72 weeks
   b. 12–72 days   d. all of these

_____ 8. A scabicide, oral antihistamines, and salicylates to reduce itching is the treatment for
   a. pediculosis   c. scabies
   b. measles   d. varicella

_____ 9. The good health habits of proper rest, nutrition, hygiene, and exercise are helpful in resisting disease and they
   a. promote circulation   c. increase heart rate
   b. destroy pathogens   d. reduce stress

_____ 10. Autoclaving is the most effective and desirable form of sterilization because it
   a. is convenient to use   c. disinfects items
   b. has an automatic timer   d. kills and destroys spores

_____ 11. All members of the health care team must remember to do ___ before and after gloving.
   a. check the patient's chart   c. inventory supplies
   b. check the day's schedule   d. proper hand washing

_____ 12. When cleaning instruments, a brush should be used to
   a. loosen and remove particles from crevices/hinges
   b. protect you from injury
   c. kill and destroy spores
   d. avoid contamination

_____ 13. Soaking instruments in ____ will help loosen material from metal.
   a. alcohol
   b. cool water
   c. zephrin chloride
   d. hot water

H. Crossword Puzzle

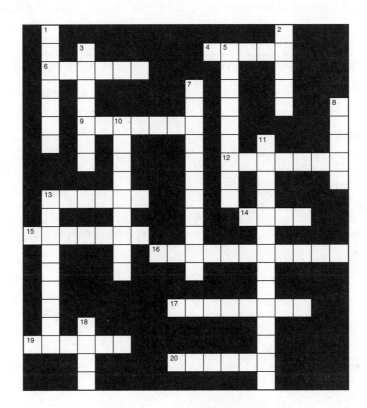

ACROSS
4. Every day
6. Latex barrier for hands
9. Regular habit
12. Free from septic matter
13. Destroyed only by autoclaving
14. Rinse used instruments in _____ water
15. Protection
16. Helps reduce the spread of diseases
17. Do over and over
19. Prior to
20. To do again

DOWN
1. Clean and sanitary
2. Circle
3. Management
5. Destroys microorganisms using steam under pressure
7. Safety measures
8. Used in washing hands/instruments
10. Global
11. Duty
13. Free of all living organisms
18. Infected person/animal

CRITICAL THINKING SCENARIOS: What would your response be in the following situations?

1. One of your co-workers is negligent about handwashing. It bothers you because you realize how easily diseases can be transmitted from person to person. _____

_____

2. You notice that there are several patients in the reception area waiting to be seen by the physician. One of them is sneezing and coughing, and appears to be very ill. _____

3. As you remove a suture pack from the autoclave, you notice that the sterilization indicator tape has not changed color. _____

4. You are checking instruments in preparation for autoclaving. You notice that two of the hemostats have loose hinges and a towel clamp is rusty. _____

_____

ACHIEVING SKILL COMPETENCY

Reread the performance objective for each procedure and then practice the skills listed below, following the procedure in your textbook.

Procedure 11-1: Hand Washing

Procedure 11-2: Wrap Items for Autoclave

When you feel you have mastered the performance of the skill, sign your name on the appropriate evaluation sheet and give it to your instructor to indicate you are prepared to perform the procedure for evaluation.

After your instructor has returned your work to you, make all necessary corrections and place in a three-ring notebook for future reference.

Chapter 12: BEGINNING THE PATIENT'S RECORD

Review the objectives and text for each unit before completing the assignment sheet for that unit. When you have completed all sheets for the chapter, remove them from this Workbook and give them to the instructor for evaluation.

Unit 1: MEDICAL HISTORY

A. Uncramble

1. _ _ _ _ _ _ _   MPYSTMO
2. _ _ _ _ _ _   RVEXET
3. _ _ _ _ _ _   YDRMEE
4. _ _ _ _ _ _   CILETI
5. _ _ _ _ _ _ _   TUSTRAE

B. Brief Answer

1. Why must assistance be given to patients in completing the medical history form? _____

2. Where should the medical assistant interview patients to obtain medical history information? _____

3. Describe how additional questions on the medical history form regarding AIDS/HIV and hepatitis should be worded. _____

4. What additional questions should be asked of patients regarding AIDS/HIV and hepatitis to determine if further investigation should be made as to the health status of that patient? _____

5. Define the following terms.
   a. CC (chief complaint) _____
   b. PI (present illness) _____
   c. ROS (review of systems) _____
   d. PH (past history) _____
   e. FH (family history) _____
   f. PSH (personal/sociocultural history) _____

6. Explain why medical history forms vary in detail and length. _____

7. What is a genogram and why is it helpful to physicians? _____

8. Why must the patient's height and weight be recorded at the initial visit? _____

9. Why is it important to keep an accurate record of the patient's weight? _____

_____

10. What is usually requested for adults when taking the chest measurement? _____

_____

C. Spelling: Each line contains four different spellings of a word. Underline the correctly spelled word and use it in a sentence.

1. measurement   measurement   measuremit   measeurment
2. stadure   statere   stateure   stature
3. infermation   informashion   information   infarmation
4. simptom   symptom   symptome   symptim
5. haight   heite   height   hieght
6. interview   intraview   innerview   inerveiw

1. _____
2. _____
3. _____
4. _____
5. _____
6. _____

D. Multiple Choice: Place the correct letter or letters on the blank line for each question.

_____ 1. The medical assistant shows respect and compassion by calling them in from the reception area by
   a. title (Mr., Ms., etc)   c. either "dear or honey"
   b. first name only   d. first and last name

_____ 2. If the patient has several chief complaints, the medical assistant should
   a. list all the questions that were asked   c. make a list of the symptoms
   b. tell the patient to tell the doctor   d. record the most serious problem

_____ 3. When a patient tells you of a significant personal change in his or her life (e.g. loss of a loved one, being fired, etc.),
   a. keep it to yourself   c. the physician should be told
   b. note it in the chart   d. just acknowledge what was said

_____ 4. A stress-inducing situation (such as mentioned above)
   a. is irrelevant   c. is the patient's business
   b. can influence treatment   d. none of these

_____ 5. If the patient gains or lose weight, this can
   a. be a hereditary trait   c. change the course of treatment
   b. be an error in the scale   d. be recorded on a genogram

CRITICAL THINKING SCENARIOS: What would your response be in the following situations?

1. A new co-worker is interviewing a new patient at the reception window, asking medical history questions and completing the form in earshot and in view of everyone in the office. What would you do? _____

_____

2. This same new worker is found erasing several items on the completed medical history form. What advice do you offer and why? _____

_____

ACHIEVING SKILL COMPETENCY

Reread the performance objectives for these procedures and then practice the skills listed below, following the procedures in your textbook.

Procedure 12-1: Interview Patient to Complete Medical History Form

Procedure 12-2: Measure Height

Procedure 12-3: Weigh Patient on Upright Scale

When you feel you have mastered performance of a skill, sign your name on the appropriate evaluation sheet and give it to your instructor to indicate you are prepared to perform the procedure for evaluation.

After your instructor has returned your work to you, make all necessary corrections and place in a three-ring notebook for future reference.

ASSIGNMENT SHEET

Chapter 12: BEGINNING THE PATIENT'S RECORD

Unit 2: TRIAGE

A. Brief Answer

1. Discuss the origin of triage. _____

2. Where in the medical office should triage be performed? _____

3. Explain phone triage. _____

4. State the purpose of progress notes in the patient chart. _____

5. What type of questioning should be used during patient interviews to obtain information regarding their medical condition? _____

6. Discuss what you should cover with patients at each office visit. _____

7. List the categories for determining the urgency of a patient's condition. _____

8. What is the best way to gain patient compliance? _____

B. Fill in the Blank

1. The French word *triage* means to _____

2. In many medical facilities, small _____ provide privacy to patients during triage.

3. In the medical office there should be a _____ of action developed regarding telephone and face-to-face triage.

4. All office personnel must be familiar with standard first aid procedures and _____

5. You should _____ patients to write down their questions to discuss with the doctor so they will not forget.

C. Matching: Match the definition in column II with the correct term in column I.

COLUMN I	COLUMN II
_____ 1. Prioritize	a. Careful; dedicated and thorough
_____ 2. Trivial	b. Permission to make decision using your own judgment
_____ 3. Dispatch	c. Sort in order of importance
_____ 4. Discretion	d. To combine together in a united whole
_____ 5. Conscientious	e. Of little importance
	f. Send; convey

After your instructor has returned your work to you, make all necessary corrections and place in a three-ring notebook for future reference.

ASSIGNMENT SHEET

Chapter 12: BEGINNING THE PATIENT'S RECORD

Unit 3: VITAL SIGNS

SUGGESTED RESPONSES TO CRITICAL THINKING CHALLENGE IN TEXTBOOK

1. What areas of the Role Delineation Chart were ignored? _____

_____

_____

_____

_____

_____

_____

2. How might this incident affect Susan's employment opportunities? _____

_____

_____

_____

3. What effect could this have on her current and future insurance coverage? _____

_____

_____

_____

_____

_____

_____

4. How might the medical assistant and the physician be affected? _____

_____

_____

_____

This unit contains many important concepts and skills to be mastered; therefore, this workbook unit is divided into four parts.

PART 1—TEMPERATURE CONTROL AND MEASUREMENT

A. Mixed Quiz

1. Identify the four vital signs, indicating what body function is being measured.

   a. _____ measures   the force of the heart.

   b. _____ measures   the body's heat.

   c. _____ measures   the action of the heart.

   d. _____ measures   action of the lungs (breathing).

2. Vital sign findings should be recorded _____

_____

3. The body loses heat through _____ and _____

4. The balance between heat production and heat loss determines the _____

167

5. Temperature is usually the _____ in the morning and the _____ in the afternoon and evening.

6. Fill in the Blank

Temperature in the body is controlled by the _____ in the _____ of the brain. When receptors sense the presence of excess heat, the _____ produce _____ which _____ from the surface of the skin, causing the body to _____ The surface blood vessels _____ which allows more blood to be in contact with the surface of the skin. The blood _____ heat, thereby _____ the blood in the vessels. When receptors sense a lack of heat, the surface blood vessels _____ to _____ heat loss. Small papillary muscles _____ producing _____ to help _____ the body. Shivering and chills will cause body heat to _____

7. Explain briefly how a fever develops (use five steps).

a. _____

_____

b. _____

c. _____

d. _____

e. _____

_____

8. Fill in the Blank

Provide the correct Fahrenheit temperature when referring to classifications of fevers.

a. Slight = _____ °F

b. Moderate = _____ °F

c. Severe = _____ °F

d. Dangerous = _____ °F

e. Fatal = _____ °F

9. The column of mercury shown on the thermometer reads a "normal" 98.6° on the Fahrenheit scale. At each arrow, read the temperature and enter the finding at the corresponding space.

a. _____   c. _____   e. _____   g. _____   i. _____

b. _____   d. _____   f. _____   h. _____   j. _____

10. The column of mercury on the thermometer reads a "normal" 37° on the Celsius scale. At each arrow, read the temperature and enter the finding at the corresponding space.

a. _____   c. _____   e. _____   g. _____   i. _____

b. _____   d. _____   f. _____   h. _____   j. _____

11. List the five thermometer types.

a. _____

b. _____

c. _____

d. _____

e. _____

12. Name situations when oral temperature measurement is contraindicated.

a. _____

b. _____

c. _____

d. _____

e. _____

13. Matching: Match the terms in column I with their meanings in column II.

COLUMN I

_____ 1. Afebrile
_____ 2. Axillary
_____ 3. Febrile
_____ 4. Oral
_____ 5. Sublingual
_____ 6. Fever
_____ 7. Celsius
_____ 8. Rectal
_____ 9. Calibration
_____ 10. Stem
_____ 11. Disinfectant
_____ 12. Contraindicated

COLUMN II

a. A metric measurement
b. By mouth
c. Numbered markings
d. Not appropriate
e. Thermometer section
f. Fever
g. Underarm
h. Germicide
i. Without fever
j. Beneath tongue
k. Elevated body heat
l. Anal
m. Fahrenheit
n. Anesthetic
o. Security

14. Convert the following Celsius temperatures to Fahrenheit.

a. 36.5°C = _____ °F   d. 35.7°C = _____ °F

b. 39.5°C = _____ °F   e. 36.8°C = _____ °F

c. 38.8°C = _____ °F   f. 37.4°C = _____ °F

15. Convert the following Fahrenheit temperatures to Celsius.

a. 96.8°F = _____ °C   d. 99.2°F = _____ °C

b. 97.4°F = _____ °C   e. 100.2°F = _____ °C

c. 98.6°F = _____ °C   f. 102.4°F = _____ °C

16. Word Search: Find the following words hidden in the puzzle.

ACCURACY DANGEROUS HOLDER SECURITY
AFEBRILE DEGREES INFECTION SEVERE
ASEPTICALLY DISINFECT INSERT SHAKE
AXILLARY ELECTRONIC INSPECT SLIGHT
BULB ELEVATION LUBRICANT STEM
BUTTOCKS FAHRENHEIT MERCURY STUBBY
CALIBRATION FATAL METRIC SUBLINGUAL
CENTIGRADE FEBRILE MODERATE SUBNORMAL
CHILLS FEVER MOUTH TEMPERATURE
CHIPPED FINDINGS NORMAL TENTHS
COLLAPSE FRAGILE ORAL THERMOMETER
COOLING GLASS RECORD
CONTRAINDICATED HEAT RECTAL

```
A G L A S S I E T V E E O F A T A L M M W Q I S T N D
C H I L L S O T B C L O B T P W I E L E V A T I O N V
O I Y T W C B N Y I C F I H E M K V Z T O P W I M G X
L G F J M I T O G P H C N E C M M I W R W S T U B B Y
L V A C C U R A C Y I U S R C V P S Y I E A S H A K E
A E A J K U R L R Y P T P M P O E E C C R V Y T Z X P
P N F A H F P U I X P B E O Q H C S R B K N L R W V C
S W E R T I C D L P E Y C M R T O W I A J L V C X I N
E N B P R R B V A G D D T E I Y Q L P U T M V X W O F
W I R C E B V X U N J H V T L W A L D I W U L W I O E
M V I M C O W G T E G H I E M C A L O E W P R T Z C V
B C L I T E N I P I U E S R C M V X U Y R W C E N L E
C F E S A I J L L Y T Q R X R S Z Y I N S E R T D E R
K H J R L N B S A W Q Z R O P U T V W L F U C B L S W
B G D O M U R B C I W R N P U F X C V N L I Y I V C S
U K O M L U B R I C A N T G H S W Q I K N A R X C V T
T C C O N T R A I N D I C A T E D E P O T B R C X I E
T D F A S C V B B N I O Y U I O R W R C E I O Y E C M
O S U B N O R M A L M T Q W E E O T C F K L H H T Y U
C E N T I G R A D E I O S D V C C S U B L I N G U A L
K E R E Y U I O O R S D D E L E I O L S D E M N V C S
S E R N K L M O U T H I S E L K L U S D R E C O R D I
U T Y T F G H C R T Y U I E R I B I O H E A T Y U I O
W E R H A S E P T I C A L L Y A K L A W E R T Y O I R
A S D S L S Z X C V B N M S D F T F I N D I N G S I A
D I S I N F E C T A N T E D E G R E E S G J K L Z X L
```

ACHIEVING SKILL COMPETENCY

Reread the performance objective for each procedure and then practice the skills listed below, following the procedures in your textbook.

Procedure 12-8:   Measure Oral Temperature with Disposable Plastic Thermometer
Procedure 12-9:   Measure Oral Temperature Electronically
Procedure 12-10: Measure Core Body Temperature with Infrared Tympanic Thermometer

When you feel you have mastered performance of a skill, sign your name on the appropriate evaluation sheet and give it to your instructor to indicate you are prepared to perform the procedure for evaluation.

PART 2—THE PULSE AND ITS MEASUREMENT

B. Mixed Quiz

1. Define *pulse* and explain how it occurs. _____
   _____

2. Name and locate the five pulse points.
   a. _____
   b. _____
   c. _____
   d. _____
   e. _____

3. How is pulse rate determined? What is the normal adult rate? _____
   _____

4. List five factors that influence heart rate.
   a. _____
   b. _____
   c. _____
   d. _____
   e. _____

5. Stimulation of the sympathetic nervous system _____ heart rate. The parasympathetic nervous system _____ the heart rate.

6. List eight situations that cause the heart rate to increase.
   a. _____ e. _____
   b. _____ f. _____
   c. _____ g. _____
   d. _____ h. _____

7. List four situations that cause the heart rate to decrease.
   a. _____ c. _____
   b. _____ d. _____

8. Name the two qualities of the heartbeat that must be observed, defining the terms and listing the words used to describe the characteristics.
   a. _____
   b. _____
   _____

9. List eight times when apical pulse measurement would be indicated.
   a. _____ e. _____
   b. _____ f. _____
   c. _____ g. _____
   d. _____ h. _____

10. True or False: Place a "T" for true or an "F" for false in the space provided. For false statements, explain why they are false.
    _____ a. A patient should be sitting or lying down when the pulse is measured.
    _____ b. The radial pulse can be found at the inner wrist area on the little finger side.
    _____ c. The radial pulse is best felt by placing your thumb over the artery.
    _____ d. The pulse that can be felt in the radial artery is caused by the contraction of the aorta.
    _____ e. Apical pulse is located at the right fifth intercostal space.
    _____ f. A quick way to estimate the location of the apex is to position the right hand over the patient's chest and listen at the point under the thumb.

11. Fill in the Blanks

Pulse deficit can be determined by measuring _____ pulse and _____

pulse at the _____ If a patient has a pulse deficit, the auscultated apical pulse rate is

_____ than the _____ pulse rate. This occurs because some of the

contractions are _____

12. Matching: Match the terms in column I with the correct meaning in column II.

COLUMN I

_____ 1. Antecubital
_____ 2. Apex
_____ 3. Arrhythmia
_____ 4. Auscultate
_____ 5. Brachial
_____ 6. Bradycardia
_____ 7. Carotid
_____ 8. Femoral
_____ 9. Palpate
_____ 10. Pulse deficit
_____ 11. Radial
_____ 12. Tachycardia

COLUMN II

a. Excessively slow heart rate
b. Feel by touching
c. Inner elbow area
d. A pulse point on the instep of the foot
e. Excessively rapid heart rate
f. A pulse point at the inner wrist
g. A pulse point near the trachea
h. Lower edge of the heart
i. To listen
j. A pulse point at the inner elbow
k. Without a regular pattern of beats
l. A pulse point at the groin
m. The difference between apical and radial pulse
n. Weak heart volume

13. Unscramble

a. _ _ _ _ _   RTEHA
b. _ _ _ _   EBTA
c. _ _ _ _ _ _ _ _   TCNTAROC
d. _ _ _ _ _ _ _ _   LYOISTSC
e. _ _ _ _ _ _   LIACAP
f. _ _ _ _ _   SLUEP
g. _ _ _ _ _ _ _ _ _ _ HRAMTIRHYA
h. _ _ _ _ _ _ _   ATCRDIO
i. _ _ _ _ _ _   ALRIDA
j. _ _ _ _ _ _ _ _   HLRAIBAC
k. _ _ _ _ _ _ _   MROAFLE
l. _ _ _ _ _ _   EYTARR
m. _ _ _ _   TREA
n. _ _ _ _ _ _   YHTRMH
o. _ _ _ _ _ _   LVEMOU

ACHIEVING SKILL COMPETENCY

Reread the performance objective for these procedures and then practice the skills listed below, following the procedures in your textbook.

Procedure 12-11: Measure Radial Pulse

Procedure 12-12: Measure Apical Pulse

When you feel you have mastered performance of a skill, sign your name on the appropriate evaluation sheet and give it to your instructor to indicate you are prepared to perform the procedure for evaluation.

PART 3: RESPIRATIONS: OBSERVATION AND MEASUREMENT

C. Mixed Quiz

1. One respiration is the combination of one total _____ and one total _____
Two other terms that are frequently used and have the same meaning are _____ and
_____

2. When are respirations usually measured? _____
_____

3. Why are respirations measured as if the pulse is being measured? _____
_____

4. The quality of respirations must be observed. Normal respirations are _____ and
_____

5. Excessively rapid and deep respirations are known as _____

6. Patients with difficult or labored breathing are said to have _____

7. Noisy respirations are called rales, and are often present with diseases such as _____
_____ and _____

8. Quality characteristics that are evaluated when respirations are measured are:
    a. Depth of inhalation which, is described as _____ _____ or
    _____
    b. Rhythm of respiration, which is described as _____ or _____

9. Absence of breathing is known as _____

10. Describe the breathing pattern known as Cheyne-Stokes. _____
_____
_____

11. Normal respiration rate for an adult is _____ per minute.

12. Respiration rate is affected by:
    a. _____
    b. _____
    c. _____
    d. _____
    e. _____

13. Fill in the temperature-pulse-respiration ratio below.

Temperature	Pulse	Respiration
99°F		
100°F		
102°F		
104°F		

14. Crossword Puzzle

ACROSS

1. Organ which pumps blood
3. Contraction phase
6. Without rhythm
9. Lower heart edge
10. Part of the verb "to be"
11. One of the vital signs
13. Heart
14. A period of time
16. Father
17. A pulse point

DOWN

1. Mercury (abbr)
2. Sudden heart failure
4. Breathe out
5. Difficult breathing
6. Auscultated heart beat
7. Prescription (abbr)
8. A plan or thought
12. Senior (abbr)
13. Anterior-posterior (abbr)
15. Solution (abbr)

15. Speling: Each line contains four different spellings of a word. Underline the correctly spelled term.

a. Cheyne-Stokes	Chain-Stokes	Cheyne-Stoakes	Chenye-Stokes
b. dispnea	dispena	dyspnea	dyspnae
c. eshale	exhale	exhail	exhaile
d. expirashun	experation	expieration	expiration
e. enhale	enhail	inhale	inhail
f. inspiration	enspiration	ensperation	insperation
g. resperation	respiration	rexpiration	rexperation

ACHIEVING SKILL COMPETENCY

Reread the performance objective for the procedure and then practice the skill listed below, following the procedure in your textbook.

Procedure 12-13: Measure Respirations

When you feel you have mastered performance of a skill, sign your name on the appropriate evaluation sheet and give it to your instructor to indicate you are prepared to perform the procedure for evaluation.

PART 4: BLOOD PRESSURE

D. Mixed Quiz

1. Name the four vital signs.
   a. _____
   b. _____
   c. _____
   d. _____

2. Define *blood pressure*. _____
   _____

3. What does blood pressure measurement evaluate?
   a. _____
   b. _____
   c. _____
   d. _____

4. Where is blood pressure measured? (be specific) _____

5. Name the two organs that maintain blood pressure in the body.
   a. _____
   b. _____

6. Explain briefly how blood pressure is maintained. _____
   _____
   _____
   _____

7. Name the two phases of the blood pressure, describing the corresponding action which occurs and the relative amount of pressure with each phase. _____
   _____

8. Blood pressure is measured in _____

9. Blood pressure is measured by a _____ which has either an _____ dial or a column of _____

10. Normal adult systolic pressure is _____ _____ _____ normal diastolic pressure is _____ _____ _____

11. Blood pressure that is consistently high is called _____

12. Blood pressure that is consistently low is called _____

13. An elevated pressure without apparent cause is said to be _____ or _____ hypertension.

14. List six possible causes of hypertension.
    a. _____   d. _____
    b. _____   e. _____
    c. _____   f. _____

15. Define *pulse pressure*. _____

16. Using the "general rule of thumb," is the pulse pressure of the following examples too low, normal, or too high? (*Note:* A normal pulse pressure does not mean the blood pressure is within a normal range.)
    a. 130/86 _____
    b. 160/90 _____
    c. 110/74 _____
    d. 200/110 _____
    e. 186/98 _____
    f. 120/100 _____
    g. 174/116 _____

17. Several equipment factors influence accurate measurement. Explain what each item indicates or would cause to occur.

    a. Leaking mercury or bubbles would cause _____

    b. Too small a cuff would cause _____

    c. Too large a cuff would cause _____

    d. Mercury meniscus below "O" indicates _____

18. True or False: Place a "T" for true or an "F" for false in the space prvoided. For false statements, explain why they are false.

    _____ a. Completely deflate the cuff before applying.

    _____ b. Blood pressure may be measured over a silky sleeve.

    _____ c. The cuff is placed around the arm with the arrow at the brachial artery.

    _____ d. Inflate cuff slowly until you no longer hear beats.

    _____ e. When you miss the systolic reading, immediately reinflate the cuff before all air pressure escapes.

    _____ f. The patient's arm should be extended straight down at the side when in sitting position.

    _____ g. Palpatory readings are done only when the pressure cannot be auscultated.

19. What does it mean to take a baseline reading? _____

_____

20. Define *auscultatory gap*. _____

21. What would cause you to think a patient might have an auscultatory gap: _____

_____

22. Crossword Puzzle

DOWN

  1. Bone

  2. Article; used in language

  3. Silver-colored liquid

  4. To take nourishment

  5. Lowered

  6. 365 days

  7. Felt in arteries

10. Contraction phase

13. Pulse point at wrist

14. Noisy respirations

16. The number of times

17. Three dimensional X ray (abbreviation)

20. Pelvic exam (acronym)

ACROSS

  2. End of prayer

  5. Difficult breathing

  8. Second word in music scale

  9. Right (abbreviation)

11. Blood _____

12. External organ of hearing

15. Most desirable option

18. Mother

19. Bottom edge of heart

21. Stories

22. Barium enema (acronym)

12. Unscramble

a. _ _ _ _ _ _ _   ENIDOAR

b. _ _ _ _ _ _ _ _ _ _ _   TUTENBLAIAC

c. _ _ _ _ _ _ _ _ _   LSAIDOTCI

d. _ _ _ _ _ _ _ _   HRABLICA

e. _ _ _ _ _ _ _ _ _   SLATSNEIE

f. _ _ _ _ _ _ _ _ _ _   ETUSLTAUAC

g. _ _ _ _ _ _ _ _ _ _ _ _   OEPTYEHRNSIN

h. _ _ _ _ _ _ _   YRUMREC

i. _ _ _ _ _ _ _ _   LTYSCOSI

j. _ _ _ _ _ _ _   TPEALPA

13. Refer to the ABHES Course Content Requirements in Appendix C of the textbook. Within the area of *Medical Office Clinical Procedures,* which content requirement is discussed in this unit? _____

_____

ACHIEVING SKILL COMPETENCY

Reread the performance objective for the procedure and then practice the skill listed below, following the procedure in your textbook.

Procedure 12-14: Measure Blood Pressure

When you feel you have mastered performance of a skill, sign your name on the appropriate evaluation sheet and give it to your instructor to indicate you are prepared to perform the procedure for evaluation.

After your instructor has returned your work to you, make all necessary corrections and place in a three-ring notebook for future reference.

ASSIGNMENT SHEET

Chapter 13: PREPARING PATIENTS FOR EXAMINATION

Review the objectives and text for each unit before completing the assignment sheet for that unit. When you have completed all sheets for the chapter, remove them from this Workbook and give them to the instructor for evaluation.

Unit 1: PROCEDURES OF THE EYE AND EAR

A. Multiple Choice: Place the correct letter or letters on the blank line for each question.

_____ 1. Patients should be screened for visual acuity

    a. wearing their corrective lenses   c. early in the morning

    b. only in natural lighting   d. without their corrective lenses

_____ 2. Patients should hold the Jaeger near vision card at what distance away from the eyes?

    a. 0.4 to 0.6 inches   c. 14 to 16 feet

    b. 4 to 6 inches   d. 14 to 16 inches

_____ 3. A person with normal hearing should be able to hear all frequencies up to ____ decibels?

    a. 0.15   c. 15

    b. 1.5   d. none of these

_____ 4. The medical assistant who will be administering the color vision acuity screening must first

    a. be tested to determine if she has normal color vision acuity

    b. take the test wearing corrective lenses

    c. tell patients to cover the right eye and test the left, then reverse, then both

    d. determine if an eye irrigation is necessary

_____ 5. It very important to administer the color vision acuity test to patients with

    a. cardiac problems   c. thyroid conditions

    b. diabetes   d. glaucoma

_____ 6. What instrument measures one's hearing ability?

    a. otoscope   c. autoclave

    b. audiometer   d. tuning fork

B. Brief Answer

1. List patient education advice you can offer during procedures of the eye and ear. _____

_____

_____

_____

2. What must the medical assistant remember to do with the ophthalmoscope and otoscope in preparing for eye and ear examinations: _____

_____

3. What types of patients will require being tested for visual acuity with the Snellen chart? _____

_____

4. Why must the patient keep both eyes open during the visual acuity screening even though one eye is covered?

_____

5. What is the Ishihara screening method, and why is it administered to patients? _____

_____

6. Why is it necessary for the medical assistant to wear latex gloves when performing procedures on the eye and ear? _____

_____

7. What is the purpose of an eye irrigation? _____

_____

8. Define instillation of eye or ear drops. _____

_____

9. What is cerumen? _____

10. Why must impacted cerumen be softened and irrigated from the ear? _____

_____

_____

11. Explain why the tip of an eye (medication) dropper or the tip of a tube of eye ointment must never touch the secretions of the eye or the eye itself. _____

_____

_____

12. Describe the Rinne test for hearing. _____

_____

_____

13. Describe the Weber test for hearing. _____

_____

14. List common behaviors that may indicate hearing loss. _____

_____

_____

15. List common complaints that may indicate visual disturbances. _____

_____

16. What is the purpose of the audiometer? _____

_____

C. Crossword Puzzle

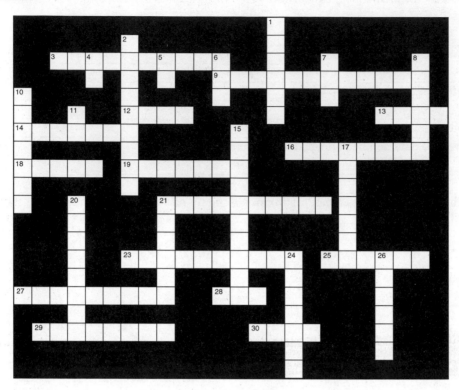

ACROSS
3. Red blindness
9. Green blindness
12. Regarding the ear
13. Please ____ the eye chart
14. Medical term for earwax
16. Another word for lavage
18. To open and close eyes fast
19. Visual acuity charts
21. Instrument used to measure hearing
23. Blue blindness
25. Used to protect hands from body fluids/standard precautions
27. Measuring intraocular pressure
28. One of a pair of the organs of sight
29. Used with otoscope to examine the ear
30. Small amount of sterile cotton (holds medication in ear)

DOWN
1. Carefully
2. Color blindness (both red and green)
4. Abbreviation for left eye
5. Abbreviation for right eye
6. To state further
7. Organ of hearing
8. Means "to wash out"
10. Unit for measuring volume of sound abbreviation for both eyes
11. Abbreviation for both eyes
15. Study of the fundus of the eye
17. To introduce a solution into a cavity
20. Instrument used to examine the ear
21. Clearness/sharpness of perception
24. The external ear
26. Capacity for sight

A. Matching: Match the definition in column II with the correct term in column I.

COLUMN I

_____ 1. Pelli-Robson chart
_____ 2. For babies
_____ 3. Numerator of 20/100
_____ 4. Ear instillation
_____ 5. For adults
_____ 6. Observe patient
_____ 7. Snellen chart
_____ 8. Eye instillation
_____ 9. Denominator of 20/100
_____ 10. Wick
_____ 11. Jaeger system

COLUMN II

a. For behaviors indicating visual disturbances
b. Pull up and back to straighten the ear canal
c. A screening for near vision acuity
d. Cotton saturated with medication for ear
e. Required distance one stands from visual acuity chart
f. To treat infection, anesthetize, dilate pupil, relieve irritation
h. Means that one stood 20 feet from chart and read the line that one should be able to read at a distance of 100 feet
g. Measure contrast sensitivity for earlier diagnosis of eye disease
i. Pull down and back to straighten the ear canal
j. Determines color vision acuity
k. To treat infection, relieve pain, soften cerumen
l. A screening for distance visual acuity

CRITICAL THINKING SCENARIOS: What would your response be in the following situations?

1. Mr. Harold tells you that his ears often get plugged up and he can't understand it because he uses a cotton-tipped applicator every day after his shower to get all the ear wax out. _____

_____

2. Myra is a teenage patient who comes in frequently to see the doctor for her allergies. She always has her head set and radio on full volume. _____

_____

ACHIEVING SKILL COMPETENCY

Reread the performance objective for the procedures and then practice the skills listed below, following the procedure in the textbook.

Procedure 13-1: Irrigate the Eye
Procedure 13-2: Irrigate the Ear
Procedure 13-3: Instill Eardrops
Procedure 13-4: Instill Eyedrops
Procedure 13-5: Screen Visual Acuity with Snellen Chart
Procedure 13-6: Screen Visual Acuity with Jaeger System

When you feel you have mastered performance of a skill, sign your name on the appropriate evaluation sheet and give it to your instructor to indicate you are prepared to perform the procedure for evaluation.

After your instructor has returned your work to you, make all necessary corrections and place in a three-ring notebook for future reference.

ASSIGNMENT SHEET

Chapter 13: PREPARING PATIENTS FOR EXAMINATION

Unit 2: POSITIONING AND DRAPING FOR EXAMINATIONS

A. Brief Answer

1. Explain the purpose of each of the following examination positions.

   a. Horizontal recumbent or supine. _____

   _____

   b. Dorsal recumbent. _____

   _____

   _____

   c. Prone. _____

   d. Standing erect or anatomical. _____

   _____

   e. Sims' or lateral. _____

   _____

   f. Knee-chest. _____

   g. Genupectoral. _____

   h. Fowler's. _____

   _____

   i. Semi-Fowler's. _____

   j. Lithotomy. _____

   _____

   k. Trendelenburg or shock _____

   _____

   _____

   l. Jackknife. _____

2. What safety precautions must be observed for protection of both the patient and the medical assistant?

   _____

   _____

3. Why is a drape used when positioning patients? _____

   _____

4. What support is used for the feet in the lithotomy position? _____

5. Name the drape used for proctological examinations. _____

B. Matching: Match the position in column II with the correct term in column I.

COLUMN I

_____ 1. Back and posterior
_____ 2. Exercise postpartum
_____ 3. Proctoscopic
_____ 4. Eye, Ear, Nose, Throat
_____ 5. Anterior
_____ 6. Pelvic
_____ 7. Shock
_____ 8. Abdominal exam
_____ 9. Gynecologist
_____ 10. GP/Internal Medicine
_____ 11. Ophthalmologist, thoracic surgeon, ENT specialist
_____ 12. Proctologist
_____ 13. No specialty
_____ 14. GP/Orthopedist/Internist
_____ 15. GP/Internal Medicine/Gynecologist

COLUMN II

a. Genupectoral
b. Sims'/knee-chest
c. Semi-Fowler's/Fowler's
d. Horizontal/recumbent/supine
e. Prone
f. Trendelenburg
g. Dorsal recumbent
h. Lithotomy

C. Multiple Choice: Place the correct letter on the blank line for each question.

_____ 1. Patient lying flat on table with buttocks at lower end of the table and feet supported in stirrups
   a. prone   c. lithotomy
   b. Sim's   d. Fowler's

_____ 2. Patient on back with feet elevated
   a. Sim's   c. prone
   b. supine   d. Trendelenburg

_____ 3. Patient sitting with head of table elevated at 45° angle
   a. lithotomy   c. semi-Fowler's
   b. lateral   d. supine

_____ 4. Patient lying flat on back with feet flat on table and knees flexed
   a. knee-chest   c. dorsal recumbent
   b. prone   d. Sim's

_____ 5. Patient flat on stomach with the head to one side
   a. Trendelenburg   c. lateral
   b. prone   d. horizontal recumbent

_____ 6. Patient on knees and chest with knees separated and head to one side
   a. dorsal recumbent   c. knee-chest
   b. Sim's   d. lateral

_____ 7. Patient on left side with left leg flexed slightly and right leg flexed sharply to the chest
   a. lithotomy   c. Sim's
   b. supine   d. supine

_____ 8. Patient lying flat on back with legs together
   a. horizontal recumbent   c. dorsal recumbent
   b. Sim's   d. prone

D. Identification: Identify the following examination positions.

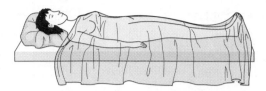

1. a _____

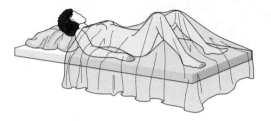

1. b _____

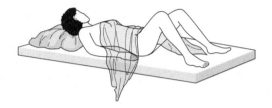

1. c _____

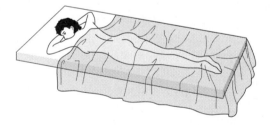

2. _____

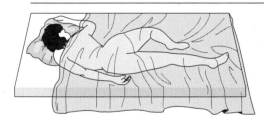

3. _____

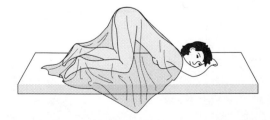

4. _____

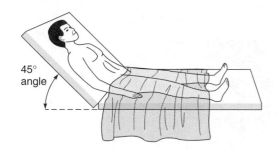

5. a _____

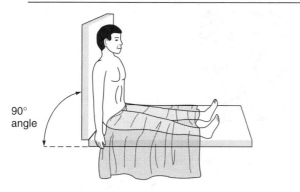

5. _____

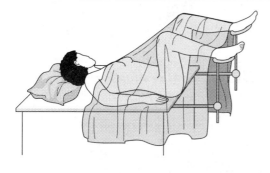

6. _____

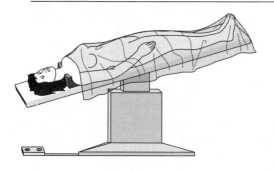

7. _____

E. Crossword Puzzle

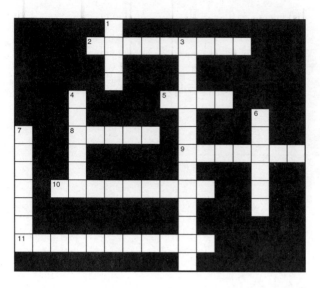

ACROSS

2. Pelvic
5. Chest, proctoscopic exam
8. Back, posterior
9. Same as Sims'
10. Same as supine
11. Eye, ear, nose, throat

DOWN

1. Proctoscopic exam
3. Shock
4. Anterior
6. Relax abdomen
7. Eye, ear, nose, throat

CRITICAL THINKING SCENARIOS: What would your response be in the following situation?

1. A female patient in her 80s seems to be very confused as you explain to her that you want her to undress and wear a gown and drape in preparation for a complete physical examination. _____

_____

ACHIEVING SKILL COMPETENCY

Reread the performance objective for each procedure and then practice the skills listed below, following the procedures in your textbook.

Procedure 13-8:   Assist Patient to Horizontal Recumbent Position
Procedure 13-9:   Assist Patient to Prone Position
Procedure 13-10: Assist Patient to Sims' Position
Procedure 13-11: Assist Patient to Knee-Chest Position
Procedure 13-12: Assist Patient to Semi-Fowler's Position
Procedure 13-13: Assist Patient to Lithotomy Position

When you feel you have mastered performance of a skill, sign your name on the appropriate evaluation sheet and give it to your instructor to indicate you are prepared to perform the procedure for evaluation.

After your instructor has returned your work to you, make all necessary corrections and place in a three-ring notebook for future reference.

ASSIGNMENT SHEET

Chapter 13: PREPARING PATIENTS FOR EXAMINATIONS

Unit 3: PREPARING PATIENTS FOR EXAMINATIONS

SUGGESTED RESPONSES TO CRITICAL THINKING CHALLENGE IN TEXTBOOK

1. What are Martina and Sylvia guilty of doing? _____
   _____

2. Should they apologize to Cassie? _____
   _____

3. Should the office manager or physician be informed of this behavior? _____
   _____

4. Do you think Sylvia and Martina meant any malice? _____
   _____

5. Is there any legal action that should be initiated in this situation? _____
   _____

6. Should Cassie have responded immediately to what she overheard? _____
   _____
   _____

7. What would you do in this situation? _____
   _____

ANSWERS TO WORKBOOK ASSIGNMENT

A. Brief Answer

1. Define *subjective* and *objective symptoms* and give three examples of each.
   _____
   _____

2. List each section of a physical examination and describe how the physician conducts the exam.
   _____

3. Describe the role of the medical assistant in the patient examination process.
   _____
   _____

4. List various patient education tips for various sections of the patient examination.
   _____

5. What are the nine sections of the abdominal cavity?
   _____

6. List the internal organs located in each of the nine sections of the abdomen.
   _____
   _____
   _____

Name _____

7. Define the Problem Oriented Medical Record (POMR) system.

_____

_____

8. Explain how data are recorded with the POMR system.

_____

_____

9. List the warning signs for adults and children.

_____

10. What are the standard physical examination schedules for adults and children?

_____

B. Matching: Match the definition in column II with the correct term in column I.

COLUMN I

_____ 1. Sphygmomanometer
_____ 2. Speculum
_____ 3. Tonometer
_____ 4. Tape measure
_____ 5. Stethoscope
_____ 6. Guaiac test paper
_____ 7. Tuning fork
_____ 8. Percussion hammer
_____ 9. Ophthalmoscope
_____ 10. Otoscope
_____ 11. Goose neck lamp
_____ 12. Tongue depressor

COLUMN II

a. Used to elicit an involuntary response
b. Provides light necessary for inspection
c. Used to view tiny capillaries behind retina
d. Used to check sense of smell
e. Instrument used to examine inner ear
f. Used for indirect auscultation
g. Instrument used to inspect a body cavity
h. Permits visual inspections of mouth/throat
i. Measures intraocular pressure to determine glaucoma
j. Physician uses this instrument to assess patient's hearing
k. Test for occult blood in stool
l. For measuring chest and extremities
m. Used to obtain blood pressure readings in both arms

188

C. Identification: Identify these instruments used in examinations.

1. _____   7. _____
2. _____   8. _____
3. _____   9. _____
4. _____   10. _____
5. _____   11. _____
6. _____

1	2	3	4	5	6

7	8	9	10	11

D. Fill in the Blank

1. Direct percussion is termed _____ and is done by striking the finger against the patient's body.
2. Pitch, quality, duration, and resonance are terms that refer to _____
3. Direct _____ is done by placing your ear directly over a body area to hear sounds within.
4. _____ of problems in the SOAP method of recording patient information means documenting measurement of the patient's symptoms.
5. Referrals, medications, surgery, therapy, exercise, or other orders to return a patient to better health are all part of the _____ in the SOAP method.

E. Matching: Match the definition in column II with the correct term in column I.

COLUMN I

_____ 1. Percussion
_____ 2. Progress notes/report
_____ 3. Palpation
_____ 4. Objective symptoms
_____ 5. Manipulation
_____ 6. First part of physical exam
_____ 7. Romberg test
_____ 8. General appearance
_____ 9. Set of procedures
_____ 10. Auscultation
_____ 11. Red ink
_____ 12. Inspection
_____ 13. Writer
_____ 14. Mensuration
_____ 15. Subjective findings

COLUMN II

a. Includes measurement, vital signs, and vision screening
b. Takes dictation during patient's exam
c. Plan of treatment
d. Visual exam of body's various parts
e. You can't see; patient feels
f. Listening to body sounds
g. Heel-to-shin test
h. Measurement of chest and extremities
i. The tapping of the fingers over a body area to produce sounds
j. The forceful passive movement of a joint to determine range of motion
k. Applying fingers/hands against the skin to feel underlying tissues/abnormalities
l. Record patient's subsequent visits on these
m. Check balance to detect muscle abnormality
n. Describes patient's overall state of health
o. Alerts of allergy or other vital information
p. Complete physical exam
q. Can be seen by all

F. Multiple Choice: Place the correct letter or letters on the blank line for each question.

_____ 1. The lack of same size, shape, and position of parts or organs on opposite sides is termed
    a. anatomical   c. acquired
    b. asymmetry   d. atypical

_____ 2. A medical term that means to empty, especially the bowels, is
    a. evoke   c. exudate
    b. emesis   d. evacuate

_____ 3. Progress notes are also referred to as
    a. chart notes   c. exam reports
    b. evaluation forms   d. progress reports

_____ 4. To help patients relax during the pelvic exam, tell them to breathe _____ through the mouth.
    a. slowly   c. deeply
    b. quickly   d. shallowly

_____ 5. The heel-to-shin test is generally performed while the patient is in the _____ position.
    a. Trendelenberg   c. prone
    b. supine   d. Fowler's

_____ 6. The Romberg test is performed by the physician to detect
    a. coordination   c. muscle abnormality
    b. flexibility   d. infection

_____ 7. Patients who are scheduled for a Pap test should be reminded that they should not engage in sexual intercourse or _____ for 24 to 48 hours before the appointment.
    a. fast   c. void
    b. douche   d. exercise

_____ 8. To detect disease and abnormalities in children, an exam every _____is recommended.
    a. 3 months   c. year
    b. 6 months   d. time child is sick

After your instructor has returned your work to you, make all necessary corrections and place in a three-ring notebook for future reference.

ASSIGNMENT SHEET

Chapter 13: PREPARING PATIENTS FOR EXAMINATION

Unit 4: ASSISTING WITH SPECIAL EXAMINATIONS

SUGGESTED RESPONSES TO CRITICAL THINKING CHALLENGE IN TEXTBOOK

1. What would you do if someone either clocked in for you or asked you to do it for them? _____
   _____

2. What did Suzanne do? Was it anything she shouldn't have done? Why? _____
   _____
   _____

3. What do you think Jackie was trying to do? _____

4. Why do you suppose that Suzanne is worried about this situation? _____
   _____
   _____

5. What should Suzanne do about this? _____
   _____

6. Why was Suzanne feeling so guilty and worried about? _____
   _____
   _____

A. Word Puzzle: Solve this word puzzle using the *Words to Know* in this unit.

```
_ _ _ _ _ _   S  _ _ _
_ _ _ _ _ _ _  P  _
        _ _  E  _ _ _ _ _ _
        _ _  C  _ _ _
      _ _ _  I  _ _ _ _ _
      _ _ _  A  _ _ _ _ _ _ _ _
    _ _ _ _  L  _ _ _ _
```

B. Multiple Choice: Place the correct letter or letters on the blank line for each question.

_____ 1. When charting the patient's LMP, you should record

      a. the last day of her period   c. the date of her period

      b. the first day of her last period   d. none of these

_____ 2. Patients are asked to wear disposable gowns and drape sheets

      a. to keep warm   c. to look nice

      b. to protect the patient's clothes   d. for privacy

_____ 3. If the physician requests a Pap and Maturation Index for a patient, she or he wants

      a. to check for diabetes   c. a pregnancy test

      b. a hormonal evaluation   d. to rule out infection

_____ 4. Because some patients get nauseated and may vomit while they are in the reception area, it is wise
to keep a disposable _____ _____ in the receptionist's drawer.

      a. trash bag   c. emesis basin

      b. box of tissues   d. paper bag

_____ 5. To reduce the possibility of accidental injury when a baby is to be transported to a scale to weigh her, the _____ should take her and place her on the scale.

    a. the physician   c. the medical assistant

    b. the PA   d. the caregiver

_____ 6. A baby's head circumference should be measured until he is

    a. 6 months   c. 24 months

    b. 12 months   d. 36 months

_____ 7. Health care professionals are responsible for reporting suspected cases of child _____ to the proper authorities.

    a. abuse   c. neglect

    b. scabies   d. growth patterns

_____ 8. Measuring a baby's recumbent length (stature) is taken from

    a. forehead to heel   c. vertex of head to heel

    b. head to toe

_____ 9. Measurements taken of infants and children should be recorded in the child's

    a. chart   c. caregiver's record book

    b. growth graph   d. all of these

_____ 10. The caregiver must sign the _____ before immunizations can be given to a child.

    a. release form   c. insurance form

    b. consent form   d. data sheet

C. True or False: Place a "T" for true or "F" for false in the space provided. For false statements, explain why they are false.

_____ 1. The sigmoidoscope is used to inspect the abdominal muscles.

_____ 2. Only patients who have used evacuants successfully can be examined with a sigmoidoscope.

_____ 3. During a sigmoidoscopy, air is sometimes introduced to distend the wall of the colon for easier placement of the lumen of the endoscope.

_____ 4. A suction pump may be necessary to remove fecal matter, blood, and mucus during a sigmoidoscopy so that the structures of the colon can be examined.

_____ 5. If a biopsy is taken during the examination of the colon, a patient information sheet should accompany the specimen to the lab.

_____ 6. The metal tip of the suction machine should be washed and dried carefully and put back for the next patient exam.

_____ 7. Patients are placed in either Sims' or knee-chest position for a sigmoidoscopy.

_____ 8. If patients complain of constipation, you should remind them to exercise, drink plenty of water, and add fruits and vegetables, grains, nuts, and cereals to their diet.

_____ 9. All patients age 50 and over should have an occult blood test every five years.

_____ 10. Patients who have a family history of cancer in their family should be alert to the warning signs of cancer and have regular checkups.

Name _____

D. Word Puzzle: Solve this puzzle using the *Words to Know* in this unit.

1.   __ __ S __ __ __ __ __
2.   __ __ __ __ I __ __ __
3.   __ __ __ __ G __ __ __ __ __
4.   __ __ __ M __ __ __ __
5.   __ __ __ O __
6.   __ __ __ __ __ I __ __ __ __ __
7.   __ __ D __ __ __ __ __ __ __ __ __
8.   __ O __ __ __ __
9.   __ __ __ __ __ __ __ __ S
10.   __ __ C __ __ __
11.   __ __ __ __ __ O __ __ __ __
12.   __ __ __ __ __ __ P __ __ __ __ __
13.   __ Y __ __ __ __ __ __

E. Brief Answer

1. What instructions must be given to patients in preparation for a sigmoidoscopy? _____

_____

2. What might result if patients are not completely informed about preparations for a diagnostic examination such as a sigmoidoscopy? _____

_____

3. What advice can you give to patients in regard to flatulence they may experience following a sigmoidoscopy?

_____

F. Identification: Identify these instruments.

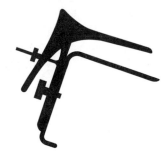

1._____

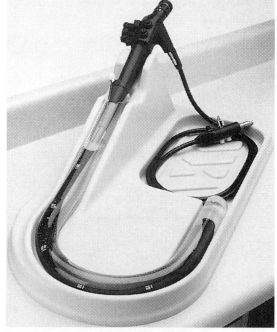

2. _____

194

G. Matching: Match the definition in column II with the correct term in column I.

COLUMN I

_____ 1. Triage
_____ 2. Pap test
_____ 3. Women age 35+
_____ 4. Proper preparation
_____ 5. Douching
_____ 6. LMP
_____ 7. Maturation index
_____ 8. Plain enema
_____ 9. Slow deep breaths
_____ 10. Flatulence
_____ 11. Constipation
_____ 12. BSE

COLUMN II

a. Necessary for successful examination
b. Relax abdominal muscles
c. Record first day of last menstrual period
d. Normally relieved with lots of fluids
e. Ascertain reason for patient's visit
f. Part of preparation for sigmoidoscopy
g. Cytological test to detect cervical cancer
h. Advise female patients to do routinely following period
i. Used to obtain a smear of interior cervix
j. Should schedule routine mammographies
k. Washes away natural vaginal secretions
l. Hormonal evaluation
m. For relief, lie in prone position with pillow across mid abdomen

H. List all necessary supplies/equipment for:

1. Pap test/pelvic examination

_____
_____
_____
_____
_____

2. Sigmoidoscopy

_____
_____
_____
_____

CRITICAL THINKING SCENARIOS: What would your response be in the following situation?

1. A female patient in her mid-30s is scheduled for a complete physical examination, including a Pap test. As you are getting the gown and drape sheet out, she tells you that she is so glad she had time this morning to douche before taking her shower because she wanted to be fresh and clean for the exam. _____

_____
_____
_____

Name _____

ACHIEVING SKILL COMPETENCY

Reread the performance objective for each procedure and then practice the skills listed below, following the procedure in your textbook.

Procedure 13-14: Assist with a Gynecological Examination and Pap Test

Procedure 13-20: Assist with Sigmoidoscopy

When you feel you have mastered performance of a skill, sign your name on the appropriate evaluation sheet and give it to your instructor to indicate you are prepared to perform the procedure for evaluation.

After your instructor has returned your work to you, make all necessary corrections and place in a three-ring notebook for future reference.

ASSIGNMENT SHEET

Chapter 14: SPECIMEN COLLECTION AND LABORATORY PROCEDURES

Review the objectives and text for each unit before completing the assignment sheet for that unit. When you have completed all sheets for the chapter, remove them from this Workbook and give them to the instructor for evaluation.

Unit 1: THE MICROSCOPE

A. Unscramble

1. _ _ _ _ _ _   TENUMI
2. _ _ _ _ _ _ _ _ _   NRBILOUCA
3. _ _ _ _ _ _ _ _ _ _   HECNTIACIN
4. _ _ _ _ _ _ _ _   NEIMPSCE
5. _ _ _ _ _ _ _   YMGNFAI
6. _ _ _ _ _ _ _ _ _ _   CPIETOIRFN

B. Fill in the Blank

1. The _____ is used to examine objects that cannot be seen with the naked eye.

2. Eyeglasses are not necessary when performing microscopic work because the microscope may be focused to _____ for all visual defects except _____

3. A monocular microscope has _____ eyepiece and a binocular microscope has _____

4. The microscope should be transported carefully by holding it by the _____ and supporting it with your other hand under the _____

5. The shortest objective lens of the microscope magnifies objects _____ larger than can be seen with the naked eye.

6. The _____ power lens of the microscope magnifies objects 40 times larger than can be seen with the naked eye.

7. The _____ regulates the amount of light directed on the magnified specimen.

8. The _____ may be raised or lowered in focusing the specimen.

9. The ocular lenses of the microscope should be cleaned with _____

10. The _____ dial helps focus the specimen in detail.

C. Identification: Label the parts of the microscope. Refer to Figure 14-2 in the textbook.

1. _____
2. _____
3. _____
4. _____
5. _____
6. _____
7. _____
8. _____
9. _____
10. _____

D. Fill in the Blank

1. Gloving is always a must when handling _____ blood or body fluid specimens.
2. When splashing of any blood/body fluids could be possible while you are working, you should wear
   _____ _____ _____ (or _____), and
   _____.
3. Basic proper handwashing _____ and _____ all procedures must
   become a habit for all health workers for self-protection from disease _____
4. Any break in the skin should be covered with a bandage after handwashing and before _____
   for self-protection against possible _____
5. It is important to recap or close bottles, jars, tubes, and the like, immediately after use to avoid _____
   _____ and _____
6. Immediate recording of lab results helps to ensure _____
7. For better _____ you should work in a well-lighted, properly ventilated, uncluttered, quiet
   area.
8. _____ should never be broken off or handled after use, but placed intact in a puncture-proof
   biohazardous container.
9. All _____ waste should be discarded in proper containers.
10. The health care worker should make _____ of all electrical appliances and equipment
    for frayed wires or faulty operation and _____ for repair if needed.
11. Accidents should be reported to your _____ immediately.
12. Emergency telephone numbers should be posted near the _____ in the lab.

13. Before using any electrical appliance or equipment, you should make sure that your hands are _____

14. First aid items should be available in the lab for _____ use.

15. Loose-fitting or bulk clothing and jewelry should not be worn when working in the lab because it could contribute to _____

16. Every lab should have an emergency _____ which is functional in preventing further damage to the eyes from chemical splashes.

17. Broken glass or any sharp, unusable item should be placed in a sturdy cardboard box or puncture-proof container marked _____ and placed in the proper waste receptacle.

18. The health care worker must _____ lean into the work area when working with flame or chemicals to avoid self-injury or accidents.

19. Chemicals should be poured at _____ to avoid injury and accidents.

20. _____ eat, drink, chew gum, smoke, or place hands or fingers to mouth or place any item in your mouth while working.

21. It is a good practice to designate a _____ and a _____ area in your lab and enforce this policy to avoid confusion about items.

E. Brief Answer

1. List the basic recommended standard precautions for health care providers.

    _____

    a. _____

    b. _____

    c. _____

    d. _____

    e. _____

    f. _____

2. How can health care providers set a good example for patients regarding health habits? _____

    _____

    _____

3. When and how and why should you clean up spills in the lab or facility? _____

    _____

    _____

4. How do you clean up spilled blood (or other body fluids)? _____

    _____

    _____

    _____

5. Why should patients be given both verbal and written instructions for procedures/tests? _____

    _____

    _____

    _____

    _____

ACHIEVING SKILL COMPETENCY

Reread the performance objective for this procedure and then practice the skill listed below, following the procedure in your textbook.

Procedure 14-1: Use a Microscope

When you feel you have mastered performance of a skill, sign your name on the appropriate evaluation sheet and give it to your instructor to indicate you are prepared to perform the procedure for evaluation.

After your instructor has returned your work to you, make all necessary corrections and place in a three-ring notebook for future reference.

ASSIGNMENT SHEET

Chapter 14: SPECIMEN COLLECTION AND LABORATORY PROCEDURES

Unit 2: CAPILLARY BLOOD TESTS

A. Word Puzzle: Use the *Words to Know* for this unit to spell out these terms.

1. _ _ _ _ _ _ _ _ E _ _ _ _ _ _ _ _ _ _
2. _ _ _ _ _ _ _ R _ _
3. _ _ _ _ Y _ _ _ _ _ _ _ _ _ _ _
4. _ T _ _
5. _ H _ _ _ _ _ _ _ _ _ _ _ _
6. _ _ R _ _ _ _ _ _ _
7. _ _ _ _ O _ _ _ _ _ _ _
8. P _ _ _ _ _
9. _ _ _ O _ _ _ _ _ _
10. I _ _ _ _ _ _ _ _ _ _ _
11. E _ _ _ _ _
12. _ _ _ _ _ S _
13. I _ _ _ _ _
14. _ _ _ _ _ _ S

B. Fill in the Blank

1. Laboratory instructions must be followed exactly in _____ _____ _____ and sending all specimens for analysis.
2. The medical assistant should alert the physician of abnormal laboratory findings by circling or underlining them in _____
3. Skin puncture is performed to obtain a _____ blood specimen.
4. Capillary blood tests are performed when _____ of blood is required.
5. _____ is a congenital disease due to a defect in the _____ of the amino acid, phenylalanine.
6. PKU tests are required by law in _____ and in _____
7. H and H is an abbreviation for _____ and _____
8. A skin puncture site should be approximately _____ deep to allow sufficient blood flow for capillary tests.
9. The microhematocrit tube fills quickly by _____
10. The three layers that blood is separated into after centrifugation in a microhematocrit tube are _____ _____ and _____
11. The hematocrit is expressed as the _____ of the total blood volume in cubic centimeters of erythrocytes packed by _____
12. When performing skin puncture procedures, the first drop of blood is blotted away because it may contain _____ or _____
13. The normal hematocrit range for adult males is _____ and for adult females _____
14. The function of the red blood cell is to transport _____ to and carry _____ from the cells.

15. Patients who complain of lack of energy or fatigue may possibly be suffering from _____
16. _____ should be worn when working with blood or any body fluids.
17. The purpose of a GGT (standard glucose tolerance test) is to determine a patient's ability to metabolize _____
18. Many physicians order a _____ GTT.
19. Patients scheduled for a GTT must _____ 8 to 12 hours before the test.
20. Patients may feel weakness and may faint during a _____
21. During a GTT, the blood glucose level falls as _____ is secreted into the blood in reaction to the glucose that has been ingested.
22. The normal blood glucose range is _____
23. The _____ is made preferably with fresh whole blood.
24. Name the five types of white blood cells in a differential count.
    a. _____
    b. _____
    c. _____
    d. _____
    e. _____
25. Draw, color, and label each of the blood cells of the differential WBC count.
26. Draw, color, and label RBCs and platelets (refer to Fig. 14-21).

C. **Labeling:** Label this centrifuged microhematocrit tube. Refer to Figure 14-10 in the textbook.

D. **True or False:** Place a "T" for true or "F" for false in the space provided. For false statements, explain why they are false.
    _____ 1. A blood smear should have an even distribution of cells and end in a feathered tip.
    _____ 2. A blood smear can be made with either venous or capillary blood.
    _____ 3. The best blood smears are those that are made with old blood from the refrigerator.
    _____ 4. Both fasting blood and urine samples are taken in a GTT.
    _____ 5. Patients may come and go during a GTT as long as they are on time every hour to have the test performed.

E. Matching: Match the definition in column II with the correct term in column I.

COLUMN I

_____ 1. Capillaries
_____ 2. 12 to 16 grams/100 ml blood
_____ 3. Hematology
_____ 4. PKU test
_____ 5. Skin puncture sites
_____ 6. Hematocrit
_____ 7. Centrifugal action
_____ 8. Fasting
_____ 9. 14 to 18 grams/100 ml of blood
_____ 10. Phenylalanine
_____ 11. Fasting blood glucose range
_____ 12. Hemoglobin
_____ 13. 5,000 to 10,000
_____ 14. Anemia
_____ 15. Differential

COLUMN II

a. Limited to neonates
b. Packed red blood cells
c. Separates blood components
d. Arteries
e. Convey blood from arteries to other venules
f. An amino acid
g. Normal hemoglobin range for females
h. Study of blood and its components
i. Ring/great finger, ear lobe, infant's heel or great toe
j. Erythrocytes
k. Decrease in the number of RBCs
l. Normal hemoglobin range for males
m. Nothing to eat or drink for specified time
n. 80 to 120 mg/100 ml of blood
o. Normal WBC count range
p. Carbon dioxide
q. Iron-carrying protein components in blood
r. Test to determine the number of each type of WBC

F. Identification: Identify these blood cells. Refer to Figure 14-21 in the textbook.

1. _____

2. _____

3. _____

4. _____

5. _____

6. _____

7. _____

G. Crossword Puzzle

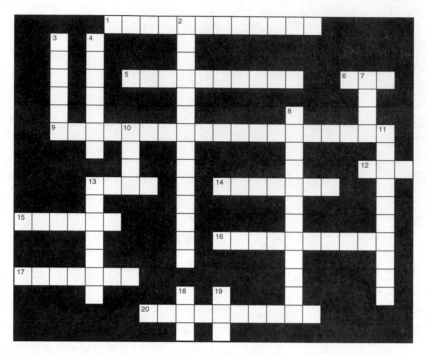

ACROSS

1. Test to determine the number and percentage of WBCs
5. Must never open while spinning
6. Physicians' office laboratory
9. The body's system that removes worn-out RBCs
12. Leukocyte
13. Immediately!
14. Sugar
15. Used for skin puncture
16. Volume of packed RBCs
17. Secreted by the Islets of Langerhans
20. Sum of all physical and chemical changes in the body

DOWN

2. Formation of RBCs
3. Relinquish; exemption
4. Newborn infant
7. Occupational Safety and Health Administration
8. Process of WBCs eating foreign cells
10. Clinical Laboratory Improvement Amendment
11. Place where diagnostic tests are performed
13. Needles used for skin puncture should be this
18. Glucose tolerance test
19. Erythrocyte

H. Brief Answer

1. What is the purpose of wearing latex gloves in performing laboratory procedures? _____
   _____

2. List the regulatory bodies that govern the POL, and explain why this is necessary. _____
   _____
   _____

3. List lab practices that yield quality assurance in the POL. _____

4. What are waivered tests? _____
   _____

5. List three laboratory tests from each of the sections in Table 14-1 of your textbook. Use reference books to explain the purpose of each test and patient preparation as indicated for each. _____

_____

6. What are the practices health care providers should follow to ensure reliable and accurate data and quality health care to patients? _____

    a. _____

    b. _____

    c. _____

    d. _____

    e. _____

7. For tests performed in the POL, what should the log book include?

    a. _____

    b. _____

    c. _____

    d. _____

    e. _____

8. Explain briefly what POCT (point of care testing) is. _____

_____

9. Explain why QA (quality assurance) and QC (quality control) are essential in laboratory procedures.

_____

_____

_____

10. Why is a GTT (glucose tolerance test) routinely performed on women in the sixth month of pregnancy?

_____

ACHIEVING SKILL COMPETENCY

Reread the performance objectives for these procedures and then practice the skills listed below, following the procedure in your textbook.

    Procedure 14-2: Puncture Skin with Sterile Lancet

    Procedure 14-3: Obtain Blood for PKU Test

    Procedure 14-4: Determine Hematocrit (Hct) Using Microhematocrit Centrifuge

    Procedure 14-5: Hemoglobin (Hb) Determination Using the Hemoglobinometer

    Procedure 14-6: Screen Blood Sugar (Glucose) Level

    Procedure 14-7: Making a Blood Smear

When you feel you have mastered performance of a skill, sign your name on the appropriate evaluation sheet and give it to your instructor to indicate you are prepared to perform the procedure for evaluation.

After your instructor has returned your work to you, make all necessary corrections and place in a three-ring notebook for future reference.

Chapter 14: SPECIMEN COLLECTION AND LABORATORY PROCEDURES

Unit 3: VENOUS BLOOD TESTS

A. Spelling: Each line contains four different spellings of a word. Underline the correctly spelled word.

1. Coageulate	Coagulate	Coagulade	Cogulate
2. Consiousness	Conseousness	Consciousness	Consciouseness
3. Elasticity	Elasticiety	Elastisity	Elosticity
4. Angorge	Engarge	Ingorge	Engorge
5. Hemolysis	Himolysis	Hemolisis	Hemolyesis
6. Hemotoma	Hematoma	Himotoma	Hemitoma
7. Legable	Ledgible	Legoble	Legible
8. Prothrombin	Prothromben	Prothrombon	Prothrambin
9. Tournequet	Tourniquiet	Tourniquet	Tournaquat
10. Venipuncture	Veniapuncture	Venapuncture	Venipunkture

B. Brief Answer

1. A means of promoting better palpation and sometimes visual position of the vein is a _____

2. Applying _____ immediately following venipuncture will reduce the possibility of a hematoma.

3. The two methods for obtaining venous blood specimens are
   a. _____
   b. _____

4. Blood drawn in blue-stoppered tubes should be tested within _____ hours.

5. Tubes used to collect whole blood for various tests contain a(n) _____

6. _____ is a clear, light yellow liquid obtained from whole blood that has been allowed to clot and then is _____

7. Information necessary to perform various blood tests for patients should contain
   a. _____
   b. _____
   c. _____
   d. _____
   e. _____
   f. _____
   g. _____
   h. _____
   i. _____

8. Cell deterioration may be prevented by _____ the blood specimen if it must be kept for over _____ hours.

9. The SED rate is useful in the diagnosis and evaluation of diseases of the _____ and in _____ _____ and collagen patients.

10. List the four most commonly used colors to code blood specimen tubes and tell what they stand for.
   a. _____
   b. _____
   c. _____
   d. _____

C. Matching: Match the commonly performed lab test in column I with normal values in column II.

COLUMN I

_____ 1. Hemoglobin
_____ 2. BUN
_____ 3. LDL cholesterol
_____ 4. Sed rate
_____ 5. CO
_____ 6. Triglyceride
_____ 7. RBC count
_____ 8. Creatinine
_____ 9. Potassium
_____ 10. Total cholesterol
_____ 11. Hematocrit
_____ 12. Uric acid
_____ 13. WBC count
_____ 14. Glucose
_____ 15. Pro time
_____ 16. HDL cholesterol
_____ 17. ESR Wintrobe method
_____ 18. Sodium
_____ 19. Platelet count
_____ 20. Chloride

COLUMN II

a. 4 to 5 mEq/L
b. 5,000 to 10,000/cu mm
c. 130 to 200 mg/dl
d. 35.5 to 49%
e. 11 to 13 sec
f. 80 to 120 mg/dl
g. 132 to 142 mEq/L
h. 3.5 to 7.5 mg/dl
i. 0 to 10 mm/hr
j. 90 to 130 mg/dl
k. 8 to 20 mg/dl
l. 12 to 16 g/dl
m. 98 to 106 mEq/L
n. 0 to 15 mm/hr
o. 40 to 150 mg/dl
p. 3.5 to 5.5 $\times$ 10/cu mm
q. 150,000 to 350,000/cu mm
r. 0.7 to 1.4 mg/dl
s. 25 to 32 mEq/L
t. 0 to 20 mm/hr
u. 45 to 65 mg/dl

D. Brief Answer

1. In compliance with quality control and quality assurance regulations, what information must be kept in the POL log book?

   a. _____
   b. _____
   c. _____
   d. _____
   e. _____
   f. _____

2. Explain how to package blood specimens for shipment to out-of-town/state laboratories. _____
   _____
   _____
   _____

3. What is the purpose of a Saf-T-Clik® shielded blood needle adapter? _____
   _____

4. How does the Saf-T-Clik® shielded blood needle adapter work? _____
   _____

E. Multiple Choice: Place the correct letter on the blank line for each question.

_____ 1. The surgical puncture of a vein is called
    a. intravenous   c. venipuncture
    b. intradermal   d. venolysis

_____ 2. The medical term for a collection of blood just under the skin is
    a. hemolysis   c. angioma
    b. hematoma   d. antigen

_____ 3. The breakdown of blood cells is called
    a. hemodialysis   c. hemolysis
    b. angioblast   d. angiosis

_____ 4. If a lab result is needed immediately, write _____ on the request form.
    a. immediately   c. same day
    b. as soon as possible   d. stat

_____ 5. The rate at which red blood cells fall in a particular calibrated tube within an hour is called a(n)
    a. analysis   c. hemoglobin
    b. sed rate   d. prothrombin

_____ 6. When an ESR is performed, you should do it within two hours with
    a. whole blood   c. blood plasma
    b. crenated blood   d. platelets

_____ 7. During the venipuncture procedure, the tourniquet should never be left on the patient's arm for more than
    a. 30 seconds   c. 2 minutes
    b. 60 seconds   d. 5 minutes

E. True or False: Place a "T" for true or "F" for false in the space provided. For false statements, explain why they are false.

_____ 1. Veins carry blood to the heart.

_____ 2. Some patients feel anxious about blood tests and may experience nausea.

_____ 3. A patient should have the arm supported for the venipuncture procedure.

_____ 4. Laws regarding venipuncture are the same everywhere.

_____ 5. Veins have some elasticity and will give somewhat when depressed.

_____ 6. Gentle mixing of blood with an anticoagulant in a figure-eight motion helps prevent hemolysis.

_____ 7. The needle guard should be kept over the needle to protect it from contamination and to prevent injuries.

_____ 8. The bevel of the needle should be down when inserting it for the venipuncture procedure.

_____ 9. Following the syringe method of venipuncture, the entire syringe and needle must be placed (intact) in a puncture-proof receptacle.

_____ 10. The same pair of gloves may be worn all day as long, as one performs proper handwashing technique before and after each procedure.

_____ 11. All breaks in the skin must be covered with a bandage to protect the health care worker from transmitting or contracting disease.

_____ 12. Health care workers should make it a habit to practice standard precaution recommendations.

ACHIEVING SKILL COMPETENCY

Reread the performance objective for this procedure and then practice the skills listed below, following the procedure in your textbook.

Procedure 14-8:   Obtain Venous Blood with Butterfly Needle Method
Procedure 14-9:   Obtain Venous Blood with Sterile Needle and Syringe
Procedure 14-10: Obtain Venous Blood with Vacuum Tube

When you feel you have mastered performance of a skill, sign your name on the appropriate evaluation sheet and give it to your instructor to indicate you are prepared to perform the procedure for evaluation.

After your instructor has returned your work to you, make all necessary corrections and place in a three-ring notebook for future reference.

ASSIGNMENT SHEET

Chapter 14: SPECIMEN COLLECTION AND LABORATORY PROCEDURES

Unit 4: BODY FLUID SPECIMENS

A. Matching: Match the terms in column I with their meanings in column II.

COLUMN I

_____ 1. Amber
_____ 2. Caustic
_____ 3. Occult
_____ 4. Crenated
_____ 5. Feces
_____ 6. Micturition
_____ 7. Dextrose
_____ 8. Random
_____ 9. Supernatant
_____ 10. Turbidity
_____ 11. Urinalysis
_____ 12. UTI
_____ 13. LMP
_____ 14. QNS

COLUMN II

a. Quantity not sufficient
b. Urination
c. Clear urine after centrifugation
d. Cloudiness
e. Examination of urine
f. Last menstrual period
g. Rusty color of urine
h. Diagnostic
i. Shrunken (RBC)
j. Hidden
k. Glucose/sugar
l. Can burn
m. Stool
n. Unplanned
o. Calibrated
p. Urinary tract infection

B. Brief Answer

1. Explain
   a. Clean-catch midstream urine specimen. _____
   _____

   b. Catheterization. _____
   _____

   c. Infant urine collection. _____
   _____

2. The three parts of a complete urinalysis are:
   a. _____
   b. _____
   c. _____

3. Distilled water has a specific gravity of _____

4. _____ is a chemically treated paper that reacts with urine to determine the presence of waste substances in the body.

5. Urine specimens should be kept _____ until analysis can be performed to avoid the growth of _____ or _____

6. Each specimen sent for laboratory analysis must have a _____ completed and attached to it for proper processing.

7. When performing urinary catheterization, the health care worker must always wear _____

8. Standard precautions state that all health care workers should wear gloves when working with any _____ and _____

C. Multiple Choice: Place the correct letter on the blank line for each question.

_____ 1. To avoid bacteria growth and decomposition of cells, urinalysis should be performed within
   a. 1 hour   c. 2 hours
   b. 45 minutes   d. 4 hours

_____ 2. Catheterization is performed
   a. to obtain a sterile urine specimen for analysis   c. to instill medication into the bladder
   b. for relief of urinary retention   d. all of these

_____ 3. The normal range of specific gravity of urine is
   a. 1.000–1.500   c. 1.020–1.025
   b. 1.010–1.025   d. 1.030–1.035

_____ 4. Urine with a strong ammonia-like odor may be alkaline from a high concentration of
   a. bacteria   c. sugar
   b. fungus   d. blood

_____ 5. The pH range for normal urine is
   a. 1 to 3   c. 5 to 7
   b. 3 to 5   d. 7 to 9

_____ 6. Ketone (acetone) bodies present in urine are the result of metabolized
   a. fat   c. starches
   b. sugar   d. bulk

_____ 7. Before performing any urine test the specimen should first be
   a. centrifuged   c. stirred
   b. heated   d. refrigerated

_____ 8. Cancer is detected from sputum specimens by the
   a. Gram stain   c. Wright stain
   b. gentian violet stain   d. Papanicolaou stain

_____ 9. Examination of fecal material (stool specimens) may determine the presence of
   a. microbial organisms   c. occult blood
   b. ova   d. all of these

D. Brief Answer

1. What patient education would you give to patients regarding:
   a. the respiratory system _____
   _____

   b. the digestive system _____
   _____

2. How do you collect a specimen for drug/alcohol analysis? _____
   _____

3. What should you make patients aware of in completing the form for substance analysis? _____
   _____

4. List all who should receive a copy of the substance analysis form.
   a. _____   d. _____
   b. _____   e. _____
   c. _____

5. What information should be included regarding samples for substance analysis?

   a. _____
   b. _____
   c. _____
   d. _____
   e. _____

6. What does the substance analysis screen for? _____

7. Refer to the ABHES Course Content Requirements in Appendix C of the textbook. Within the area of *Medical Office Clinical Procedures,* which two content requirements are discussed in this unit? _____

_____

CRITICAL THINKING SCENARIOS: What would your response be in the following situations?

1. A 10-year-old patient needs to have his hemoglobin checked. He wants you to use his little finger to obtain the blood sample. _____

_____

2. A patient calls to ask if she can run errands in between the times that you take blood and urine samples for her GTT scheduled for tomorrow morning. _____

_____

3. A patient calls to inform you that the scheduled first morning urine sample will have to be dropped off after work tomorrow. _____

_____

ACHIEVING SKILL COMPETENCY

Reread the performance objectives for these procedures and then practice the skills listed below, following the procedure in your textbook.

Procedure 14-11: Catheterize Urinary Bladder
Procedure 14-12: Test Urine with Multistix® 10 SG
Procedure 14-13: Determine Glucose Content of Urine with Clinitest Tablet
Procedure 14-14: Obtain Urine Sediment for Microscopic Examination
Procedure 14-15: Instruct Patient to Collect Sputum Specimen
Procedure 14-16: Instruct Patient to Collect Stool Specimen

   When you feel you have mastered performance of a skill, sign your name on the appropriate evaluation sheet and give it to your instructor to indicate you are prepared to perform the procedure for evaluation.

   After your instructor has returned your work to you, make all necessary corrections and place in a three-ring notebook for future reference.

Chapter 14: SPECIMEN COLLECTION AND LABORATORY PROCEDURES

Unit 5: BACTERIAL SMEARS AND CULTURES

SUGGESTED RESPONSES TO CRITICAL THINKING CHALLENGE IN TEXTBOOK

1. What was Judy's thinking when she realized there were no gloves in the room? _____

_____

2. What should she have done? _____

3. Why was she in such a hurry? _____

4. How do you think she felt when she realized that she could have been at risk? _____

_____

5. Should the doctor be notified? _____

6. What would you have done in this situation? _____

_____

A. Fill in the Blank

1. _____ is a gelatinlike substance, mixed with sheep's blood that encourages the growth of microorganisms in a petri dish.

2. Gram-positive bacteria take a _____ color from the gram-stain procedure.

3. _____ bacteria take a red or pink color from the counterstain in the gram-stain procedure.

4. The purpose of gram-staining is to make heat-fixed bacteria visible for _____ examination.

B. Brief Answer

1. Explain how to obtain a bacteriological smear. _____

_____

_____

2. Explain how to heat-fix a bacteriological smear for staining. _____

_____

3. Why is heat-fixing necessary? _____

_____

4. What is the purpose of culturing? _____

_____

5. Why are culture plates placed upside down in the incubator? _____

_____

6. Name the diseases caused by gram-positive bacteria. _____

7. Name the diseases caused by Gram-negative bacteria. _____

_____

_____

8. Why is it necessary to stain bacteria? _____

_____

9. How are bacteria identified? _____

_____

10. Why must all solutions be recapped immediately after each use? _____

_____

11. Why must gloves be worn when working with bacterial smears and cultures? _____

_____

_____

_____

12. What patient education could you offer a patient while preparing or obtaining a throat culture? _____

_____

_____

_____

_____

C. Matching: Match the term in column II with the correct definition in column I.

COLUMN I

_____ 1. Breaks infection cycle
_____ 2. Staphylococci
_____ 3. Nasopharyngeal culture
_____ 4. Diplococci
_____ 5. Streptococci
_____ 6. Incubation period for cultures
_____ 7. Blue flame
_____ 8. Alcohol/acetone
_____ 9. Destroys specimen
_____ 10. Spore-forming bacteria

COLUMN II

a. Bacteria that form pairs
b. 23–48 hours
c. Hottest
d. Proper handwashing and sterile technique
e. Excessive heating
f. Form grapelike clusters
g. NPC
h. Bacteria appearing in chains
i. Crystal violet
j. Helpful in removing dye
k. Immersion oil
l. Have capsule-like coverings

D. Crossword Puzzle

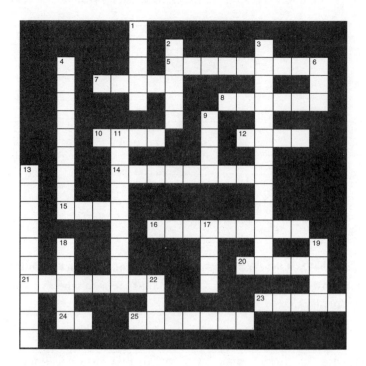

Across

5. Means passed through a flame
7. Nutrient for microorganisms
8. Gram-positive bacteria stain
10. Gram-negative bacteria stain
12. Cultures streaked with a fine wire _____
14. Means of isolating disease-causing organisms
15. Must be sterile to obtain sample
16. Clear plastic dish with lid
20. Wear latex gloves to obtain a bacteriological
_____
21. Have certain characteristic formations and shapes
23. Blue part is the hottest
24. Acronym for identification
25. Fill with dye for gram stain

Down

1. What a bacteriological smear is made on
2. Bacteria are classified by
3. Purpose of the bacteriological smear is to identify
_____
4. Take care in handling
6. Crystal violet
9. Gelatin-like substance
11. Provides proper growth temperature for cultures
13. Roll specimen onto slide to _____
microorganisms
17. Use in gram-stain procedure
18. Bacteria in clusters
19. Purpose of procedure is for identification of
bacteria
22. Allow specimens to _____ dry

E. Identification: Identify these bacterial shapes. Refer to Figure 14-52 in the textbook.

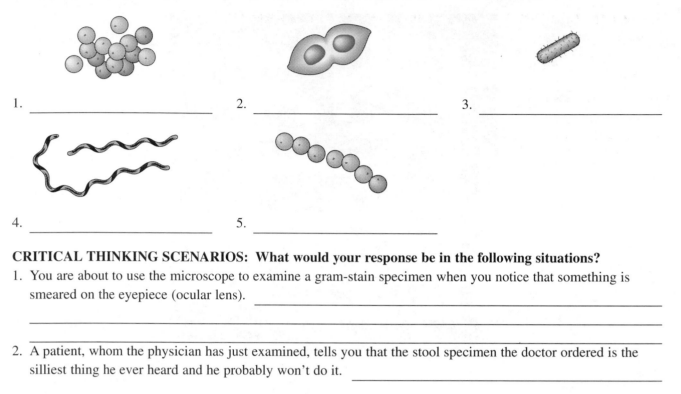

1. _____   2. _____   3. _____

4. _____   5. _____

CRITICAL THINKING SCENARIOS: What would your response be in the following situations?

1. You are about to use the microscope to examine a gram-stain specimen when you notice that something is smeared on the eyepiece (ocular lens). _____

_____

_____

2. A patient, whom the physician has just examined, tells you that the stool specimen the doctor ordered is the silliest thing he ever heard and he probably won't do it. _____

_____

_____

_____

ACHIEVING SKILL COMPETENCY

Reread the performance objectives for these procedures and then practice the skills listed below, following the procedure in your textbook.

Procedure 14-18: Prepare Bacteriological Smear

Procedure 14-19: Obtain a Throat Culture

Procedure 14-20: PrepareGram Stain

When you feel you have mastered performance of a skill, sign your name on the appropriate evaluation sheet and give it to your instructor to indicate you are prepared to perform the procedure for evaluation.

After your instructor has returned your work to you, make all necessary corrections and place in a three-ring notebook for future reference.

ASSIGNMENT SHEET

Chapter 15: DIAGNOSTIC TESTS, X-RAYS, AND PROCEDURES

Review the objectives and text for each unit before completing the assignment sheet for that unit. When you have completed all sheets for the chapter, remove them from this Workbook and give them to the instructor for evaluation.

Unit 1: DIAGNOSTIC TESTS

A. Word Search: Find the words hidden in the puzzle.

ALLERGY	HISTAMINE
INJECTION	SERUM
DILUTE	ADRENALINE
INTERPRET	ITCH
ANTIBODY	SYMPTOM
HYPERSENSITIVE	WHEAL
EXTRACT	SYSTEMATIC
CONTACT DERMATITIS	VENOM
NOTE	GAUGE
EOSINOPHIL	TIME
KIT	SHOCK

```
G E D C A R T J P F J K T G K L B T
A O I N J E C T I O N M U N G J L H
L R L K R A O A J L S V D H L K B W
L K U C J S N B I N T E R P R E T C
E X T R A C T E J P Z N P F L O B P
R Z E C R H A N T I B O D Y D S R W
G L V A M B C R D O A M K A B I F D
Y B Q D P T T N S E R U M W G N C C
N S T R B C D A J T J T W H C O U K
H Y P E R S E N S I T I V E K P I Z
I N S N A P R S Y Z L T I A D H U O
S R E A G K M K M K Y C O L P I H K
T I M L L R A B P M E H T K F L N T
A L O I O H T C T O G A G O W O R I
M S Y N T D I F O E A B C S E S U M
I B K E Z N T N M Z U H I H O H H E
N O T E D E I G R E G K Z O A O E K
E V E S B O S Y S T E M A T I C E C
K I Q T Z L P C R E O D U P N K I T
```

Name _____

B. True or False: Place a "T" for true or "F" for false in the space provided. For false statements, explain why they are false.

_____ 1. A positive allergic reaction to a skin test is shown by a raised area on the skin called a wheal.

_____ 2. Wheals are measured in inches.

_____ 3. Reactions to scratch tests usually occur within the first 20 minutes.

_____ 4. Intradermal tests are sometimes used by physicians to determine medicine sensitivity or immunization needs.

_____ 5. The patch test is read after a 12-hour and a 20-hour time period.

_____ 6. Cockroaches, their egg casings, and fecal matter are major sources of allergens in large cities.

_____ 7. Patients may have allergies only from irritants such as tobacco smoke, perfumes, cleaning supplies, and paint fumes.

_____ 8. Patients who have food allergies should read the content label of all foods and over-the-counter medications before ingesting.

_____ 9. If a patient is to report a skin test reaction by phone after the usual time it should react, explain that the size of the wheal/welt should be compared to a well-known item.

C. Fill in the Blank

1. _____ are utilized to determine allergic reactions in patients.

2. Desirable sites for the _____ test are the arms and back.

3. The _____ test is done to determine the cause of contact dermatitis.

4. In performing the intradermal test, the antigen is introduced into the dermal layer of skin in dosages of _____ to _____ by sterile technique.

5. For accurate test results, the expiration date of the _____ should be checked each time before use.

6. It may be necessary to _____ small children to perform skin tests successfully.

7. A life-threatening allergic reaction must be counteracted with an injection of _____ to prevent anaphylactic shock.

8. Symptoms of _____ initially include intense anxiety, weakness, sweating, and shortness of breath.

9. Patients refer to desensitizing injections of allergy serum as _____

10. It is a good practice to alternate arms of patients who have frequent allergy serum injections to prevent _____

11. The medical assistant's role in diagnostic tests and procedures is to _____ and _____ patients.

D. Matching: Match the definition in column II with the correct term in column I.

COLUMN I

_____ 1. Antibody
_____ 2. Immune
_____ 3. Venom
_____ 4. Histamine
_____ 5. Systemic
_____ 6. Antigen
_____ 7. Extract

COLUMN II

a. Released in allergic/inflammatory reactions
b. Of or pertaining to the whole body
c. Immunizing agent that produces antibodies
d. Protected or exempt from a disease
e. A protein substance carried by cells to counteract effects of an antigen
f. Pertaining to tissue
g. A poisonous secretion
h. A substance distilled or drawn out of another substance

E. Brief Answer

1. Describe patient education regarding allergy injections.

_____

_____

_____

2. Explain how you would advise a new allergy patient about scheduling desensitizing injections and other instructions.

_____

_____

_____

_____

ACHIEVING SKILL COMPETENCY

Reread the performance objectives for these procedures and then practice the skills listed below, following the procedure in your textbook.

Procedure 15-1: Perform a Scratch Test

Procedure 15-2: Apply a Patch Test

When you feel you have mastered the performance of the skill, sign your name on the appropriate evaluation sheet and give it to your instructor to indicate you are prepared to perform the procedure for evaluation.

After your instructor has returned your work to you, make all necessary corrections and place in a three-ring notebook for future reference.

ASSIGNMENT SHEET

Chapter 15: DIAGNOSTIC TESTS, X-RAYS, AND PROCEDURES

Unit 2: CARDIOLOGY PROCEDURES

A. Matching: Match the definition in column II with the correct term in column I.

COLUMN I

_____ 1. Artifacts
_____ 2. Somatic
_____ 3. Segment
_____ 4. Repolarization
_____ 5. Purkinje
_____ 6. Augmented
_____ 7. Sedentary
_____ 8. Galvanometer
_____ 9. Precordial
_____ 10. Voltage
_____ 11. Interval
_____ 12. Electrode
_____ 13. Standardization
_____ 14. Impulse
_____ 15. Stylus

COLUMN II

a. Enlarged
b. Electrocardiogram
c. Little activity
d. Additional electrical activity
e. Changes impulses into mechanical motion
f. Chest leads
g. Difference in electrical potential
h. Fibers that cause muscles of the ventricle to contract
i. Momentary surge of current
j. Provides a reliable reading
k. Muscle voltage artifacts
l. Provides printed representations of ECG paper
m. Period when heart momentarily relaxes
n. Bectrolyte
o. Metal sensors that pick up electrical impulses
p. Portion of EKG between two waves
q. Length of a wave

B. Multiple Choice: Place the correct letter on the blank line for each question.

_____ 1. The ECG is interpreted by the _____ .

a. lab technician   c. physician
b. medical assistant   d. nurse practitioner

_____ 2. The routine ECG consists of _____ leads.

a. 6   c. 8
b. 10   d. 12

_____ 3. The patient must be _____ for a good tracing to be obtained.

a. sleeping   c. relaxed
b. standing   d. unconscious

_____ 4. Metal electrodes should be cleaned with _____ .

a. mild detergent/scouring powder   c. baking soda/water
b. alcohol/ether   d. mild detergent/silver polish

_____ 5. A proper amount of _____ must be used with each metal electrode to provide maximum electrical conduction.

a. alcohol   c. oil
b. electrolyte   d. powder

_____ 6. The _____ of the ECG is necessary to enable a physician to judge deviations from the standard.

a. length   c. standardization
b. quality   d. augmentation

_____ 7. The usual standardization mark is _____ in size.
      a. 1 mm wide and 10 mm high   c. 1 mm wide and 5 mm high
      b. 2 mm wide and 5 mm high   d. 2 mm wide and 10 mm high

_____ 8. If the tracing is too large, the _____ button should be turned down to one half.
      a. sensitivity   c. selector
      b. stylus   d. on/off

_____ 9. The tracing paper is normally run at a speed of _____ mm/second.
      a. 15   c. 50
      b. 25   d. 75

C. Labeling: Label these diagrams of the ECG cycle.

1. Place the correct letter for each wave of the ECG tracing on the line next to the number in the following. Refer to Figure 15-17 in the textbook.

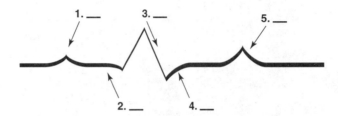

2. Label the numbered lines below with the correct name of each area of the electrical conduction through the heart. Refer to Figure 15-16 in the textbook.

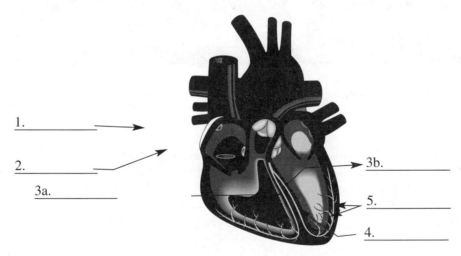

D. Fill in the Blank

1. All muscle movement produces _____
2. The current enters the electrocardiograph through the wires to reach the _____
3. The amplifier _____ the electrical impulses.
4. Electrical impulses are transformed into mechanical motion by the _____
5. A _____ produces printed representations on ECG paper.
6. An electrical impulse originates in the modified myocardial tissue in the _____
7. The first impulse recorded on the ECG paper from the atrial contraction is known as the _____
8. When the muscles of the ventricles contract, the _____ of waves is produced on the ECG paper.
9. During the recovery of the ventricles, the _____ is produced.
10. A routine ECG consists of _____ leads.

11. _____ means to make larger.
12. Chest leads are also called _____ leads.
13. AC or _____ current interference is caused by additional electrical activity.
14. The standardization mark is included in an EKG to provide a _____ reading.

E. Crossword Puzzle

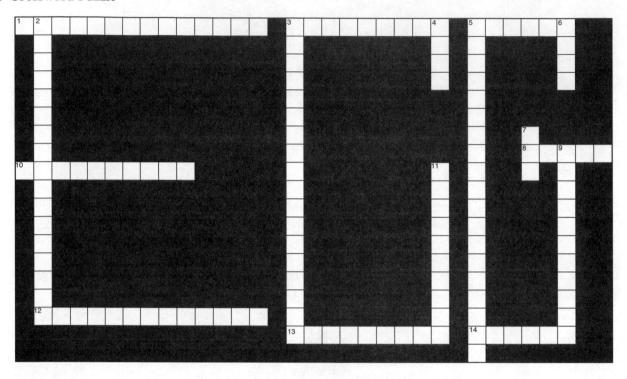

ACROSS
 1. Time of recovery before heart contracts again
 3. Pick up electrical current from patient
 5. Produces a printed representation on ECG paper
 8. Precordial is another name for _____ leads
10. Irregular heartbeat
12. Ambulatory ECG
13. Inactivity
14. Slight/distant

DOWN
 2. Instrument used to record electrical impulses of the heart
 3. Permanent record of heart's electrical activity
 4. An ECG tech does lots of these
 5. These provide a basis for physicians to judge deviations from the standard
 6. Immediately!
 7. Acronym for electrocardiogram
 9. Used to provide maximum electrical conduction
11. Study of the heart

F. True or False: Place a "T" for true or "F" for false in the space provided. For false statements, explain why they are false.

_____ 1. In the electrical conduction system, the first area of the heart to receive the electrical impulse is the Purkinje fibers.

_____ 2. Shivering from being nervous or cold can cause somatic tremor.

_____ 3. A rhythm strip indicates to the physician the size of a patient's heart.

_____ 4. For better electrode contact, the skin sites should be rubbed vigorously to increase circulation.

_____ 5. For single- and multi-channel computerized electrocardiographs, you simply press "auto" to run a 12-lead ECG.

_____ 6. It is necessary to shave dense chest hair for placement of electrodes.

_____ 7. Stress test ECGs are performed routinely on all patients.

_____ 8. A fetal monitor is a walking or 24-hour ECG.

_____ 9. Patients should keep a diary of their activities and symptoms during a 24-hour electrocardiogram.

_____ 10. It is important to check the batteries and proper working order of the Holter monitor before applying the device to a patient.

G. Labeling: Fill in the missing information from this diagrammatic representation of cardiac impulses on EKG tracing: (A) course of electrical impulses, (B) cardiac muscle reaction to impulses, (C) ECG tracing of impulse waves, (D) phases of cardiac cycle. Refer to Figure 15-17 in the textbook.

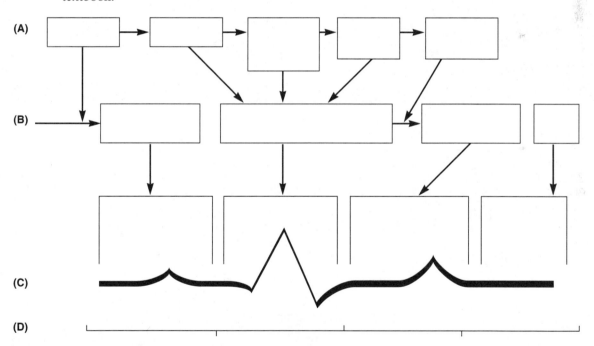

H. Labeling: Label the ECG Tracings. Are they abnormalities or interference artifacts?

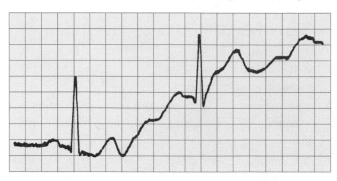

1. _____

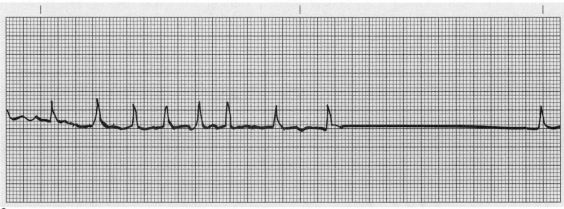

2. _____

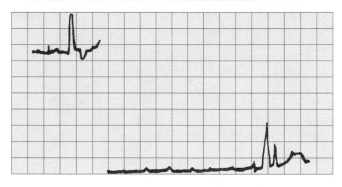

3. _____

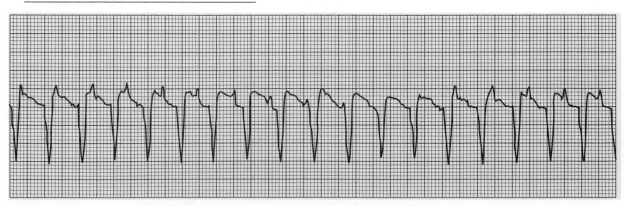

4. _____

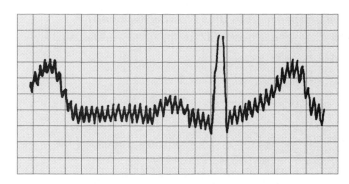

5. _____

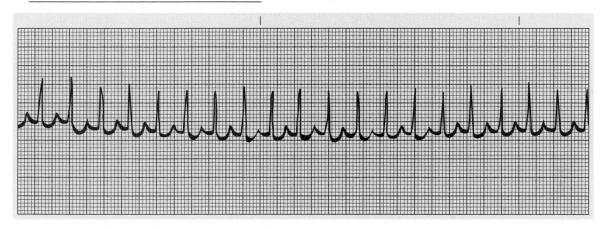

6. _____

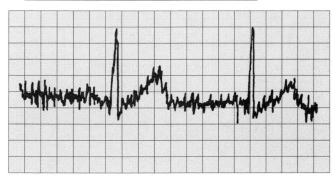

7. _____

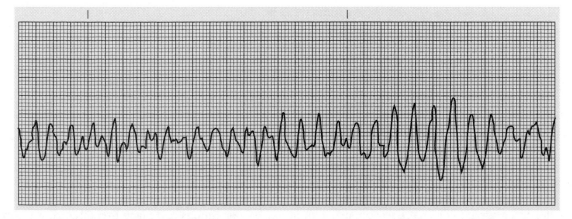

8. _____

CRITICAL THINKING SCENARIOS: What would your response be in the following situation?

1. A patient is being prepped for an ECG and appears to be very apprehensive. She is apparently intimidated by the machine and the wires and expresses a great fear of electric shock.

   _____

   _____

ACHIEVING SKILL COMPETENCY

Reread the performance objective for this procedure and then practice the skill listed below, following the procedure in your textbook.

Procedure 15-3: Obtain a Standard 12-Lead Electrocardiogram

When you feel you have mastered the performance of the skill, sign your name to the evaluation sheet and give it to your instructor to indicate you are prepared to perform the procedure for evaluation.

After your instructor has returned your work to you, make all necessary corrections and place in a three-ring notebook for future reference.

ASSIGNMENT SHEET

Chapter 15: DIAGNOSTIC TESTS, X-RAYS, AND PROCEDURES

Unit 3: DIAGNOSTIC PROCEDURES

A. Fill in the Blank

1. Vital capacity should equal _____ capacity plus _____ reserve.
2. _____ mouthpieces are used with vital capacity tests to prevent disease transmission.
3. Advising patients to list their concerns and bring them to their next appointment will _____ the number of phone consultations.
4. In the performance of procedures, the medical assistant must be aware of explaining what is _____ of the patient, for cooperation is essential in successful completion of the procedure.
5. As a _____ patients should be made aware of the expected amount of time a procedure will take so that their transportation can be planned accordingly.

B. Matching: Match the definition in column II with the correct term in column I.

COLUMN I

_____ 1. Dyspnea
_____ 2. Maturity
_____ 3. Ultrasound
_____ 4. Intermittent
_____ 5. Spirometry
_____ 6. Resonance
_____ 7. Expirations
_____ 8. Patient education
_____ 9. Claustrophobia

COLUMN II

a. Coming and going
b. To sound again
c. Breathing out; exhaling air
d. Fear of being enclosed
e. Yields more accurate test results
f. Full development
g. Difficulty breathing
h. Measures hearing
i. Measurement of air capacity of lungs
j. Vibrations of sound waves

C. Word Search: Find the words hidden in the puzzle. After you complete the puzzle, use the words numbered 5, 7, 8, 9, 11 in a sentence.

1. TEST
2. CONTRAST
3. EARLY
4. POLYPS
5. INVASIVE
6. PATIENT
7. ECHOES

8. CLAUSTROPHOBIA
9. SPIROMETER
10. IMPLANTS
11. MAGNETIC
12. IMAGE
13. SONOGRAM

```
C  M  H  M  M  M  R  E  S  A  D  A  S  D  O  S  A  C  P  F
J  S  S  A  R  B  R  M  S  P  I  R  O  M  E  T  E  R  B  S
I  M  A  G  E  H  R  B  G  L  A  L  D  J  T  N  D  H  L  K
L  J  A  N  I  T  K  A  L  C  P  T  I  N  V  A  S  I  V  E
Y  A  C  E  X  N  L  M  P  D  H  J  T  F  R  L  F  C  L  R
C  P  A  T  I  E  N  T  O  Q  A  H  C  F  B  P  Y  C  M  B
M  H  M  I  F  G  S  B  M  S  N  Y  C  P  L  M  E  G  M  C
R  E  C  C  L  A  U  S  T  R  O  P  H  O  B  I  A  P  D  W
T  K  L  A  B  E  T  V  A  U  G  C  Q  Z  N  P  F  E  R  K
S  O  N  O  G  R  A  M  H  U  R  B  C  A  T  T  A  W  B  C
W  M  K  B  P  C  T  A  A  G  A  S  D  U  S  R  R  A  J  T
P  L  B  T  L  S  G  I  R  S  P  M  H  D  L  C  B  A  P  E
Z  T  F  L  O  K  A  S  H  O  H  M  I  Y  Q  T  C  F  S  S
R  S  E  O  H  C  E  Z  S  P  Y  L  O  P  K  L  H  B  K  T
```

5. Invasive _____
7. Echoes _____
8. Claustrophobia _____
9. Spirometer _____
11. Magnetic _____

D. True or False: Place a "T" for true or "F" for false in the space provided. For false statements, explain why they are false.

_____ 1. In the spirometry procedure a clip is placed on some patients' noses to encourage them to breathe in deeply through the mouth.

_____ 2. One of your important duties in performing spirometry is to coach patients to expel completely all the air from their lungs quickly.

_____ 3. An oscilloscope is an instrument that shows a picture of converted electrical impulses from the patient during echocardiography.

_____ 4. High-frequency sound waves are conducted through the use of a transducer in ultrasonic scanning.

_____ 5. Thermography is a measurement of heat patterns given off by the skin.

_____ 6. Diaphanography is performed by transillumination.

CRITICAL THINKING SCENARIOS: What would your response be in the following situation?

1. The patient that you just scheduled for an MRI lets you know in no uncertain terms that she is extremely claustrophobic and just might not go if she's having a bad day.

_____
_____
_____
_____

After your instructor has returned your work to you, make all necessary corrections and place in a three-ring notebook for future reference.

ASSIGNMENT SHEET

Chapter 15: DIAGNOSTIC TESTS, X-RAYS, AND PROCEDURES

Unit 4: DIAGNOSTIC RADIOLOGICAL PROCEDURES

SUGGESTED RESPONSES TO CRITICAL THINKING CHALLENGE IN TEXTBOOK

1. What was Johnetta's first mistake? _____

_____

2. When should she have made the appointment? _____

_____

3. Did she even look at the chart before filing it? _____

_____

4. Why didn't she tell the physician? _____

_____

5. How serious is this situation? _____
6. What should Johnetta do? _____

_____

_____

7. Is the clinical supervisor at fault for anything? _____

_____

8. What would you have done in this situation? _____

_____

ANSWERS TO WORKBOOK ASSIGNMENT

A. Word Puzzle: Use the *Words to Know* to spell out these terms.

1. _ _ _ _ _ _ _ M _ _ _ _ _ _ _ _
2. _ _ _ _ A _ _ _ _
3. _ _ M _ _ _ _ _ _ _
4. _ _ _ M _ _ _ _ _
5. _ _ _ O _ _ _ _ _ _ _
6. _ _ _ _ G _ _ _
7. _ _ R _ _ _
8. _ _ _ _ _ A _ _ _ _ _
9. _ _ _ _ _ _ P _ _ _ _ _
10. _ _ H _ _ _ _ _
11. _ _ _ Y

B. Brief Answer

1. What are roentgen rays?

_____

_____

2. What are therapeutic x-rays used for?

_____

3. What type of symptoms do patients experience if the gallbladder malfunctions?

_____

4. What food should patients avoid if they have gallbladder trouble?

_____

5. Why must the digestive tract be free of foods during an upper GI series?

_____

_____

6. Why is air contrast sometimes ordered with a barium enema examination?

_____

_____

7. What is an IVP?

_____

_____

8. What is another term for KUB?

_____

9. How are patients x-rayed for mammography?

_____

_____

10. Describe the method of radiology called a CAT (computerized axial tomography) scan.

_____

_____

11. Describe echocardiography.

_____

_____

12. List the steps to prepare patients for a barium enema.

_____

_____

_____

13. Describe a barium swallow or upper Gl Series.

_____

_____

_____

14. Explain why pregnant women should not have x-rays.

_____

15. List x-ray procedures that do not require patient preparation.

_____

16. Refer to the ABHES Course Content Requirements in Appendix C of the textbook. Within the area of *Medical Office Clinical Procedures,* which two content requirements are discussed in this unit? _____

_____

C. Matching: Match the definition in column II with the correct term in column I.

COLUMN I

_____ 1. Therapeutic x-rays
_____ 2. Mammography
_____ 3. Evacuants
_____ 4. UGI series
_____ 5. CAT scan
_____ 6. Bone studies
_____ 7. IVP
_____ 8. KUB
_____ 9. Contrast media
_____ 10. Retrograde pyelogram

COLUMN II

a. Defines structures of the urinary system
b. Do not require patient preparation
c. Barium and water mixture
d. Flat plate of abdomen
e. Breast self-examination
f. Performed with sterile catheter in conjunction with cystoscopy
g. Laxatives and enemas
h. x-ray of different angles of breast tissue
i. Used to treat cancer
j. Generates images of tissue in slices about one centimeter thick
k. Barium swallow

D. Multiple Choice: Place the correct letter on the blank line for each question.

_____ 1. A diagnostic aid frequently requested by physicians that needs no patient preparation is the:
　　a. IVP　　　　　　　　　　　c. UGI
　　b. chest x-ray　　　　　　　　d. cholecystogram

_____ 2. Diagnostic x-rays are _____ in pregnant female patients, especially during the first trimester.
　　a. contraindicated　　　　　　c. important
　　b. indicated　　　　　　　　　d. common

_____ 3. Carbonated and alcoholic beverages should be avoided prior to x-rays of the visceral organs because they produce
　　a. rashes　　　　　　　　　　c. delays
　　b. stones　　　　　　　　　　d. flatus

_____ 4. A voiding cystogram may be ordered along with a(n)
　　a. UGI　　　　　　　　　　　c. IVP
　　b. KUB　　　　　　　　　　　d. BaE

_____ 5. Nuclear medicine is the branch of medicine that uses _____ in the diagnosis and treatment of patients.
　　a. xeroradiography　　　　　　c. radioactive materials
　　b. radionuclides　　　　　　　d. both b and c

_____ 6. Which x-ray is helpful in determining the position of an IUD?
　　a. IVP　　　　　　　　　　　c. MRI
　　b. UGI　　　　　　　　　　　d. KUB

_____ 7. Breast self-examination is recommended for women of all ages
　　a. daily　　　　　　　　　　　c. monthly
　　b. weekly　　　　　　　　　　d. yearly

_____ 8. All women should have a baseline mammography between the ages of
　　a. 25 and 39　　　　　　　　　c. 45 and 49
　　b. 35 and 39　　　　　　　　　d. 55 and 59

_____ 9. To reduce the possible effects of swelling and soreness often caused by compression of the breasts during mammography you should instruct patient to omit _____ from their diets 7 to 10 days prior to the examination.

    a. salt   c. fats

    b. caffeine   d. cholesterol

_____ 10. Compression of the breasts during mammography allows a much clearer picture of breast tissue and also requires less

    a. analgesics   c. radiation

    b. time   d. flatus

CRITICAL THINKING SCENARIOS: What would your response be in the following situation?

1. A male patient in his late 50s phones to tell you of his discomfort following his barium enema this morning. He says he feels bloated and constipated.

_____

_____

_____

    After your instructor has returned your work to you, make all necessary corrections and place in a three-ring notebook for future reference.

ASSIGNMENT SHEET

Chapter 16: MINOR SURGICAL PROCEDURES

SUGGESTED RESPONSES TO CRITICAL THINKING CHALLENGE IN TEXTBOOK

1. Who was at fault here? _____

2. What was Barry's first mistake? _____
_____

3. Was Renita responsible for any problems? _____
_____

4. What should Barry have done? _____
_____
_____

5. Do you think Barry handled the reprimand from the doctor well? _____
_____

6. Since Barry didn't know that there were no sterile packs in the drawer, should the doctor blame him?
_____
_____

7. Did Renita really do Barry a favor? _____
_____
_____

ANSWERS TO WORKBOOK ASSIGNMENT

A. Word Puzzle: Use the list of *Words to Know* from this unit to spell out these terms.

1. _ _ _ _ _ _ _ I _ _ _ _ _ _ _

2. _ C _ _ _ _ _ _

3. _ _ _ _ S _ _ _ _ _

4. _ _ _ _ O _ _ _ _

5. _ _ _ _ _ _ _ _ A _ _ _ _

6. R

7. A _ _ _ _ _ _ _ _ _ _

_ _ _ _ _ _ _ I _ _ _

8. N

_ _ _ _ _ _ _ A _ _ _ _

9. G

_ _ E _ _ _ _ _ _ _

B. Brief Answer

1. List what you must tell a patient in preparation for minor office surgery.

   a. _____

   b. _____

   c. _____

   d. _____

2. What two things should the medical assistant do the day before the scheduled surgery?

   a. _____

   b. _____

3. What is the purpose of the skin preparation before a surgical procedure?

   a. _____

   b. _____

4. Why must the medical assistant be extremely careful to avoid nicking the patient's skin when performing a skin preparation? _____

5. What must the medical assistant do if asked to assist directly with a surgical procedure? _____

6. Other than directly assisting with a surgery procedure, when else should the medical assistant wear surgical gloves, and why? _____

7. List the items included in the basic setup for most minor surgical procedures. _____

_____

_____

8. What types of surgical procedures may the medical assistant be asked to assist with in the medical office/clinic? _____

_____

_____

9. What is the usual recommended post-op diet? _____

10. Why are follow-up visits necessary in patient care? _____

11. Other than the scheduled post-op visit, what can the medical assistant do to follow up with patients? _____

12. What, in general, can the medical assistant advise patients to do following minor surgery? _____

_____

13. How should the medical assistant instruct patients to care for the site of surgery? _____

_____

14. What is the purpose of an electrocautery device in minor office surgical procedures? _____

_____

15. Give pre-op instructions to a patient scheduled for a minor surgical procedure. _____

    a. _____

    b. _____

    c. _____

    d. _____

    e. _____

    When the patient arrives for the appointment:

    a. _____

    b. _____

    c. _____

    d. _____

16. Give post-op instructions to a patient following a minor office surgery.

    a. _____

    b. _____

    c. _____

    d. _____

    e. _____

    f. _____

    g. _____

17. List standard precaution barriers that must be worn by health care providers for invasive procedures.

_____

18. Explain how to care for surgical instruments before and following use. _____

_____

19. List the important information that must be recorded on the patient's chart regarding a surgical procedure.

_____

20. List the items needed for a skin prep tray. _____

_____

21. Explain how to remove sutures properly and why. _____

_____

_____

_____

_____

22. Describe how to remove skin staples. _____

_____

23. Describe skin closures and how they are applied. _____

24. Refer to ABHES Course Content Requirements in Appendix C of the textbook. Within the area of *Medical Office Clinical Procedures*, which content requirements are discussed in this chapter?

_____

_____

C. Matching: Match the definition in column II with the correct term in column I.

COLUMN I

_____ 1. Local anesthetic
_____ 2. Medical history
_____ 3. I & D
_____ 4. Before surgery
_____ 5. Formalin solution
_____ 6. Necessary
_____ 7. 30° angle
_____ 8. Application of antiseptic
_____ 9. Sterile transfer forceps
_____ 10. After surgery
_____ 11. 6 minutes
_____ 12. IUD
_____ 13. Antiseptic
_____ 14. D & C
_____ 15. Contaminated

COLUMN II

a. Preoperative
b. Used to place specimen in formalin solution
c. Surgical consent form
d. Dilation and curettage
e. Postoperative
f. Incision and drainage
g. Skin preparation
h. Administered by physician
i. May help in determining possible allergic reactions
j. Reduces microbial growth
k. Used to preserve tissue specimen
l. Expiration date
m. Angle of shaving surgery site
n. Intrauterine device
o. Circular motions
p. Unsterile
q. Thorough surgical scrub

D. Identification: Identify the following surgical instruments. Refer to Table 16-1 in the textbook.

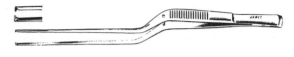

1. _____

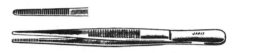

2. _____

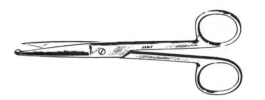

3. _____

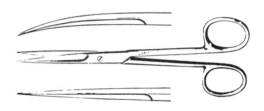

4. _____

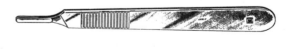

5. _____

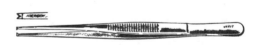

6. _____

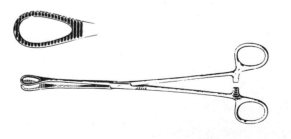

7. _____

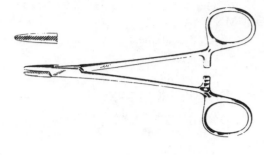

8. _____

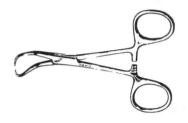

9. _____

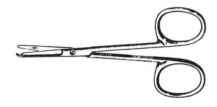

10. _____

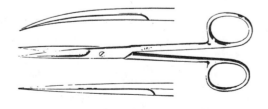

11. _____

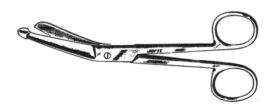

12. _____

E. Multiple Choice: Place the correct letter on the blank line for each question.

_____ 1. This process uses subfreezing temperature to destroy/remove tissue.

   a. electrocautery   c. diathermy

   b. cryosurgery   d. chemotherapy

_____ 2. Electrocoagulation is performed with a(n)

   a. cryo unit   c. hyfrecator

   b. autoclave   d. scalpel

_____ 3. A fenestrated sheet is one that has a(n)

   a. fold   c. stain

   b. pleat   d. opening

_____ 4. Autoclaved items remain sterile if they have been properly processed and protected from moisture
           for

   a. 3 days   c. 3 weeks

   b. 30 days   d. 3 months

_____ 5. Reducing the possibility of infection for a surgical procedure skin preparation includes

   a. cleaning the site with a soapy solution   c. applying antiseptic solution

   b. shaving the skin   d. all of these

_____ 6. A serious hereditary blood clotting disease that occurs mostly in males is called

   a. hemophilia   c. hematuria

   b. hemophobia   d. hemiplegia

_____ 7. A thorough initial surgical scrub must be performed for _____ minutes.

   a. two   c. six

   b. four   d. eight

_____ 8. Assisting with surgical procedures not only requires knowledge and skill, but

   a. self-discipline   c. empathy

   b. personal integrity   d. all of these

_____ 9. Tell patients who are to have skin staples removed that it is normal to feel a _____ sensation during
           the procedure.

   a. burning   c. nauseating

   b. tugging   d. stinging

_____ 10. Patients are normally requested to fast before surgical procedures because it lessens the possibility of
           the patient

   a. bleeding a lot   c. being late

   b. talking too much   d. becoming nauseated

_____ 11. Included in the list of symptoms following a surgical procedure that should be reported to the
           physician are

   a. unusual pain, burning, or uncomfortable sensation   c. fever, nausea, and vomiting

   b. bleeding or discharge   d. all of these

_____ 12. The use of sterile needles to stimulate the energy force (chi) of the body is

   a. debridement   c. electrocautery

   b. cryosurgery   d. acupuncture

_____ 13. The process of using sterile technique with sterile instruments to remove necrotic tissue from a wound or a burn is called

    a. cauterization   c. debridement

    b. dermabrasion   d. diathermy

_____ 14. The medical term for the healing of a wound commonly known as a scab is

    a. erythroderma   c. esthesia

    b. eschar   d. extima

_____ 15. Medical/surgical scissors are labeled as _____ to describe the points of the blades.

    a. sharp-sharp   c. blunt-blunt

    b. sharp-blunt   d. all of these

_____ 16. You should always check the patient's emergency room report for the following information regarding suture removal:

    a. the date and the number of sutures put in   c. the length of time the sutures were to be left in

    b. date of patient's tetanus booster   d. all of the above

_____ 17. An ace wrap is a supportive bandage that

    a. gives an attractive appearance to the injury   c. gives support to the injured limb

    b. increases circulation of the injured area   d. b and c

F. Word Search: Find the following words hidden in the puzzle.

PATIENT	ELECTROCAUTERY
GLOVES	SUTURE
BIOPSY	HISTOLOGY
AUTHORIZE	WART
PRE-OP	FENESTRATED
CAUTERIZE	ANTISEPTIC
HEMOPHILIA	CRYOSURGERY
POLYP	TAUT
ANESTHESIA	POST-OP

```
G L E X A T R E P A T I E N T R E A
L Q M L Q K B I O P S Y N L R E A S
O Z A B S M Z T L B S R A T K M F D
V K Z N U P A R Y T Z E D G F R B H
E R P K T H O T P M A G M K E B J I
S E W O U I B T G I E R P W N L A S
L Z F Q R H S S S F G U L B E R T T
K I H C E T G E T O L S B F S K C O
P R E O P W H M P X P O D P T S E L
Z O T S A T A U T T K Y N L R F C O
P H W B S G L R O Z I R Z S A X B G
Q T X E E L E C T R O C A U T E R Y
S U N O P Y A I L I H P O M E H E P
C A U T E R I Z E T X C M J D O F D
```

G. Fill in the Blank: **Fill in what's missing in this list of sterile items used in a basic setup for most minor surgical procedures.**

1. scalpel handle and _____
2. hemostats
3. _____
4. needles and _____
5. suture scissors
6. _____
7. probe
8. gauze squares
9. vial of _____ medication
10. _____
11. _____
12. towels
13. _____
14. tray

CRITICAL THINKING SCENARIOS: **What would your response be in the following situations?**

1. As you are performing a skin prep on a patient for removing a sebaceous cyst from his scalp, he tells you that he is rather nervous about this procedure because he is a hemophiliac. _____
   _____
   _____

2. A young lady returns to have sutures removed. As you take the bandage off you notice that the sutured laceration site is infected. _____
   _____

3. You have not been able to clean and sterilize the instruments on the counter because you have been so busy with patient care. A co-worker picked up these instruments and says the doctor needs them for a surgical procedure stat! _____
   _____
   _____

4. You have set up the suture tray for the physician to suture a 7-year-old's laceration of the right forearm. This child is curious about everything he sees and asks many questions. The child's mother is with him. You must leave the room to answer a phone call. When you return, the child's mother is in the rest room and the child is touching some of the instruments on the suture tray. _____
   _____
   _____
   _____

ACHIEVING SKILL COMPETENCY

Reread the performance objectives for these procedures and then practice the skills listed below, following the procedure in your textbook.

Procedure 16-1: Prepare Skin for Minor Surgery

Procedure 16-2: Put on Sterile Gloves

Procedure 16-3: Assist with Minor Surgery

Procedure 16-4: Assisting with Suturing a Laceration

Procedure 16-5: Remove Sutures

When you feel you have mastered the performance of the skill, sign your name on the appropriate evaluation sheet and give it to your instructor to indicate you are prepared to perform the procedure for evaluation.

After your instructor has returned your work to you, make all necessary corrections and place in a three-ring notebook for future reference.

ASSIGNMENT SHEET

Chapter 17: ASSISTING WITH MEDICATIONS

Review the objectives and text for each unit before completing the assignment sheet for that unit. When you have completed all sheets for the chapter, remove them from this Workbook and give them to the instructor for evaluation.

Unit 1: PRESCRIPTION AND NONPRESCRIPTION MEDICATIONS

A. Word Puzzle: Use the clues below to spell out these terms.

1. __ D __ — Medication reference
2. __ __ __ __ R __ __ __ __ — Mastery
3. __ __ __ __ __ U __ __ — To plan
4. __ __ G __ __ __ __ __ __ __ — Rule
5. __ __ __ __ E __ __ __ — Distribute
6. __ __ __ __ N __ — Quantity
7. __ __ __ __ __ __ F __ __ __ __ __ __ __ — Categorize
8. __ __ __ __ __ O __ __ __ __ — Monitored
9. __ __ __ __ __ R __ __ __ — Correct
10. __ __ __ __ __ __ C __ __ __ __ __ — Study of medicines/drugs
11. __ __ __ __ E __ __ __ __ __ __ __ __ __ — To shorten
12. __ __ __ __ M __ __ __ __ __ — One show fills prescriptions
13. __ __ E __ __ __ __ __ __ __ __ __ — Written order for medicine
14. __ __ __ __ N __ __ — A permit
15. __ __ T __ — Numerical calculations
16. __ __ __ __ __ A __ __ __ __ — Medicines
17. __ __ D __ __ __ — Command
18. __ __ __ __ M __ __ __ __ __ __ __ __ __ — Big word for drugs/medicines
19. __ __ __ __ __ I __ __ — Highly controlled substances
20. __ __ __ __ __ __ N __ __ — Consultation
21. __ __ __ I __ __ __ __ — Enrollment
22. __ __ __ S __ __ __ __ __ — To write an order for medicine
23. __ __ __ __ T __ __ __ __ __ — Chemical
24. __ __ __ __ __ R __ __ — Means
25. __ __ __ A __ __ — Amount of medicine to take
26. __ T __ — Needs no prescription
27. __ __ __ __ __ I __ __ __ __ — To give
28. __ __ O __ __ — Call
29. __ __ __ N __ __ __ — Caution

B. Matching: Match the definition in column II with the correct term in column I.

COLUMN I   COLUMN II

_____ 1. Schedule I   a. Low potential for addiction
_____ 2. Schedule II   b. Subject to state/local regulations
_____ 3. Schedule III   c. Special instructions on prescription
_____ 4. Schedule IV   d. Produces lack of feeling
_____ 5. Schedule V   e. High potential for addiction
_____ 6. Hypnotic   f. Increases excretion of urine
_____ 7. Warning labels   g. High psychological dependency
_____ 8. Antipyretic   h. Not refilled without prescription
_____ 9. Diuretic   i. Produces sleep
_____ 10. Anesthetic   j. Relaxes skeletal muscles
                            k. Reduces fever

C. Fill in the Blank

1. The _____ is a valuable resource that the medical assistant should keep handy in the medical office.

2. The medical assistant should keep abreast of the newest _____ approved by the FDA.

3. The _____ is a legal document.

4. When phoning in a prescription, to assure accuracy, you should ask the pharmacist to _____ the information to avoid dangerous misunderstandings.

5. All physicians who prescribe, dispense, or administer medication in the United States must register annually with the United States Department of Justice, _____ under the Controlled Substance Act of 1970.

6. Commonly used medications must be rotated according to their _____

7. One of the most sensitive and important duties the medical assistant performs is _____

8. You must check with your employer regarding the _____ in your state before administering medications.

9. The OTC-PDR is a valuable reference to help you identify medicines that patients use for _____

10. When the physician moves the medical practice, it must be reported to the nearest _____

11. DEA registration must be renewed every _____ years.

12. Physicians must be in compliance with the DEA requirements of the _____ to administer, dispense, or prescribe any controlled substance.

13. _____ prescriptions are primarily prohibited since there is very limited medical use for them.

14. For convenience in writing several medication orders at once, many physicians use the _____ medication prescription pads.

15. If the physician does not want a generic substituted for a medication prescribed for a patient, this will be written on the prescription as _____

16. _____ are assigned by manufacturers to each batch of the products they produce so that any unusual side effects or problems of patients can be traced to the source.

17. A _____ routine check of the refrigerator and freezer temperatures is in compliance with the MSDS regulations.

D. Math Review: Solve the following problems. Show all work and place the answer on the provided line.

Addition

1. $0.2 + 0.35 + 0.0037 =$ _____
2. $0.4 + 0.003 + 0.421 =$ _____
3. $0.222 + 0.0003 + 0.216 =$ _____
4. $3.15 + 0.237 =$ _____
5. $3.007 + 0.2 =$ _____

Subtraction

6. $0.2 - 0.03 =$ _____
7. $0.37 - 0.205 =$ _____
8. $2.5 - 1.8 =$ _____
9. $4.5 - 0.127 =$ _____
10. $5.5 - 5.017 =$ _____

Multiplication

11. $5 \times 0.4 =$ _____
12. $7 \times .137 =$ _____
13. $5 \times 3.5 =$ _____
14. $10 \times 0.07 =$ _____
15. $100 \times 0.0238 =$ _____

Division

16. $0.2 \div 100 =$ _____
17. $0.35 \div 25 =$ _____
18. $2.5 \div 3 =$ _____
19. $1.45 \div 15 =$ _____
20. $3.15 \div 10 =$ _____

Fractions

21. $^2/_5 + ^1/_8 =$ _____
22. $2 ^1/_2 - 1 ^3/_4 =$ _____
23. $^2/_3 \times ^1/_4 \times ^3/_5 =$ _____
24. $^1/_8 \div ^3/_5 =$ _____
25. (change to decimal) $^3/_4 =$ _____

Percentages

26. 25% of $4.8 =$ _____
27. 30% of $17 =$ _____
28. 15% of $36 =$ _____
29. 75% of $74 =$ _____
30. 63% of $97 =$ _____

Ratio/Proportion: Find x in the following

31. $5:200 :: x:40$ _____
32. $^1/_2:2 :: ^1/_4:x$ _____
33. $x:30 :: 4:10$ _____
34. $0.05:x :: 0.15:30$ _____
35. $20:60 :: x:50$ _____

E. Translation: Translate the following abbreviations into sentence form.

1. Rx$\overline{s}$ aq po pc qd PRN _____

2. Rx ss tab po tid $\overline{c}$ aq com ac _____

3. alt noc rep ad lib _____

4. pt DC Fe caps STAT _____

5. Give 2 T emul qid alt dieb _____

6. qns sol _____

7. G 1 tsp. H2O2 hs. _____

8. dil pulv /c aq ferv et f sat sol _____

9. Div dos et adde aq bull, 1 m elix, m et sig. _____

10. pt NPO/am Ba po/GI studies. _____

F. Multiple Choice: Place the correct letter on the blank line for each question.

_____ 1. A medication that slows the blood clotting process is called a(n)

   a. anorexic   c. anticoagulant

   b. sedative   d. hormone

_____ 2. Bronchodilators are medications used to

   a. treat anemia   c. neutralize stomach acid

   b. stop diarrhea   d. promote easier breathing

_____ 3. Physicians prescribe antipyretics to

   a. prevent convulsions   c. elevate mood

   b. reduce fever   d. relieve tension

_____ 4. Medications that promote sleep/sedation are called

   a. antiemetics   b. antacids

   c. sedatives   d. vitamins

_____ 5. Antihistamines are prescribed to

   a. relieve cold/allergy symptoms   c. reduce heartbeat rate

   b. suppress coughing   d. increase urinary output

_____ 6. Antitussives are medications that are used to

   a. treat hormonal disorders   c. fight infection

   b. suppress coughing   d. supplement vitamin deficiencies

_____ 7. To fight infection a physician may prescribe a(n)

   a. tranquilizer   c. bronchodilator

   b. cathartic   d. antibiotic

_____ 8. A heart depressant will

   a. reduce heart rate   c. prevent convulsions

   b. suppress appetite   d. stop vomiting/nausea

_____ 9. To promote evacuation of the bowel tract, a physician may prescribe a(n)

   a. sedative   c. cathartic

   b. antidiarrheal   d. tranquilizer

_____ 10. Respiratory stimulants are used to treat

   a. convulsions   c. vitamin deficiencies

   b. shock and drug poisoning   d. muscle/bone conditions

_____ 11. Iron compounds are prescribed to treat

      a. anemia   c. appetite disorders

      b. muscle/bone conditions   d. tension/anxiety

_____ 12. Analgesics are medications prescribed to

      a. promote sleep/sedation   c. relieve pain

      b. reduce fever   d. relieve tension/anxiety

_____ 13. An anticonvulsant is a medication that is used to

      a. suppress appetite   c. suppress coughing

      b. prevent convulsions   d. relieve anxiety

_____ 14. Muscle/bone conditions are often treated with

      a. tranquilizers   c. vitamins

      b. antibiotics   d. musculoskeletal relaxants

_____ 15. Antacids are prescribed to

      a. neutralize stomach acid   c. stop vomiting/nausea

      b. suppress appetite   d. supplement vitamin deficiencies

G. Matching: Match the color in column I with the corresponding section of the *Physicians' Desk Reference* in column II.

COLUMN I

_____ 1. Yellow

_____ 2. Pink

_____ 3. White

_____ 4. Blue

_____ 5. Green

COLUMN II

a. Products in alphabetical order according to their classification

b. Current information about diagnostic products

c. Brand or (if desired) generic names of products

d. Generic or chemical names of products

e. Picture identification

f. Complete product information

H. Math Review: Solve the following word problems.

1. Jessica, a medical assistant, earns $7.50 per hour for the first 40 hours per week. When she exceeds 40 hours in any work week, she is paid time and a half. One week during the winter flu season she worked 53 hours. When she received her paycheck, the gross amount was $397.53

   a. When Jessica works overtime, what is the hourly rate of pay?

   _____

   b. Based on the 53 hours, 13 of which were overtime, what should the gross amount be on her paycheck?

   _____

   c. Is the gross amount on the paycheck she received correct?

   _____

2. The Medical Supply Company is offering a 15% discount on sterile gloves purchased during their anniversary month. The regular cost of the sterile gloves is $37.50 per 100 gloves.

   a. What is the cost of 300 gloves without the discount?

   _____

   b. What is the cost of 300 gloves with the discount?

   _____
   _____

   c. How much is saved with the discount?

   _____

3. A medical assistant can type 250 words in 3 minutes. At the same rate, how long would it take this medical assistant to type 5000 words?

   _____
   _____
   _____

4. Two of Mrs. Smith's children have been diagnosed with conjunctivitis. The physician wrote a prescription for an antibiotic ophthalmic solution. It reads: 2 gtts TID in each affected eye for 5 days.

   a. If each child needs drops instilled in each eye, how many drops would be needed?

   _____
   _____
   _____

   b. How many household teaspoons would this be? _____

Name _____

5. A medical assistant was asked by her physician-employer to check over a small order from the medical supply house that had arrived while the staff was out to lunch. To expedite the task, the physician handed the medical assistant a copy of the original order (see illustration following):

THE ORIGINAL ORDER

ITEMS	PER UNIT	TOTAL
2 boxes disposable gloves; 100 ct.	$3.75	$7.50
3 boxes syringes; 50 ct.	25.00	75.00
10 thermometers	1.50	10.50
12 boxes tissues	0.25	3.00
5 cartons tongue dep.; 100 ct.	1.38	6.90
6 bottles hand soap	1.77	17.70
		$130.60

THE FINAL BILL

ITEMS	PER UNIT	TOTAL
2 ctns., surg. gloves	$5.75	$11.50
3 ctns., disp. syr.	25.00	75.00
100 thermometers	1.50	150.00
12 boxes tissues	0.25	3.00
5 cartons tongue dep.	1.38	6.90
19 bottles, hand soap	1.77	17.70
		$264.15

The first obvious problem is that the totals do not match on the order and on the bill. An item count further reveals some discrepancies between the quantities shown on the bill and the items actually received. Specifically, only 10 boxes of tissues and 4 cartons of tongue depressors were delivered.

a. Double check each item on the original order; if any mathematical errors are found, correct them.

THE ORIGINAL ORDER

ITEMS	PER UNIT	TOTAL

b. Double check the final bill as shown: if any mathematical errors are found, correct them.

_____

c. Still working with the bill as shown, are there any further discrepancies beyond mathematical errors?
   1. _____

   2. _____
   3. _____
   4. _____

d. Now reconcile the count discrepancies with the corrected amounts shown on the bill.

_____

_____

_____

_____

_____

_____

_____

e. What procedure should be followed in paying the supplier for items actually ordered and received? What should be done with overages? with shortages? with incorrect items?

_____

_____

_____

6. Mrs. Brown, a patient of Dr. Johnston, has been diagnosed as suffering from refractory rickets. Dr. Johnston has prescribed the following treatment:

Ergocalciferol USP, Vitamin D_2 Tab, 100,000 USP units q6h for 14 days.

Ergocalciferol USP, Vitamin D_2 is available in either 50,000 USP units tablets or 8,000 USP units/ml drops. Dr. Johnston has decided to start Mrs. Brown on tablets. After 14 days of treatment, Dr. Johnston will test to determine if Mrs. Brown's serum calcium levels have returned to within normal limits. If so, therapy may be continued at a lower dosage.

a. How many tablets should be given q6h?

_____

b. How many tablets should be given Qid? _____

c. How many tablets should be ordered for the 14-day treatment? _____

7. After the 14-day treatment that Mrs. Brown took in problem 6, Dr. Johnston finds that her serum calcium levels are returning to normal limits. He decides to continue her on a treatment of Ergocalciferol USP, Vitamin D_2 at a reduced level for a period of one month. However, instead of tablets, the medication will be administered in liquid form. His new prescription is as follows:

Ergocalciferol USP, Vitamin D_2 gtt, 48,000 USP units, Bid for 30 days.

As stated in problem 6, Ergocalciferol USP, Vitamin D_2, is available in 8,000 USP units/ml drops; 60 ml bottle with dropper.

a. How many drops will be required for each dosage?

_____

b. How many drops are required for Mrs. Brown's daily dosage? _____

c. How many bottles of Ergocalciferol USP, Vitamin D_2, will be needed to fill the entire prescription?

_____

_____

8. Bill Jones, a young boy weighing 73 $\frac{1}{4}$ pounds, has a mild ulcerative colitis condition which has been bothering him for several weeks. The physician recommended a treatment of Azulfidine and wrote the following prescription:

   Azulfidine 30mg/kg, q6h for 7 days.

   Azulfidine is available in 500 mg 100s tablets.

   a. How many ml of Azulfidine will Bill receive per day?

      1. _____

      2. _____

   b. How many tablets will be needed per dosage? For the whole prescription?

      1. _____
         _____

      2. _____

      _____

9. Brad has a history of chronic asthma. As a treatment of first choice, Brad's doctor has prescribed theophylline anhydrous. Since this is a rather strong medication, the dosage is individualized for Brad based on his body weight and age. Brad is 15 years old and weighs 121 pounds. The recommended dosage for ages 12–16 years is 18mg/kg/day. The prescription is as follows:

   18mg/kg/day p.o., not to exceed 900 mg/day.

   Theophylline is available in 125 mg capsule form.

   a. How many mg of theophylline would Brad receive based on 18mg/kg/day p.o.?

      _____
      _____
      _____
      _____

   b. Would this amount be the proper dosage?

      _____

   c. If not, what would be the amount of theophylline in mg Brad would receive per day based on the prescription?

      _____

10. Bobby, a 10-year-old boy, was diagnosed as having strep throat. The physician ordered penicillin G potassium U 5,000,000 IM, stat. The recommended pediatric dosage is U 3,000,000–1,200,000 per day. Penicillin G potassium is available in U 5,000,000/ml. How many ml has the doctor prescribed for Bobby?

   _____

CRITICAL THINKING SCENARIOS: What would your response be in the following situations?

1. A patient stops in your office to pick up a prescription for his allergy. He mentions that if it's the same thing he got the last time, he might as well not take it. _____

   _____

2. One of your elderly patients calls to tell you that all of the prescriptions that she had filled at the pharmacy look different from what she usually takes. She mentions that they didn't cost as much and she's not going to take any of them because she thinks the doctor made a mistake. _____

   _____

   _____

   _____

After your instructor has returned your work to you, make all necessary corrections and place in a three-ring notebook for future reference.

ASSIGNMENT SHEET

Chapter 17: ASSISTING WITH MEDICATIONS

Unit 2: METHODS OF ADMINISTERING MEDICATIONS

SUGGESTED RESPONSES TO CRITICAL THINKING CHALLENGE IN TEXTBOOK

1. What should be done in this situation? _____

_____

2. Is it that critical that a patient take a prescribed medication? _____

_____

3. Do you need an interpreter to help make the patient understand? _____

_____

4. Can you go to the physician and ask him to take this problem? _____

_____

5. What might an option to his treatment be? _____

_____

6. Should you have printed instructions? In what language? _____

_____

7. What would you do in order of importance? _____

_____

_____

_____

A. Fill in the Blank

1. Most oral medications are intended for absorption in the _____
2. The _____ method of administering medication involves placing the medication under the tongue.
3. Sublingual and buccal methods of administration introduce medication immediately into the _____ through membranes.
4. _____ medications are supplied as creams, suppositories, tablets, douches, foams, ointments, tampons, sprays, and salves.
5. Medications that are applied in various forms to the skin are termed _____
6. _____ medications are breathed into the respiratory tract.
7. _____ medications are given by means of injection.
8. The _____ is the most convenient method of medication.
9. The dosage of _____ drugs is determined by the body surface area of the patient.
10. Allergies and other vital information are noted on a patient's chart in _____ ink.

B. Matching: Match the definition in column II with the correct term in column I.

COLUMN I

_____ 1. Buccal
_____ 2. Oxygen
_____ 3. Package insert
_____ 4. Transdermal patch
_____ 5. Patient education
_____ 6. Oral medication
_____ 7. Topical
_____ 8. Prescription
_____ 9. Sublingual
_____ 10. Sample medications

COLUMN II

a. Placed on a fleshy body part
b. Most common medication method
c. Applied to the skin
d. Require categorized storage
e. Placed in mouth between cheek and gums
f. Contains medication information
g. Inhalation treatment in emergencies
h. Gains compliance with treatment plan
i. Requires physician's signature
j. Big part of medical assistant's job
k. Placed under tongue

C. Brief Answer

1. List the points of the standard format checklist for administering medications. _____
_____

2. How many times should you check a medication before you administer it and why? _____
_____

3. Why is it a good idea to always check the medication container after administering medication? _____
_____

4. What does *technique* mean regarding medications? _____
_____

5. Explain what time has to do in regard to medications. _____
_____

6. Why is it important to check the expiration date on medications? _____
_____

7. Do the same guidelines apply to sample packets of medicines the same as to prescriptions?   Explain your
answer. _____
_____

After your instructor has returned your work to you, make all necessary corrections and place in a three-ring
notebook for future reference.

ASSIGNMENT SHEET

Chapter 17: ASSISTING WITH MEDICATIONS

Unit 3: INJECTIONS AND IMMUNIZATIONS

SUGGESTED RESPONSES TO CRITICAL THINKING CHALLENGE IN TEXTBOOK

1. What happened here? _____

_____

2. What do you suppose will happen when Darlene returns from lunch? _____

_____

3. What is Darlene guilty of? _____

_____

4. Will Darlene be fired for doing what she did? _____

_____

5. What do you think Mrs. Jackson will do? _____

_____

6. Is Mrs. Jackson at fault for this situation? Why or why not? _____

_____

_____

_____

_____

7. Who is responsible if the baby has a serious reaction? _____

_____

8. Do you think Darlene noticed the baby's fever? _____

_____

9. What would you do about this situation? _____

_____

A. Fill in the Blank

1. In order to mix insulin within the vial (bottle) you should gently _____ it between your fingers (hands).

2. The amount of air injected into the vial should be _____ to the insulin dose.

3. Too large an air bubble in the syringe will _____ the insulin dose.

4. Insulin injections should be administered at a(n) _____ angle.

5. It should take one less than _____ seconds to inject the insulin dose.

6. There is always a possibility of _____ shock when administering any medication.

7. Medication should only be administered to patients when a physician is available nearby should the patient exhibit any _____

8. The term _____ simply means "under the skin."

9. _____ injections are used in allergy and tuberculin testing.

10. A small _____ will develop at the site of the intradermal injection, giving evidence that the medication is in the dermal layer of the skin.

11. Following the intradermal injection, the patient must be observed for at least _____ minutes.
12. Subcutaneous injections are administered at a _____ angle of insertion.
13. Medications injected into the muscle tissue are termed _____
14. The purpose of the _____ method of injection is to inject irritating substances deep into the muscle layer of tissue and prevent leakage from following the path of the needle.
15. In the Z-track and subcutaneous methods of injection, the injection site should not be _____ after medication is administered.
16. The medical assistant is not qualified to administer _____ injections.

B. Labeling: Label the parts of this syringe. Refer to Figure 17-10 in the textbook.

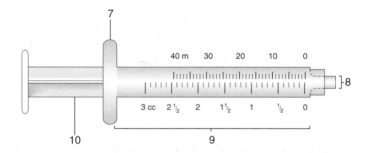
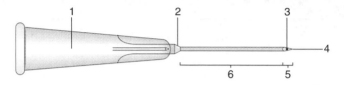

1.   1. _____
     2. _____
     3. _____
     4. _____
     5. _____
     6. _____
     7. _____
     8. _____
     9. _____
    10. _____

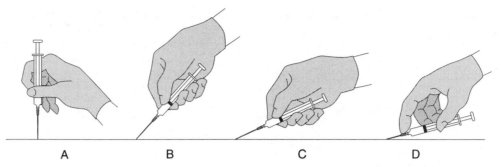

2. Labeling: Label the angles of injection in these pictures. Refer to Figure 17-11 in the textbook.

   a. _____

   b. _____

   c. _____

   d. _____

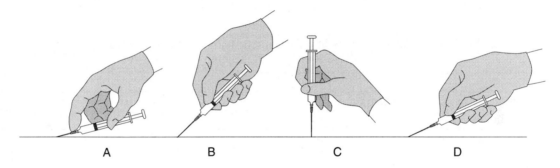

3. Labeling: Identify the types of injections that these pictures indicate. Refer to Figure 17-11 in the textbook.

   a. _____

   b. _____

   c. _____

   d. _____

C. Brief Answer

1. Name the tissue layers and sites of injection for intradermal, intramuscular, and subcutaneous. _____

   _____

   _____

   _____

   _____

2. Explain how to reassure a patient in preparing for an injection. _____

   _____

   _____

3. What is the proper way to dispose of used syringes and needles? _____

   _____

4. If a needle must be recapped, how should it be done? _____

   _____

   _____

Name _____

5. Why must patients be given written information and sign authorization forms before immunizations are administered? _____

_____

_____

_____

6. Explain how to give insulin injections. _____

_____

_____

_____

_____

7. List the various sites for insulin injections. _____

8. List symptoms of anaphylactic shock. _____

_____

_____

9. How long should a patient wait after receiving an injection? Why? _____

_____

10. Explain why you should not rub medications into tissues following a Z-tract injection. _____

_____

_____

11. What is immunity? List the different types. _____

_____

_____

_____

_____

_____

D. Brief Answer

1. At what age is the immunization schedule routinely begun? _____

2. What are the first three immunizations (vaccines) given to infants? _____

3. How long should the ideal time period be between immunizations in a series? _____

4. Assuming an infant has had a regular routine immunization schedule, at what age will the child be at the completed primary series of DTP, OPV, and Hib? _____

5. What immunization does a child receive at age 18 months? _____

6. At ages four to six years, what booster immunization should a child receive? _____

7. Td is given to what age group of children? _____

8. How often should adult tetanus and diphtheria toxoids be repeated? _____

9. Besides oral polio vaccine, there is a higher-potency polio vaccine, IPV (inactivated polio vaccine), which is administered by _____

10. Bacterial meningitis is a highly contagious disease that can cause serious and long-lasting effects on the _____ system.

11. Infectious hepatitis can be prevented with the hepatitis A vaccine, which consists of _____ injections _____ apart and is recommended for those who are traveling to distant continents.

12. Refer to ABHES Course Content Requirements in Appendix C of the textbook. Within the area of *Medical Office Clinical Procedures,* which content requirements are discussed in this chapter? _____

Name _____

E. Brief Answer

1. Discuss the drugs that are under federal regulation according to category or Schedules I through V.

_____
_____
_____
_____
_____
_____
_____
_____
_____
_____
_____

2. What is the Hib vaccine? Who should receive it? _____

_____

F. True or False: Place a "T" for true or "F" for false in the space provided. For false statements, explain why they are false.

1. You should take *only* the medicine that has been prescribed for you by the physician.
2. Prescribed medicine may be shared with family members.
3. Taking more (extra) doses of prescribed medicine will make you get better faster.
4. Any reaction to or side effect of any medicine must be reported to the physician immediately.
5. You do not need to instruct patients to tell you of any OTC medications they take on their own.
6. It is important to advise patients if the physician has prescribed medications that could interfere with their concentration or make them sleepy.
7. After six months, medicines should be thrown away (flushed down the toilet).
8. Patients should be made aware that generic and brand name products (prescriptions) are the same.
9. The medical assistant should instruct patients to refrain from consuming alcoholic beverages while taking medications.
10. It is not necessary for female patients to report whether they plan to become pregnant, are pregnant, or are nursing mothers before taking medication.

G. Matching: Match the disease in column I with the common symptoms in column II.

COLUMN I

_____ 1. Tetanus
_____ 2. Measles
_____ 3. Hepatitis B
_____ 4. Diphtheria
_____ 5. Influenza
_____ 6. Pertussis
_____ 7. Mumps
_____ 8. Haemophilus type B
_____ 9. Pneumonia
_____ 10. Rubella

COLUMN II

a. Headache, malaise, fever, sore throat with yellowish-white or gray membrane

b. Chills, fever, headache, pain and swelling below and in front of ears

c. Begins with fever, malaise, headache, nausea/vomiting, abdominal discomfort, generalized paralysis

d. Abrupt onset, severe chills, high fever, headache, chest pain/dyspnea, rapid pulse, cyanosis, cough/blood-stained sputum

e. Slow onset of fever, malaise, no appetite, nausea/vomiting, jaundice

f. Slight fever, sore throat, drowsiness, malaise, swollen glands/lymph nodes, diffuse fine red rash

g. Fever, malaise, runny nose, cough, sore throat, Koplik's spots

h. Sudden onset of fever, chills, sore throat, cough, muscle aches/pains, weakness, general malaise

i. Stiffness of jaw/esophageal muscles sometimes neck muscles, fever, painful spasms of all muscles, irritability, headache

j. High WBC count, respiratory drainage, slight fever, irritability, dry cough, whooping inspiration sounds

k. Sudden onset of fever, sore throat, cough, muscle aches, weakness and general malaise

H. Multiple Choice: Place the correct letter on the blank line for each question.

_____ 1. Common flu is a disease that affects the
a. kidneys
b. respiratory tract
c. liver
d. spinal column

_____ 2. In addition to bed rest, fluids, analgesics, and antipyretics, pneumonia is sometimes treated with
a. muscle relaxants
b. vitamins
c. oxygen
d. sedatives

_____ 3. Haemophilus influenza type B affects
a. infants/small children
b. elementary school children
e. the elderly
c. adolescents
d. adults

_____ 4. Complications of measles can result in deafness, brain damage, and
a. paralysis
b. pneumonia
c. baldness
d. myopia

_____ 5. The incubation period for mumps is
a. 14–28 hours
b. 14–28 days
c. 14–28 weeks
d. 14–28 months

_____ 6. Rubella is a most dangerous disease that can cause severe abnormalities to a(n)
a. pregnant female
b. teenager
c. infant
d. the fetus

_____ 7. A tracheostomy is sometimes necessary to perform in which of these diseases?
a. tetanus
b. mumps
c. diphtheria
d. pneumonia

_____ 8. A trace cough may last for several months to two years following
  a. pertussis   c. diphtheria
  b. influenza   d. tetanus

_____ 9. A disease that is commonly transmitted in puncture wounds is
  a. polio   c. haemophilus
  b. diphtheria   d. tetanus

_____ 10. Alcohol and fats should especially be eliminated from the diet of one who has
  a. mumps   c. hepatitis
  b. tetanus   d. influenza

_____ 11. An acute infection and inflammation of the gray matter of the spinal cord is
  a. polio   c. tetanus
  b. hepatitis   d. diphtheria

CRITICAL THINKING SCENARIOS: What would your response be in the following situations?

1. One of your adult patients comes in for his first allergy injection. He says to use his left arm because that's the one he always had his allergy shots in before where he used to live. He is also in a hurry and wants to be somewhere in 10 minutes. _____

_____

_____

_____

ACHIEVING SKILL COMPETENCY

Reread the performance objective for each procedure and then practice the skills listed below, following the procedure in your textbook.
  Procedure 17-1: Obtain and Administer Oral Medication
  Procedure 17-2: Withdraw Medication from Ampule
  Procedure 17-3: Withdraw Medication from Vial
  Procedure 17-4: Administer Intradermal Injection
  Procedure 17-5: Administer Subcutaneous Injection
  Procedure 17-6: Administer Intramuscular Injection
  Procedure 17-7: Administer Intramuscular Injection by Z-Tract Method

When you feel you have mastered the performance of the skill, sign your name on the appropriate evaluation sheet and give it to your instructor to indicate you are prepared to perform the procedure for evaluation.

After your instructor has returned your work to you, make all necessary corrections and place in a three-ring notebook for future reference.

ASSIGNMENT SHEET

Chapter 18: EMERGENCIES, ACUTE ILLNESS, ACCIDENTS, AND RECOVERY

Review the objectives and text for each unit before completing the assignment sheet for that unit. When you have completed all sheets for the chapter, remove them from this Workbook and give them to the instructor for evaluation.

Unit 1: MANAGING EMERGENCIES IN THE MEDICAL OFFICE

Mixed Quiz

1. What is a universal emergency medical identification symbol and what does it do?

   _____

   _____

2. Identify five medical conditions for which a patient should wear an identification symbol.

   a. _____

   b. _____

   c. _____

   d. _____

   e. _____

3. When is a situation considered to be an emergency? _____

   _____

4. List the 16 items identified in the text that should be included in an emergency kit or cart.

   a. _____

   b. _____

   c. _____

   d. _____

   e. _____

   f. _____

   g. _____

   h. _____

   i. _____

   j. _____

   k. _____

   l. _____

   m. _____

   n. _____

   o. _____

   p. _____

5. What is an AED unit, and what three functions can it perform?

   _____

   _____

6. Refer to the CAAHEP Standards in Appendix B of the textbook. Within the area of *Medical Assisting Clinical Procedures,* which curriculum standard is discussed in this unit? _____

7. True or False: Answer the following statements with "T" for True or "F" for False, where true indicates the data is necessary to document in an emergency situation and false indicates the data is *not* necessary to document in an emergency situation.

    a. _____ Name of injured patient or employee

    b. _____ Date of incident

    c. _____ Social Security number of person injured

    d. _____ Time of injury or emergency

    e. _____ Name and phone number of next-of-kin

    f. _____ Location of accident or injury

    g. _____ Description of condition surrounding accident or injury

    h. _____ Description of past like incidences

    i. _____ Employer's name, address, and phone number

    j. _____ Identification of accident or incident witnesses

    k. _____ Signature of examining physician

    l. _____ Description of action taken, including disposition of the patient

    m. _____ Signature of person filing report

8. Enter below the phone number for emergency medical services in your location. (Don't assume the universal 911 number is in effect in your area. Be certain!

_____

9. Determine the procedure to follow in your area when an individual dies without benefit of recent medical attention either within a physician's office or at another site.

_____

10. What follow-up record-keeping action is necessary following death of a patient?

_____

_____

11. Word Puzzle: Using the *Words to Know,* spell out the following terms.

_ _ E _ _ _	An emetic
_ _ _ _ M _	Injury
_ E _ _ _ _ _ _ _ _ _ _ _	Revive
_ _ R _ _ _ _	A physician
_ _ _ _ _ G _	A dressing
_ _ E _ _ _	Cause vomiting
_ _ _ _ _ _ N _	A happening
_ _ C _ _ _ _ _	Unexpected injury
_ Y _ _ _ _	An emblem

12. Unscramble

_____	EULNRISVA
_____	IANRCOTITFECI
_____	OCRERON
_____	TIDNICNE
_____	OLYSBM
_____	CTICEAND

After your instructor has returned your work to you, make all necessary corrections and place in a three-ring notebook for future reference.

ASSIGNMENT SHEET

Chapter 18: EMERGENCIES, ACUTE ILLNESS, ACCIDENTS, AND RECOVERY

Unit 2: ACUTE ILLNESS

Mixed Quiz

1. Matching: Match the common term used to describe the severity of illness in column I with the correct meaning in column II.

COLUMN I   COLUMN II

_____ Chronic   a. Occurring quickly and without warning

_____ Insidious   b. Extensive, advanced

_____ Urgent   c. May cause death

_____ Sudden   d. Long, drawn out, not acute

_____ Acute   e. Hidden, not apparent

_____ Severe   f. Requires intervention as soon as possible

_____ Life-threatening g. Rapid onset, severe symptoms, and short course

2. List the nine steps or stages that might occur with a major seizure.

a. _____

b. _____

c. _____

d. _____

e. _____

f. _____

g. _____

h. _____

i. _____

3. Fill in the Blank: Listed below are symptoms of diabetic coma and insulin shock. Enter "C" for coma or "S" for shock before the symptom to indicate which condition may be present.

_____ a. Drooling

_____ b. Perspiration

_____ c. Dry mouth

_____ d. Not hungry

_____ e. Full, bounding pulse

_____ f. Dry, flushed skin

_____ g. Fruity odor to breath

_____ h. Weak, rapid pulse

_____ i. Intense thirst

_____ j. Double vision

4. Fill in the Blank

A temporarily diminished supply of _____ to the _____ may cause _____
The medical term for this condition is _____ A patient should be positioned with
_____ to improve circulation to the _____ Symptoms of approaching syncope
are _____ and complaints of _____ or _____
When using aromatic spirits of ammonia capsules, it is important to _____

_____

5. List the prime symptoms of heart attack.

   a. _____

   b. _____

   c. _____

   d. _____

   e. _____

   f. _____

   g. _____

   h. _____

   i. _____

6. Fill in the Blank: Indicate whether the following symptoms are possible heat stroke (S) or heat exhaustion (E). Place an "S" or "E" in front of the symptoms.

   _____ Pale, cool skin

   _____ Profuse perspiration

   _____ Rapid pulse, possible Cheyne-Stokes respirations

   _____ Dry, red face

   _____ Body temperature above average

   _____ Dilated pupils

   _____ Hypertension

   _____ Headache

   _____ Mental confusion, giddiness

   _____ Thirst, nausea, vomiting

7. List the six successive symptoms of frostbite and identify the most often damaged body parts.

   a. _____

   b. _____

   c. _____

   d. _____

   e. _____

   f. _____

8. Name the three types of visible bleeding and the characteristics of each type.

   a. _____

   b. _____

   c. _____

9. Labeling: Label the pressure points where severe arterial bleeding can be controlled. Refer to Figure 18-5 in the textbook.

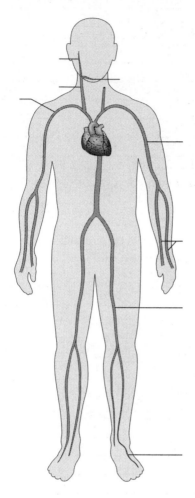

10. What are the symptoms of internal bleeding, and how is it initially and eventually treated?

   a. _____

   b. _____

   c. _____

   d. _____

   e. _____

   f. _____

   g. _____

   h. _____

   i. _____

11. Identify six routes by which poison can enter the body.

   a. _____

   b. _____

   c. _____

   d. _____

   e. _____

   f. _____

12. Determine the phone number for your local poison control center. Write it on the line below and add it to the emergency medical service number on your personal reference card.

_____

13. List the seven most common causes of obstructed airway.

    a. _____
    b. _____
    c. _____
    d. _____
    e. _____
    f. _____
    g. _____

14. What are the three names for the method used to relieve an obstructed airway?

    a. _____
    b. _____
    c. _____

15. List six conditions that may cause respiratory distress.

    a. _____
    b. _____
    c. _____
    d. _____
    e. _____
    f. _____

16. Name the components of the AED unit. _____

17. What three things need to be examined in a scheduled equipment check? _____
_____

18. List the sequence of events required for survival of cardiac arrest.

    a. _____
    b. _____
    c. _____
    d. _____
    e. _____
    f. _____

19. What is the critical concern in cases of cervical spinal injury?
_____

20. Identify the six symptoms of shock.

    a. _____
    b. _____
    c. _____
    d. _____
    e. _____
    f. _____

21. What are the usual causes of shock?
_____
_____

22. What is anaphylactic shock?
_____

23. Name substances that can cause anaphylactic shock.

a. _____

b. _____

c. _____

d. _____

e. _____

f. _____

g. _____

h. _____

i. _____

j. _____

24. What are the symptoms of stroke?

a. _____

b. _____

c. _____

d. _____

e. _____

f. _____

g. _____

h. _____

i. _____

23. Spelling: Each line contains three different spellings of a word. Underline the correctly spelled word.

asperation	aspirashun	aspiration
diaphoresis	diephoresis	diaforesis
incidious	insidious	insideous
profalatic	profalytic	prophylatic
exhaustion	eghaustion	egaustion
ammonea	ammonia	amoania
seezure	seazure	seizure

24. Refer to the Role Delineation Chart in Appendix A of the textbook. Within the area of *Patient Care,* which role relates to the content of this unit? _____

ACHIEVING SKILL COMPETENCY

Reread the performance objectives for the procedures and then practice the skills listed below, following the procedure in your textbook.

Procedure 18-1: Give Mouth-to-Mouth Resuscitation

Procedure 18-2: Give Cardiopulmonary Resuscitation (CPR) to Adults

Procedure 18-3: Give Cardiopulmonary Resuscitation (CPR) to Infants and Children

When you feel you have mastered the performance of a skill, sign your name on the appropriate evaluation sheet and give it to your instructor to indicate you are prepared to perform the procedure for evaluation.

After your instructor has returned your work to you, make all necessary corrections and place in a three-ring notebook for future reference.

ASSIGNMENT SHEET

Chapter 18: EMERGENCIES, ACUTE ILLNESS, ACCIDENTS, AND RECOVERY

Unit 3: FIRST AID IN ACCIDENTS AND INJURIES

Mixed Quiz

1. How is a bee stinger removed?

   _____

2. When is anti-rabies serum required following an animal bite?

   _____

3. Name the three types of burns, and give examples of each.

   a. _____

   _____

   b. _____

   c. _____

4. What is the first priority in the treatment of burns?

   _____

5. Compare the first aid treatment for the three degrees of burns

   _____

   _____

   _____

   _____

   _____

6. Describe the symptoms of a dislocation.

   _____

7. What is the benefit of adding moisture to a heat treatment?

   _____

8. What action does the application of cold treatments have on the body?

   _____

9. What action does the application of heat treatments have on the body?

   _____

   _____

10. Name four types of wounds.

    a. _____

    b. _____

    c. _____

    d. _____

11. Refer to the CAAHEP Standards in Appendix B of the textbook. Within the area of *Medical Assisting Clinical Procedures,* which three curriculum standards are discussed in this unit? _____

    _____

12. Word Puzzle: Use the *Words to Know* to spell out these terms.

_ _ _ A _ _ _ _	A scrape or scratch
_ _ _ _ _ C _ _	Acid or alkaline substance
_ _ _ C _ _ _ _ _ _	Having a current
_ _ _ _ _ _ I _ _ _ _	Prevent from moving
_ _ _ _ D	An injury
_ _ _ E _ _ _ _ _	A tear
_ _ N _ _ _ _	A hole
_ _ _ _ T _ _ _	Rub briskly
_ _ _ _ S _ _ _	Smooth cut

12. Word Search: Find the following words hidden in the puzzle.

ANAPHYLACTIC
BANDAGE
BITE
BURN
CHEMICAL
ELECTRICAL
FRICTION
IMMOBILIZE
INCISION
INJURIES
LACERATION

MOLTEN
PUNCTURE
SHOCK
SPLINTER
SPRAIN
STINGS
STRAIN
SUPERFICIAL
THERMAL
WOUND

```
S U P E R F I C I A L E
R I P D J V S H O C K L
L I W N I S P R A I N E
A N A P H Y L A C T I C
C C C H E M I C A L M T
E I P S T I N G S C M R
R S F R I C T I O N O I
A I M O L T E N Q O B C
T O M T H E R M A L I A
I N J U R I E S V X L L
O Q W O U N D B P B I H
N I W S T R A I N U Z P
W R G P U N C T U R E Y
X B A N D A G E P N I U
```

After your instructor has returned your work to you, make all necessary corrections and place in a three-ring notebook for future reference.

ASSIGNMENT SHEET

Chapter 18: EMERGENCIES, ACUTE ILLNESS, ACCIDENTS, AND RECOVERY

Unit 4: RECOVERING FUNCTION AND MOBILITY

SUGGESTED RESPONSES TO CRITICAL THINKING CHALLENGE IN TEXTBOOK

1. What factors might be involved in Mary's problem with using a cane? _____
_____

2. What options does Shelly have to help Mary with her mobility? _____
_____
_____

3. Does Shelly have an obligation to question the physician's order? _____
_____

4. What risk factors may be involved in this situation? _____
_____

5. Are there any options at home to be considered? _____
_____
_____
_____
_____
_____

Mixed Quiz

1. Identify seven situations when the use of some form of device may be indicated to assist patients with mobility.
   a. _____
   b. _____
   c. _____
   d. _____
   e. _____
   f. _____
   g. _____
2. Identify six basic benefits from regular exercise.
   a. _____
   b. _____
   c. _____
   d. _____
   e. _____
   f. _____
3. What is a range-of-motion exercise? _____
_____
4. What is a flexibility exercise? _____
_____

5. What two precautions must be observed when applying a sling? _____
_____

6. Identify two guidelines concerning fitting a cane. _____
_____

7. Explain the proper height for crutches. _____
_____

8. List four factors that will increase safety for the patient at home. _____
_____
_____

9. Matching: Match the definition in column II with the correct term in column I.

COLUMN I		COLUMN II
_____	1. Ambulate	a. A type of cane
_____	2. Axilla	b. Manner of walking
_____	3. Balance	c. Extent of movement
_____	4. Flexibility	d. To walk
_____	5. Gait	e. To hold secure
_____	6. Mobility	f. Area under arm
_____	7. Quad-base	g. The ability to twist and bend
_____	8. Range-of-motion	h. Equilibrium
_____	9. Stabilize	i. Move about freely

10. Using the text, practice the range-of-motion exercises to become familiar with the movements.

11. Refer to the ABHES Course Content Requirements in Appendix C of the textbook. Within the area of *Medical Office Clinical Procedures,* which content requirement is discussed in this unit? _____

ACHIEVING SKILL COMPETENCY

Reread the performance objective for each procedure and then practice the skills listed below, following the procedure in your textbook.

Procedure 18-1: Apply Arm Sling
Procedure 18-2: Use a Cane
Procedure 18-3: Use Crutches
Procedure 18-4: Use a Walker
Procedure 18-5: Assist Patient from Wheelchair to Examination Table
Procedure 18-6: Assist Patient from Examination Table to Wheelchair

When you feel you have mastered the performance of the skill, sign your name on the appropriate evaluation sheet and give it to your instructor to indicate you are prepared to perform the procedure for evaluation.

After your instructor has returned your work to you, make all necessary corrections and place in a three-ring notebook for future reference.

ASSIGNMENT SHEET

Section 4: BEHAVIORS AND HEALTH

Chapter 19: BEHAVIORS INFLUENCING HEALTH

Review the objectives and text for each unit before completing the assignment sheet for that unit. When you have completed all sheets for the chapter, remove them from this Workbook and give them to the instructor for evaluation.

Unit 1: NUTRITION, EXERCISE, AND WEIGHT CONTROL

SUGGESTED RESPONSES TO CRITICAL THINKING CHALLENGE IN TEXTBOOK

1. Why was Mrs. Fletcher so interested in those pamphlets? _____

_____

2. How did Darlene encourage the interest in the pamphlets without even knowing it? _____

_____

_____

3. What should Darlene have done about Mrs. Fletcher's complaint of a stiff back? _____

_____

_____

_____

4. Why did Mrs. Fletcher's back complaint disappear? _____

_____

5. Did Mrs. Fletcher disclose another problem? What is it? _____

_____

6. What should Darlene have done in response to Mrs. Fletcher's request for her to explain each pamphlet?

_____

_____

_____

7. What would you have done? _____

_____

A. Unscramble

1. _ _ _ _ _ _ _   LEACIRO
2. _ _ _ _ _ _ _ _   EPTVOIIS
3. _ _ _ _ _ _   YSRUCV
4. _ _ _ _ _ _ _ _   RAAIOXNE
5. _ _ _ _ _ _ _ _ _   IIANDTTI
6. _ _ _ _ _ _ _   KTRSCIE
7. _ _ _ _ _ _ _ _   ERBBIIRE
8. _ _ _ _ _ _   TONMOI
9. _ _ _ _ _   NREGA
10. _ _ _ _ _ _   ETHALH
11. _ _ _ _ _ _ _ _   RIOUNTNTI
12. _ _ _ _ _ _ _ _ _   FNYMIIRTI
13. _ _ _ _ _ _ _ _ _ _ _   PHECUTATERI
14. _ _ _ _ _ _ _   LCEBMUI

Name _____

B. Brief Answer

1. Explain the significance of diet and exercise to health. _____
   _____

2. Name the food groups in the food guide pyramid and the amounts recommended daily for each. _____
   _____
   _____
   _____

3. Name the fat-soluble vitamins. _____

4. Name the water-soluble vitamins. _____

5. Name the essential minerals that are most often missing from the average diet. _____

6. How might you encourage patients to comply in weight control? _____
   _____

7. What is the purpose of flexibility or stretching exercises? _____
   _____

8. List four things one can do to improve one's health. _____
   _____

9. List the guidelines for promoting good health. _____
   _____
   _____

10. Why is sleep and a positive outlook important to good health? _____
    _____

11. Why is it helpful especially for weight reduction to eat slowly? _____

12. What is the reason for eating several small meals a day instead of the traditional three meals a day? _____
    _____

13. What is anorexia nervosa? _____
    _____

14. Discuss health concerns in regard to adolescents in general. _____
    _____
    _____

C. Labeling: Label this food guide pyramid. Refer to Figure 19-2 in the textbook.

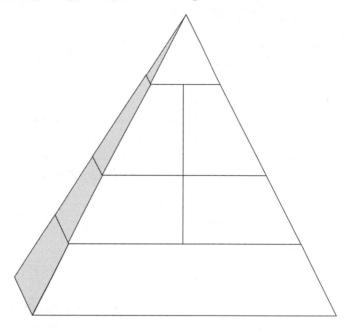

D. Fill in the Blank

1. A deficiency of vitamin A could cause _____

2. The main source of vitamin D is _____

3. Prothrombin formation and normal blood coagulation is the function of _____

4. Growth cessation and dermatosis is due to a deficiency of _____

5. Vegetable oil, wheat germ, leafy vegetables, egg yolk, margarine, and legumes are the principal sources of the _____

6. Carbohydrate metabolism, central and peripheral nerve cell function, and myocardial function are attributed to sufficient amounts of _____ or _____ in the diet.

7. Nicotinic acid and niacinamide are the other terms for the micronutrient, _____

8. The usual therapeutic dosage of folic acid is _____

9. Scurvy, hemorrhages, loose teeth, and gingivitis are caused by a deficiency of _____ or _____

10. Some sources of potassium include whole and skim milk, _____ prunes, and raisins.

11. Magnesium is necessary in bone and _____ formation.

12. One who is diagnosed as having anemia has a(n) _____

13. Simple goiter and cretinism are due to a deficiency of _____

14. A deficiency in _____ may cause growth retardation.

15. People who weigh more than _____ of their ideal body weight are considered to be _____

16. Generally, a _____ diet is recommended at least every 2 hours for the first 24 hours for patients who have diarrhea.

17. What do the letters of the BRAT diet stand for? _____

18. The _____ diet is recommended for patients who have tolerated the 24-hour clear liquid diet.

19. Those who have been sick and are just getting over an intestinal virus may find the _____ diet to be tolerated.

20. Patients who wish to reduce their weight should exercise at least _____ times a week and follow a _____ diet.

21. Patients who have special dietary needs should consult with a _____
22. _____ is a term used to describe not being able to sleep.
23. Lack of sleep is termed _____
24. Research shows that a person needs both REM and _____ stages of sleep.
25. People who sleep at least six hours at a time generally feel good because they benefit from the effects of the proper _____ of sleep.

CRITICAL THINKING SCENARIOS: What would your response be in the following situations?

1. A female patient in her late 20s calls to tell you that she just read about a diet plan in a new magazine that promises a weight loss of 20 pounds in two weeks. She wants to get the physician's permission for her to lose 20 pounds before her class reunion in three weeks. She has not been seen by the doctor for almost a year.

   _____
   _____

2. A male patient in his mid-40s is recovering from gall bladder surgery four weeks ago. He tells you that he's going to the health spa to work out because he's bored with sitting around. _____

   _____

3. A worried mother of three grade school children tells you as she is leaving the office that her children aren't eating well at dinner time anymore. She says that they eat so much junk food when they come home from school that they can't finish the meals she prepares. _____

   _____
   _____
   _____

After your instructor has returned your work to you, make all necessary corrections and place in a three-ring notebook for future reference.

ASSIGNMENT SHEET

Chapter 19: BEHAVIORS INFLUENCING HEALTH

Unit 2: HABIT-FORMING SUBSTANCES

A. Brief Answer

1. List the most commonly abused major groups of drugs and give an example of each. _____
   _____
   _____
   _____

2. What are the effects of depressants? _____
   _____

3. What are the effects of hallucinogens? _____
   _____

4. What are the effects of narcotics? _____

5. What are the effects of stimulants? _____
   _____

6. List behaviors that are indicators of drug/alcohol abuse. _____
   _____
   _____
   _____
   _____

7. Describe the difference between an alcoholic-dependent drinker and an alcoholic. _____
   _____

8. Describe research efforts into the causes of alcoholism. _____
   _____

9. How can the medical assistant be influential in assisting the drug addict or the alcoholic toward rehabilitation?
   _____

10. List organizations and facilities that assist in the rehabilitation of drug addicts and alcoholics. _____
   _____
   _____

11. Describe the effects that tar, nicotine, and carbon monoxide have on the body. _____
   _____
   _____
   _____
   _____
   _____

12. List ways a person can stop smoking.

a. _____
b. _____
c. _____
d. _____
e. _____
f. _____
g. _____
h. _____
i. _____
j. _____
k. _____

13. Name the diseases that smokers are more likely to acquire. _____

_____

_____

14. Describe the effects of passive or involuntary smoking. _____

_____

15. What health problems do young children have as a result of being exposed to second-hand smoke of caretakers?

_____

B. Matching: Match the definition in column II with the correct term in column I.

COLUMN I

_____ 1. Euphoria
_____ 2. Synergism
_____ 3. Addiction
_____ 4. Bizarre
_____ 5. Narcolepsy
_____ 6. Al-Ateen
_____ 7. Barbiturate
_____ 8. Hallucinogen
_____ 9. Al-Anon
_____ 10. Depressant
_____ 11. Amphetamine
_____ 12. Alcoholic
_____ 13. Stimulant
_____ 14. Traumatic
_____ 15. Psychedelics

COLUMN II

a. The habitual use of drugs
b. Stimulates the central nervous system
c. Support group for adolescent family members of alcoholics
d. Induce sleep
e. Mixing two or more drugs
f. Refers to a painful emotional experience
g. Exaggerated good feeling
h. A drinker who has become totally dependent on alcohol
i. Referred to as mind-expanding chemicals
j. Support group for family members and close friends of alcoholics
k. Uncontrollable desire to sleep
l. Hallucinogens
m. Strange; odd in manner
n. Used in treatment of patients who need sedation
o. Comprehensive rehabilitation
p. Taken to stay awake, feel more energetic

C. True or False: Place a "T" for true or "F" for false in the space provided. For false statements, explain why they are false.

_____ 1. Men have a higher risk of premature death due to smoking cigarettes than women.

_____ 2. Of the 2000 substances identified in tobacco smoke, most of the harm is done by tar, nicotine, and carbon monoxide.

_____ 3. Nicotine stimulates the appetite.

_____ 4. Approximately 10% of the blood supply in smokers is in the form of carboxyhemoglobin.

_____ 5. Smokers need to become thoroughly educated on the facts about smoking before they can eliminate their habit.

_____ 6. Tobacco contains poisons that could be fatal to toddlers and pets if swallowed.

_____ 7. Cigarette smoking is dangerous to your health.

CRITICAL THINKING SCENARIOS: What would your response be in the following situations?

1. One of your high-school patients comes in, hanging on her mother's shoulder to help her stand up. Her speech is slurred and she is nauseated. The visit, of course, is unexpected. _____

_____

_____

_____

2. A concerned parent has found some strange pills in her son's room and calls to ask you what to do. She says her son's behavior has changed recently and she is worried about him. _____

_____

After your instructor has returned your work to you, make all necessary corrections and place in a three-ring notebook for future reference.

ASSIGNMENT SHEET

Chapter 19: BEHAVIORS INFLUENCING HEALTH

Unit 3: STRESS AND TIME MANAGEMENT

A. Word Puzzle: Use the list of *Words to Know* to spell out these terms.

1. __ __ __ __ P __ __ __ __ __ __
2.   __ __ S __ __ __ __
3.   __ __ Y __ __ __ __ __ __
4.   __ __ C __ __ __ __ __
          H
5.   __ __ __ O __ __ __ __ __ __
6   __ __ S __ __ __ __ __ __
7.   __ O __ __ __ __ __ __
8.   __ M __ __ __ __ __ __ __
9.   A __ __ __ __ __ __ __
10. __ __ __ T __ __ __
11.   I __ __ __ __ __ __ __ __
12. __ __ __ C __ __ __ __ __ __

B. Brief Answer

1. Describe the phenomenon of stress. _____
_____
_____
_____

2. List the physical effects of stress. _____
_____
_____

3. What is "good stress"? _____

4. What is "bad stress"? _____

5. Describe the Type-A personality. _____

6. Describe the Type-B personality. _____

7. List the four basic human physical needs. _____

8. List the four basic human development needs. _____

9. What can be done to eliminate unnecessary stress? _____
_____

10. List methods for dealing with stress. _____
_____
_____

11. List possible mental health resources for patient referrals. _____

_____

12. List and discuss ways to relax and cope with daily stress. _____

_____

_____

13. What is the purpose of time management? _____

14. List some of the benefits of time management. _____

_____

C. Matching: Match the definition in column II with the correct term in column I.

COLUMN I

_____ 1. Exercise
_____ 2. Perspective
_____ 3. Implement
_____ 4. Eustress
_____ 5. Psychosomatic
_____ 6. Psychosis
_____ 7. Prioritizing
_____ 8. Flexible
_____ 9. Conflict
_____ 10. Anxiety
_____ 11. Depression

COLUMN II

a. Low spirits; sadness
b. Impairment of normal intellectual and social functioning
c. Arranging in order of importance
d. Constant state of worry
e. Clash, be in opposition
f. To put into effect
g. Support group
h. Real symptoms, not imagined
i. Positive effect in reducing stress
j. Able to bend without breaking
k. Proper evaluation/consideration
l. Planned stress; it motivates

D. Brief Answer

1. Make a list of the good and bad stress in your life.

_____

_____

_____

_____

E. Use the following words in a complete sentence.

Anxiety _____

Discretion _____

Exemplify _____

Flexible _____

Nurture _____

Perspective _____

Prioritize _____

After your instructor has returned your work to you, make all necessary corrections and place in a three-ring notebook for future reference.

ASSIGNMENT SHEET

Chapter 19: BEHAVIORS INFLUENCING HEALTH

Unit 4: RELATED THERAPIES

SUGGESTED RESPONSES TO CRITICAL THINKING CHALLENGE IN TEXTBOOK

1. Discuss how you think Renita felt during this situation. _____
   _____

2. Who should she call? Why? _____
   _____
   _____

3. Should she call the doctor? _____

4. How should she speak to this patient? Why? _____
   _____
   _____

5. Should she continue the calls? _____
   _____

6. Is there any potential legal problem here? _____
   _____
   _____
   _____
   _____

7. What would you do in this situation? _____
   _____
   _____

Mixed Quiz

1. Define and give four examples of complementary therapy. _____
   _____

2. Define and give three examples of alternative therapy. _____
   _____

3. Why should a person using a related therapy inform her or his physician? _____
   _____

4. List six guidelines to follow when using related therapies. _____
   _____
   _____

5. Identify nine specific goods with documented health benefits. _____
   _____

6. Name the nine common herbal products that may have some benefits. _____
   _____

7. Matching: Match the therapy in column I with its description in column II.

COLUMN I   COLUMN II

_____ Accupuncture   a. Uses the Low of Similiars
_____ Aromatherapy   b. Uses a trance state
_____ Ayurvedic   c. Uses laughter
_____ Biofeedback   d. Used to treat neuropathy and pain
_____ Faith   e. Stinulates points on the hand
_____ Homeopathy   f. Uses thin, sterile needles inserted into the skin
_____ Humor   g. Uses diet, rest, relaxation, exercise, and herbal products
_____ Hypnosis   h. Uses brain activities to influence the nervous system
_____ Magnet therapy   i. Teaches how to control involuntary body functions
_____ Massage   j. Uses a series of fluid movements
_____ Naturopathy   k. Uses the power of prayer
_____ Reflexology   l. Uses extracted plant oils for message and inhalation
_____ Visualization   m. Uses hands to manipulate muscles
_____ Yoga   n. Uses brain control meditation, stretching and strengthening exercises
_____ Tai Chi   o. Traditional healing system from India

8. Refer to the ABHES Course Content Requirements in Appendix C of the textbook. Within the area of *Psychology of Human Relations,* which content requirement is discussed in this unit? _____

_____

9. Word Puzzle: Use the clues to spell out these terms.

```
    _ _ R _ _ _              From plants
    _ _ _ E _ _ _ _ _        Dilute mixtures
    _ _ _ _ L _ _ _ _ _ _ _  Supplemental
    _ _ _ _ A _ _ _ _        Treatments
    _ _ T _ _ _ _ _ _ _ _    Instead of
    _ _ _ _ _ _ E _ _ _ _    Beneficial
    _ _ _ _ _ _ D _ _        Oldest medicine
```

CRITICAL THINKING SCENARIOS: What would your response be in the following situations?

1. Your neighbor, Mrs. Slovosky, has just told you that she is probably dying. She said her doctor told her that her lung scan indicated she has a fairly large mass in her left upper lobe that appears to be malignant. He wants her to see a surgical oncologist as quickly as possible. She has heard people say that when they open up your body to do surgery it just makes the cancer spread. Because she is afraid, she has neglected to make arrangements to see the surgeon. However, she has been taking some pills she ordered over the Internet because the Web site had testimonials from a lot of cured people. She feels her chances are better with the medication than with surgery. _____

_____

_____

_____

_____

_____

2. Charlie Kantor has tried several times to quit smoking. He even chewed the gum and wore a patch for a while, but he couldn't break his habit. He has heard about hypnosis but is afraid the practitioner will make him do silly things while he's hypnotized, like he's seen on television. _____

_____

_____

_____

_____

After your instructor has returned your work to you, make all necessary corrections and place in a three-ring notebook for future reference.

ASSIGNMENT SHEET

Section 5: EMPLOYABILITY SKILLS

Chapter 20: ACHIEVING SATISFACTION IN EMPLOYMENT

Review the objectives and text for each unit before completing the assignment sheet for that unit. When you have completed all sheets for the chapter, remove them from this Workbook and give them to the instructor for evaluation.

Unit 1: THE JOB SEARCH

SUGGESTED RESPONSES TO CRITICAL THINKING CHALLENGE IN TEXTBOOK

1. How do you think Anthony got the idea he had the job? _____
_____

2. What should he do about this situation? _____
_____
_____

3. Does Anthony have a reason to seek legal counsel? _____
_____
_____

4. Why do you suppose Anthony wasn't hired? _____
_____

5. What do you think of having a new person at the reception desk who is not qualified? _____
_____
_____
_____

6. What would you do in this situation? _____
_____
_____
_____
_____

A. Brief Answer

1. What is the purpose of a resumé? _____
_____

2. Why should a cover letter accompany a resumé? _____
_____

3. List the different types of resumés and the purpose of each.
   a. _____
   b. _____
   c. _____
   d. _____
   e. _____

4. Describe the services of an employment agency. _____
_____

5. List three contacts to assist the medical assistant in the job search. _____

_____

6. What is a classified ad? _____

_____

7. Where can the medical assistant find additional information abut job opportunities? _____

_____

B. Fill in the Blank

1. The job search begins with the _____ to work.
2. The _____ should be complete, accurate, and neatly organized.
3. Preparation of a resumé requires you to list systematically experiences that show your valuable

   _____
4. In listing your educational background, you should note that a _____ can be furnished
   upon request.
5. Permission should be obtained from those persons listed as _____
6. Personal data are _____ on a resumé.
7. The resumé should be _____ and _____ as needed to document additional
   employment experience, educational achievements, awards, and personal development.
8. All states offer assistance in locating jobs through the state _____
9. Many potential jobs are _____ meaning that the employer pays the agency's fees.
10. The job search takes patience, persistence, and _____
11. _____ a resumé should be done only when an employer requests it.

C. Matching: Match the acronym in column I with the correct term in column II.

COLUMN I		COLUMN II
_____	1. SAL	a. Position(s)
_____	2. PT	b. License
_____	3. INT	c. Beginning
_____	4. REQ	d. Necessary
_____	5. POS	e. Negotiable
_____	6. LIC	f. Education
_____	7. FB	g. Immediate
_____	8. BGN	h. Words per minute
_____	9. NEG	i. Experience
_____	10. COL	j. Required
_____	11. IMMED	k. Interview
_____	12. EDUC	l. Part-time
_____	13. NEC	m. Salary
_____	14. WPM	n. College
_____	15. EXP	o. Fringe benefits

D. Fill in the Blank: **Grouped below are some of the qualities that employers expect from their employees. After the brief definition of each, place the appropriate quality on the line provided.**

initiative	dependability	courteous	responsible
reliability	cooperative	time management skill	
punctuality	enthusiasm	interest	

1. To excite the attention or curiosity of: _____
2. Trustworthy: _____
3. Answerable; accountable: _____
4. The ability to think and act without being urged: _____
5. Organization by priority: _____
6. Intense or eager interest: _____
7. Considerate toward others; well-mannered: _____
8. Working together for a common purpose: _____
9. Being on time: _____
10. Can be depended on: _____

E. Ads/Cover Letter
In the space below, paste a want ad from your local paper for a medical assistant position. Below it respond with the cover letter about yourself that you would send. Show it to your instructor to evaluate when you are finished.

_____
_____
_____
_____
_____
_____
_____
_____
_____
_____
_____
_____
_____
_____
_____
_____
_____
_____

F. Crossword Puzzle

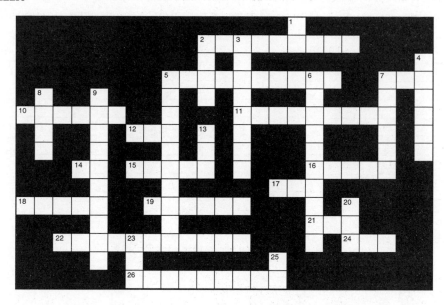

ACROSS

2. A quality
5. It's said to be the best teacher
7. Words per minute (acronym)
10. A wish
11. Schooling
12. Salary (abbreviation)
14. High school (abbreviation)
15. Refers to form or _____ of resumé
16. Immediately (abbreviation)
17. Reference (abbreviation)
18. Type of letter sent with resumé
19. Outlined summary of your abilities and experience
21. Equal opportunity employer (acronym)
22. Strong ambition
24. College (abbreviation)
26. Capable for position

DOWN

1. Fringe benefit (abbreviation)
2. Appointment (abbreviation)
3. Aimed
4. To hire or _____
5. Work
6. Employment ads
7. Newspaper ad listings that say "help _____"
8. Skillful and precise
9. You may furnish on request
13. Payment for services
20. Secretary (abbreviation)
23. Required (abbreviation)
25. Advertisement (abbreviation)

CRITICAL THINKING SCENARIOS: What would your response be in the following situations?

1. Planning ahead to allow spare time for traffic, you are on your way to an interview for a position you really want. Traffic is unusually congested because a truck is stalled on the freeway. You realize that you will most likely be late. _____

   _____

   _____

   _____

2. During an interview, the employer asks you if you have ever been late to work. This employer also asks for references. _____

   _____

After your instructor has returned your work to you, make all necessary corrections and place in a three-ring notebook for future reference.

ASSIGNMENT SHEET

Chapter 20: ACHIEVING SATISFACTION IN EMPLOYMENT

Unit 2: GETTING THE JOB AND KEEPING IT

SUGGESTED RESPONSES TO CRITICAL THINKING CHALLENGE IN TEXTBOOK

1. What is the first thing that Juanita should have done? _____

_____

2. Do you think Juanita will get a good reference from her former employer when she applies for a job?

_____

3. What do you think of Juanita? Do you understand what she did? Why? _____

_____

4. What do you think was the reaction of the office manager? the physician(s)? _____

_____

5. What should Juanita have done? _____

_____

_____

6. What would you tell Juanita? _____

_____

7. What would you have done in her situation? _____

_____

A. Matching: Match the definition in column II with the correct term in column I.

COLUMN I

_____ 1. Contemporary
_____ 2. Negate
_____ 3. Demeanor
_____ 4. Competent
_____ 5. Arbitrary
_____ 6. Affiliate
_____ 7. Apprise

COLUMN II

a. Well-qualified
b. To connect or associate
c. To inform or notify
d. To discriminate
e. Modern
f. Conduct; outward behavior
g. To make ineffective
h. Not fixed by rules; based on one's preference
i. An attitude or system

B. Brief Answer

1. What information should you be prepared to provide on an application for employment? _____

_____

2. What important factor must the medical assistant remember when completing a job application? _____

_____

3. Why is appearance so important when interviewing for a job? _____

_____

4. What is the purpose of a job interview? _____

_____

5. Why must one be prompt and courteous at a job interview? _____

_____

6. Explain why it is a good idea to send a follow-up letter to the interviewer after the job interview. _____

_____

_____

7. What is the best way to close an interview. Why? _____

_____

8. How may a medical assistant demonstrate pride in the profession of medical assisting? _____

_____

9. How should you dress when applying for a job or when returning an application form? Why? _____

_____

_____

10. List areas of concern employers have regarding (prospective) employees. _____

_____

_____

_____

_____

11. What documents are employers required to ask for of prospective employees and why? _____

_____

_____

_____

12. How can time management skills be applied to the work day? _____

_____

13. Explain what "work ethics" is and why it is important regarding employment. _____

_____

_____

14. What is the value of an employment evaluation review? _____

_____

15. What are some of the subjects you should discuss with your employer during an evaluation review?

_____

_____

_____

16. Discuss the purpose and advantages of a job description. _____

_____

_____

17. Refer to ABHES Course Content Requirements in Appendix C of the textbook. Within the area of *Medical Office Clinical Procedures,* which four content requirements are discussed in this chapter? _____

_____

_____

C. Fill in the Blank

1. An employer will expect you to perform with increasing _____ in your position as you continue to gain experience.

2. One particular quality that the medical assistant must keep in mind is _____

3. Your _____ will probably follow you throughout your working life.

4. Advancement will depend largely upon your _____ in performing administrative and clinical tasks.

5. In terminating employment, the employee has major responsibility of giving the employer at least a _____

6. The usual cause for termination initiated by the employer is _____ to perform job responsibilities.

D. Letters

1. In the space below write a follow-up letter thanking an employer who interviewed you for a job. Show it to your instructor for evaluation.

_____
_____
_____
_____
_____
_____
_____
_____

2. Write a letter of resignation below and show it to your instructor for evaluation.

_____
_____
_____
_____
_____
_____

E. Word Search: Find the following words hidden in the puzzle.

WORK

ON TIME

TACT

VALUES

SMILE

THANK

ACTIVE

ETHICS

REVIEW

PROMPT

GOALS

HONEST

RESPONSIBILITY

ENTHUSIASM

RELIABILITY

INITIATIVE

COOPERATION

GRAMMAR

COMMUNICATION

ADVANCEMENT

OPPORTUNITY

COMPETENT

QUESTIONS

FORM

SKILL

MANNERS

FOLLOW UP

```
Y T I L I B A I L E R L P T E V O J K T
T C A J N P U T A J E N T H U S I A S M
I A D H O N E S T S S M D A J B S D B R
N R R M I P B M N T P K C N N F L V K B
U T A C T F P K P Y O K I K C G O A L S
T N C Q A R V M S L N G C L K Z M N K M
R O T U R E O B J T S H J F L J S C S I
O C K H E R A G I N I T I A T I V E S L
P C F D P F G J D A B W J B N S M M D E
P R C F O C R C S T I G S C I H T E R Y
O H O R O S A A E C L M A D P S F N A P
J N M C O M M U N I C A T I O N T M U
A Z P W L B M Y L O T M J N L C R L B W
F W E S C Z A F A I Y B O Y N S W F L O
B Q T A M G R E V I E W T N G E O K V L
J K E R D T L E F W K V Q R A I R I T L
C W N L L F Z I O Q U E S T I O N S V O
O N T I M E A W T W K I A L W R B M A F
```

CRITICAL THINKING SCENARIOS: What would your response be in the following situations?

1. You have just started to work on some reports, of which you are behind schedule in mailing, when your employer brings the new employee to you for a tour of the clinic. You are also asked to explain the office policy and duties to this person. _____

_____

2. You have been employed at the clinic for almost three months. You know that your three-month (90-day) evaluation is scheduled for next week. Since you have done well, you feel you will be eligible for a promotion and raise. You have overheard that the supervisor is thinking about hiring a new person for the job. _____

_____

_____

    After your instructor has returned your work to you, make all necessary corrections and place in a three-ring notebook for future reference.

PERFORMANCE EVALUATION CHECKLIST

Name _____

Date _____ Score* _____

PROCEDURE 5-1   Open the Office

PERFORMANCE OBJECTIVE—Follow all the steps in the procedure, role-play the actions necessary to prepare a medical office to see patients. Verbally describe actions while performing.

PROCEDURE STEPS	STEP PERFORMED	POINTS POSSIBLE	COMMENTS
EVALUATOR: Place check mark in space following each step performed satisfactorily			
NOTE TIME BEGAN _____			
1. Unlocked the reception room door.	_____	10	
2. Adjusted heat or air conditioning for the comfort of the patients.	_____	5	
3. Checked for safety hazards in the office.			
a. Checked electrical wires	_____	15	
b. Checked furniture condition	_____	15	
c. Checked floor	_____	15	
4. Checked magazines for condition and date.	_____	5	
5. Checked the telephone answering device or call the answering service for any messages.	_____	10	
6. Pulled the charts of patients to be seen.	_____	15	
7. Wrote or stamped today's date.	_____	15	
8. Checked for previously ordered studies and filed in chart.	_____	15	
9. Checked examining rooms to be sure they were clean and stocked with supplies.	_____	10	
10. If it is the policy of the office, prepared a list of the patients to be seen and the times of their appointments and placed this list on the physician's desk.	_____	5	
EVALUATOR: NOTE TIME COMPLETED _____			

ADD POINTS OF STEPS CHECKED   _____ EARNED

TOTAL POINTS POSSIBLE   135 POSSIBLE

Points assigned reflect importance of step to meeting objective: Important = (5)   Essential = (10)   Critical = (15)
Automatic failure results if any of the critical steps are omitted or performed incorrectly.

DETERMINE SCORE (divide points earned by total points possible, multiply results by 100)   _____ SCORE*

Evaluator's Name (print) _____ Signature _____

Comments _____

PERFORMANCE EVALUATION CHECKLIST

Name _____

Date _____ Score* _____

PROCEDURE 5-2   Obtain New Patient Information

PERFORMANCE OBJECTIVE—In a simulated situation, clearly communicate instructions and complete the steps designated in the procedure within acceptable time limits.

PROCEDURE STEPS	STEP PERFORMED	POINTS POSSIBLE	COMMENTS
EVALUATOR: Place check mark in space following each step performed satisfactorily			
NOTE TIME BEGAN _____			
1. Took new patient to private area to ask preliminary questions.	_____	10	
2. Instructed new patient to complete a data sheet.	_____	10	
a. Provided clipboard and pen	_____	10	
b. Requested return when completed	_____	10	
3. Checked form for completeness.	_____	15	
4. Prepared a patient folder by typing the patient's name on a label and attaching it to the tab of the folder.	_____	5	
5. Transferred information from the data sheet to the chart sheet.	_____	10	
6. Copied the insurance card and returned to patient.	_____	15	
7. Inserted the chart, data sheets, and insurance card copy in folder.	_____	15	
8. Placed any referral material in chart.	_____	15	
9. Prepared charge slip.	_____	10	
10. Placed the folder in the area reserved for charts of patients to be seen.	_____	5	
11. Completed within established time limit.	_____	15	
EVALUATOR: NOTE TIME COMPLETED _____			

ADD POINTS OF STEPS CHECKED   _____ EARNED
TOTAL POINTS POSSIBLE   145 POSSIBLE

Points assigned reflect importance of step to meeting objective: Important = (5)   Essential = (10)   Critical = (15)
Automatic failure results if any of the critical steps are omitted or performed incorrectly.

DETERMINE SCORE (divide points earned by total points possible, multiply results by 100)   _____ SCORE*

Evaluator's Name (print) _____ Signature _____

Comments _____

PERFORMANCE EVALUATION CHECKLIST

Name _____

Date _____ Score* _____

PROCEDURE 5-3   Close the Office

PERFORMANCE OBJECTIVE—Following all the steps in the procedure, role-play the actions required to close the office. Actions must be verbally described while performing the procedure.

PROCEDURE STEPS	STEP PERFORMED	POINTS POSSIBLE	COMMENTS
EVALUATOR: Place check mark in space following each step performed satisfactorily			
NOTE TIME BEGAN _____			
1. Checked to see that records were collected and filed in locked cabinets.	_____	15	
2. Placed any money received in safe or took to the bank to be deposited.	_____	15	
3. Turned off all electrical appliances.	_____	15	
4. Checked that rooms were cleaned and supplied for the next day.	_____	10	
5. Straightened reception room if time allowed.	_____	5	
6. Pulled charts for the next day if time allowed.	_____	5	
7. Activated answering device on phone or called answering service with information about when the office would reopen.	_____	15	
8. Turned off lights.	_____	10	
9. Activated alarm system.	_____	15	
10. Securely locked doors.	_____	15	
EVALUATOR: NOTE TIME COMPLETED _____			

ADD POINTS OF STEPS CHECKED   _____ EARNED
TOTAL POINTS POSSIBLE   120 POSSIBLE

Points assigned reflect importance of step to meeting objective: Important = (5)   Essential = (10)   Critical = (15)
Automatic failure results if any of the critical steps are omitted or performed incorrectly.

DETERMINE SCORE (divide points earned by total points possible, multiply results by 100)   _____ SCORE*

Evaluator's Name (print) _____ Signature _____

Comments _____

PERFORMANCE EVALUATION CHECKLIST

Name _____

Date _____ Score* _____

PROCEDURE 6-1 Answer the Office Phone

PERFORMANCE OBJECTIVE—In a simulated (or actual) situation, using proper grammar, answer the telephone by the third ring, identifying the office and yourself.

PROCEDURE STEPS	STEP PERFORMED	POINTS POSSIBLE	COMMENTS
EVALUATOR: Place check mark in space following each step performed satisfactorily			
NOTE TIME BEGAN _____			
1. Answered the phone promptly (by third ring) in a polite and pleasant manner.	_____	10	
2. Identified the office and self by name.	_____	15	
a. Voice clear, distinct, moderate rate of speaking	_____	10	
3. Listened to and recorded the name of the caller.	_____	15	
4. Recorded:			
a. Date	_____	5	
b. Time	_____	5	
c. Reason for call	_____	5	
5. a. Spelled name correctly	_____	10	
b. Processed emergency call immediately	_____	15	
c. Waited for response before placing on hold	_____	15	
d. Checked with caller on hold once each minute	_____	5	
e. Completed interrupted on-hold calls	_____	5	
6. Screened and completed as many calls as possible before adding to the physician's call-back list.	_____	10	
7. Responded to an untimely request to speak to physician by taking a message.	_____	10	
EVALUATOR: NOTE TIME COMPLETED _____			

ADD POINTS OF STEPS CHECKED   _____ EARNED
TOTAL POINTS POSSIBLE   135 POSSIBLE

Points assigned reflect importance of step to meeting objective: Important = (5)   Essential = (10)   Critical = (15)
Automatic failure results if any of the critical steps are omitted or performed incorrectly.

DETERMINE SCORE (divide points earned by total points possible, multiply results by 100)   _____ SCORE*

Evaluator's Name (print) _____ Signature _____

Comments _____

303

Name _____

Date _____ Score* _____

PROCEDURE 6-2   Process Phone Message

PERFORMANCE OBJECTIVE—In a simulated situation (or actual situation) receive, evaluate, and document a phone message.

PROCEDURE STEPS	STEP PERFORMED	POINTS POSSIBLE	COMMENTS
EVALUATOR: Place check mark in space following each step performed satisfactorily			
NOTE TIME BEGAN _____			
1. Answered the phone properly.	_____	10	
2. Listened carefully and determined caller's needs.	_____	15	
3. Documented information regarding message (including date/time) on message pad/phone call log—included:			
a. Whom the request was for	_____	15	
b. What it concerned	_____	15	
c. When information was needed	_____	15	
d. Where to return call	_____	15	
4. Repeated message to caller to verify the contents.	_____	10	
5. Closed conversation politely.	_____	5	
6. Allowed caller to hang up first.	_____	5	
7. Signed initials after the message.	_____	5	
8. Pulled patient's chart and recorded or attached message.	_____	10	
EVALUATOR: NOTE TIME COMPLETED _____			

ADD POINTS OF STEPS CHECKED   _____ EARNED
TOTAL POINTS POSSIBLE   120 POSSIBLE

Points assigned reflect importance of step to meeting objective: Important = (5)   Essential = (10)   Critical = (15)
Automatic failure results if any of the critical steps are omitted or performed incorrectly.

DETERMINE SCORE (divide points earned by total points possible, multiply results by 100)   _____ SCORE*

Evaluator's Name (print) _____ Signature _____

Comments _____

PERFORMANCE EVALUATION CHECKLIST

Name _____

Date _____ Score* _____

PROCEDURE 6-3   Record Telephone Message on Recording Device

PERFORMANCE OBJECTIVE—In a simulated situation (or actual situation) procedure, with all necessary information in a pleasant tone of voice, a clear, accurate, and precise phone message on the telephone message device.

PROCEDURE STEPS	STEP PERFORMED	POINTS POSSIBLE	COMMENTS
EVALUATOR: Place check mark in space following each step performed satisfactorily			
NOTE TIME BEGAN _____			
1. Assembled necessary items away from noise and distractions.	_____	10	
a. Determined amount of time allowed on recording device for message before beginning	_____	10	
2. Wrote out appropriate message.			
a. Checked for completeness and accuracy	_____	10	
b. Read and determined the amount of time of message	_____	10	
3. Recorded message following directions of answering device.	_____	15	
a. Spoke in a pleasant, clear, and articulate tone of voice	_____	5	
b. Sat up straight and projected voice into the speaker	_____	5	
c. Identified the office	_____	10	
d. Was not too wordy or overly friendly	_____	5	
e. Complete and accurate information	_____	10	
4. Played message back and evaluated quality of message.	_____	5	
a. Listened and determined if the message was of good quality	_____	5	
b. Appropriate for all callers	_____	5	
5. Set the device to play messages when unavailable to answer phone.	_____	15	
EVALUATOR: NOTE TIME COMPLETED _____			

ADD POINTS OF STEPS CHECKED   _____ EARNED

TOTAL POINTS POSSIBLE   120 POSSIBLE

Points assigned reflect importance of step to meeting objective: Important = (5)   Essential = (10)   Critical = (15)
Automatic failure results if any of the critical steps are omitted or performed incorrectly.

DETERMINE SCORE (divide points earned by total points possible, multiply results by 100)   _____ SCORE*

Evaluator's Name (print) _____ Signature _____

Comments _____

Name _____

Date _____ Score* _____

PROCEDURE 6-4   Obtain Telephone Message from Phone Recording Device

PERFORMANCE OBJECTIVE—In a simulated situation (or actual situation), obtain necessary and pertinent information from all phone messages from the phone message recording device.

PROCEDURE STEPS	STEP PERFORMED	POINTS POSSIBLE	COMMENTS
EVALUATOR: Place check mark in space following each step performed satisfactorily			
NOTE TIME BEGAN _____			
1. Assembled necessary items in an area away from noise and distractions.	_____	5	
2. Listened to recordings and wrote message(s) accurately.	_____	15	
3. Repeated listening to difficult messages to obtain complete information.	_____	5	
4. Signed initials after message(s).	_____	5	
5. Noted date and time of the message(s).	_____	10	
6. Listed all patients who left messages and pulled their charts.	_____	15	
7. Prioritized messages according to their seriousness.	_____	15	
8. Distributed messages to appropriate staff member/ department to be processed.	_____	10	
EVALUATOR: NOTE TIME COMPLETED _____			

ADD POINTS OF STEPS CHECKED   _____ EARNED

TOTAL POINTS POSSIBLE   80 POSSIBLE

Points assigned reflect importance of step to meeting objective: Important = (5)   Essential = (10)   Critical = (15)
Automatic failure results if any of the critical steps are omitted or performed incorrectly.

DETERMINE SCORE (divide points earned by total points possible, multiply results by 100)   _____ SCORE*

Evaluator's Name (print) _____ Signature _____

Comments _____

Name _____

Date _____ Score* _____

PROCEDURE 6-5   Schedule Appointments

PERFORMANCE OBJECTIVE—In a simulated situation, schedule an appointment for a patient according to accepted medical standards with consideration for the physician, staff, and needs of the patient.

PROCEDURE STEPS	STEP PERFORMED	POINTS POSSIBLE	COMMENTS
EVALUATOR: Place check mark in space following each step performed satisfactorily			
NOTE TIME BEGAN _____			
1. Determined the means of scheduling: appointment book or computer entry.	_____	10	
2. Marked off hours when the physician was unable to see patients.	_____	15	
3. Attempted to give patients two appointment choices.	_____	5	
4. Recorded names in black ink with phone number(s).	_____	10	
5. Asked patient(s) to schedule next appointment before leaving office.	_____	5	
6. Wrote patients' names in the schedule book.	_____	10	
7. Recorded appointment first in appointment book and then on appointment card.	_____	15	
8. Completed appointment card and gave to patient.	_____	15	
9. Left sufficient time for work-ins in appointment book.	_____	10	
10. Allowed time for return phone calls to be made by the doctor.	_____	5	
EVALUATOR: NOTE TIME COMPLETED _____			

ADD POINTS OF STEPS CHECKED   _____ EARNED

TOTAL POINTS POSSIBLE   100 POSSIBLE

Points assigned reflect importance of step to meeting objective: **Important = (5)   Essential = (10)   Critical = (15)**
Automatic failure results if any of the critical steps are omitted or **performed incorrectly.**

DETERMINE SCORE (divide points earned by total points possible, multiply results by 100)   _____ SCORE*

Evaluator's Name (print) _____ Signature _____

Comments _____

Name _____

Date _____ Score* _____

PROCEDURE 6-6   Arrange Referral Appointment

PERFORMANCE OBJECTIVE—In a simulated situation, schedule a referral appointment for a patient by phoning the requested medical facility according to accepted medical standards with consideration for the physician, staff, and needs of the patient.

PROCEDURE STEPS	STEP PERFORMED	POINTS POSSIBLE	COMMENTS
EVALUATOR: Place check mark in space following each step performed satisfactorily			
NOTE TIME BEGAN _____			
1. Obtained patient's chart with request for referral to another facility.	_____	15	
2. Used phone directory to obtain phone number and address of referral office.	_____	10	
3. Placed the call to referral office and provided receptionist with:			
a. Your name/physician's name and address	_____	15	
b. Patient's name, address, etc., and reason for appointment	_____	15	
c. Indicated that confirmation letter will be mailed/faxed	_____	5	
d. Recorded appointment information on patient's chart	_____	10	
e. Gave complete information to patient (time, day, date, name, address, etc.)	_____	10	
4. Gave patient printed instructions regarding appointment as appropriate.	_____	5	
a. Initialed patient's chart signifying completion of request	_____	5	
EVALUATOR: NOTE TIME COMPLETED _____			

ADD POINTS OF STEPS CHECKED   _____ EARNED

TOTAL POINTS POSSIBLE   90 POSSIBLE

Points assigned reflect importance of step to meeting objective: Important = (5)   Essential = (10)   Critical = (15)
Automatic failure results if any of the critical steps are omitted or performed incorrectly.

DETERMINE SCORE (divide points earned by total points possible, multiply results by 100)   _____ SCORE*

Evaluator's Name (print) _____ Signature _____

Comments _____

Name _____

Date _____ Score* _____

PROCEDURE 6-7   Compose a Business Letter

PERFORMANCE OBJECTIVE—Given access to equipment and supplies, complete a mailable letter following the steps in the procedure within the number of attempts and time frame specified by the instructor. The final copy must meet mailable standards described in the text.

PROCEDURE STEPS	STEP PERFORMED	POINTS POSSIBLE	COMMENTS
EVALUATOR: Place check mark in space following each step performed satisfactorily			
NOTE TIME BEGAN _____			
1. Moved cursor down at least three lines below letterhead.	_____	5	
2. Entered the date in appropriate location for letter style.	_____	10	
3. Moved to the fifth line below the date.	_____	5	
4. Entered the inside address in appropriate location for letter style.	_____	5	
a. Entered name as received on letter or listed in a directory	_____	15	
5. Double spaced after the last line of the address.	_____	5	
6. Entered the appropriate salutation followed by a colon.	_____	10	
7. Double spaced.	_____	5	
8. a. Entered the reference line in the location appropriate for letter style	_____	5	
b. Entered RE: Entered patient's name or person about whom the letter was written	_____	10	
9. Double spaced.	_____	5	
10. Prepared the body of letter.			
a. Paragraph style appropriate to the style of the letter	_____	5	
b. Double spaced between paragraphs	_____	5	
11. (When second page)—			
a. Entered second page heading at 7th line	_____	—	
b. Entered name, page number, date	_____	—	
c. At least two lines of paragraph were on first page	_____	—	
d. Last word on first page not divided	_____	—	
(Note: Subtract 10 points for each step a–e if omitted)			
12. Continued body of letter	_____	—	

PROCEDURE 6-7   Compose a Business Letter—continued

PROCEDURE STEPS	STEP PERFORMED	POINTS POSSIBLE	COMMENTS
13. Complimentary closing entered in letter style format.	_____	10	
14. Four spaces entered.	_____	5	
15. Sender's name entered in letter style format exactly as printed on letterhead;	_____	15	
a. Title followed name after comma or			
b. Title entered below name			
16. Double space.	_____	5	
17. Entered reference initials to indicate typist.	_____	15	
18. Single or double spaced if enclosed materials.	_____	—	
19. "cc" and recipient's name entered	_____	—	
a. Numbered and identified if more than one.	_____	—	
20. Double spaced (if needed)	_____	—	
(Subtract 10 points if omitted in error)			
21. PS for postscript if applicable	_____	—	
(Subtract 10 points if omitted in error)			
EVALUATOR: NOTE TIME COMPLETED _____			
Completed within specified time		15	
Meets mailable standard		15	

ADD POINTS OF STEPS CHECKED   _____ EARNED
TOTAL POINTS POSSIBLE   170 POSSIBLE

Points assigned reflect importance of step to meeting objective: Important = (5)   Essential = (10)   Critical = (15)
Automatic failure results if any of the critical steps are omitted or performed incorrectly.

DETERMINE SCORE (divide points earned by total points possible, multiply results by 100) _____ SCORE*

Evaluator's Name (print) _____ Signature _____

Comments _____

Name _____

Date _____ Score* _____

PROCEDURE 6-8   Total Charges on Calculator

PERFORMANCE OBJECTIVE—Provided with necessary equipment and materials, calculate a list of 20 charges, performing any necessary mathematical functions, and correctly determine the total amount. The same correct answer must be obtained twice within a maximum of three attempts.

PROCEDURE STEPS	STEP PERFORMED	POINTS POSSIBLE	COMMENTS
EVALUATOR: Place check mark in space following each step performed satisfactorily			
NOTE TIME BEGAN _____			
1. Turned on calculator.	_____	5	
2. Cleared machine.	_____	15	
3. Accurately entered figures from list.	_____	15	
4. Totaled fees.	_____	10	
5. Refigured to see if the same answer was obtained twice.	_____	15	
6. Recorded correct total. _____	_____	15	
EVALUATOR: NOTE TIME COMPLETED _____			

ADD POINTS OF STEPS CHECKED   _____ EARNED
TOTAL POINTS POSSIBLE   75 POSSIBLE

Points assigned reflect importance of step to meeting objective: Important = (5)   Essential = (10)   Critical = (15)
Automatic failure results if any of the critical steps are omitted or performed incorrectly.

DETERMINE SCORE (divide points earned by total points possible, multiply results by 100)   _____ SCORE*

Evaluator's Name (print) _____ Signature _____

Comments _____

PERFORMANCE EVALUATION CHECKLIST

Name _____

Date _____ Score* _____

PROCEDURE 6-9   Operate Copy Machine

PERFORMANCE OBJECTIVE—Given access to necessary equipment and supplies, demonstrate adjustment of settings in order to
produce the specified copy or copies, while operating the copy machine accurately following the steps in the procedure.

PROCEDURE STEPS	STEP PERFORMED	POINTS POSSIBLE	COMMENTS
EVALUATOR: Place check mark in space following each step performed satisfactorily			
NOTE TIME BEGAN _____			
1. Assembled material to be copied.	_____	10	
2. Determined number of copies needed.	_____	10	
3. Turned on copy machine.	_____	5	
4. Adjusted settings to produce desired copy.			
a. Paper size	_____	15	
b. One/two sided	_____	15	
c. Regular/reduced/enlarged size	_____	15	
d. Number of copies	_____	15	
5. Checked paper supply.	_____	15	
6. Raised lid and placed material to be copied, one sheet at a time, face down on glass, or in feeder.	_____	10	
7. Closed lid, if appropriate.	_____	—	
8. Pressed button or key pad to activate copier.	_____	5	
9. Removed original(s) and copy/copies.	_____	10	
10. Removed special paper, if used, from supply.	_____	10	
11. Returned machine to "standard" settings if changed.	_____	5	
12. Turned off machine (if policy).	_____	5	
EVALUATOR: NOTE TIME COMPLETED _____			

ADD POINTS OF STEPS CHECKED   _____ EARNED

TOTAL POINTS POSSIBLE   145 POSSIBLE

Points assigned reflect importance of step to meeting objective: Important = (5)   Essential = (10)   Critical = (15)
Automatic failure results if any of the critical steps are omitted or performed incorrectly.

DETERMINE SCORE (divide points earned by total points possible, multiply results by 100)   _____ SCORE*

Evaluator's Name (print) _____ Signature _____

Comments _____

Name _____

Date _____ Score* _____

PROCEDURE 6-10   Operate Transcriber

PERFORMANCE OBJECTIVE—Given access to equipment and supplies, operate the transcriber, correctly following all steps in the procedure. Complete an accurate transcription within a specified time period.

PROCEDURE STEPS	STEP PERFORMED	POINTS POSSIBLE	COMMENTS
EVALUATOR: Place check mark in space following each step performed satisfactorily			
NOTE TIME BEGAN _____			
1. Turned on the transcriber.	_____	5	
2. Attached headset with earphones and the foot control to the unit.	_____	10	
3. Selected tape; chose rush reports or oldest dictation first.	_____	10	
4. Adjusted headset with earphones.	_____	5	
5. Inserted tape. Pressed play tab or the pedal to listen for the beginning of the dictation.	_____	10	
6. Adjusted volume, tone, and speed controls for clearest communication reception.	_____	10	
7. Listened for physician's instructions.	_____	15	
8. Set word processor or computer margins and tabulator stops.	_____	10	
9. Selected appropriate paper for transcription.	_____	10	
10. Brought up blank screen on computer.	_____	5	
11. Alternately pressed and released foot pedal to listen and transcribe the recorded message.	_____	10	
12. Turned off the machine and placed accessory items in proper storage space.	_____	5	
13. Completed transcript is accurate copy of recorded message, on appropriate paper, within specified time period.	_____	15	
EVALUATOR: NOTE TIME COMPLETED _____			

ADD POINTS OF STEPS CHECKED   _____ EARNED
TOTAL POINTS POSSIBLE   120 POSSIBLE

Points assigned reflect importance of step to meeting objective: Important = (5)   Essential = (10)   Critical = (15)
Automatic failure results if any of the critical steps are omitted or performed incorrectly.

DETERMINE SCORE (divide points earned by total points possible, multiply results by 100)   _____ SCORE*

Evaluator's Name (print) _____ Signature _____

Comments _____

PERFORMANCE EVALUATION CHECKLIST

Name _____

Date _____ Score* _____

PROCEDURE 6-11   Operate Office Computer

PERFORMANCE OBJECTIVE—Given access to equipment and material to be entered, operate system following steps in the procedure to produce an accurate print copy of a schedule.

PROCEDURE STEPS	STEP PERFORMED	POINTS POSSIBLE	COMMENTS
EVALUATOR: Place check mark in space following each step performed satisfactorily			
NOTE TIME BEGAN _____			
1. Turned on power to computer.	_____	5	
2. Positioned cursor on appropriate program on main menu, keyed "ENTER" or clicked mouse.	_____	5	
3. Positioned cursor on scheduling software program, keyed "ENTER" or clicked mouse.	_____	5	
4. Positioned cursor or clicked on first cell to be completed.	_____	5	
5. Entered 1:00 P.M. appointment for first patient on list.	_____	10	
6. Entered remaining names at 15-minute intervals.	_____	15	
7. Saved data.	_____	15	
8. Exited scheduling program to main menu.	_____	10	
9. Exited from main menu.	_____	10	
10. Re-entered main menu.	_____	10	
11. Brought up scheduling software.	_____	10	
12. Located cursor at 2:30, entered patient as work-in who was currently scheduled for 1:30.	_____	10	
13. Located cursor at 1:30, canceled appointment.	_____	5	
14. Scrolled through schedule to view and proofread.	_____	10	
15. Turned on printer.	_____	5	
16. Allowed time for test sheet. (If appropriate; subtract 10 points if omitted)	_____	—	
17. Checked paper supply.	_____	5	
18. Keyed or clicked on print.	_____	10	
19. Selected from options.	_____	10	
20. Printed document.	_____	15	
21. Exited program.	_____	10	

PROCEDURE 6-11 Operate Office Computer—continued

PROCEDURE STEPS	STEP PERFORMED	POINTS POSSIBLE	COMMENTS
22. Exited main menu.	_____	10	
23. Turned off power to printer.	_____	5	
24. Turned off power to computer.	_____	5	

EVALUATOR: NOTE TIME COMPLETED _____

ADD POINTS OF STEPS CHECKED   _____ EARNED
TOTAL POINTS POSSIBLE   200 POSSIBLE

Points assigned reflect importance of step to meeting objective: Important = (5)   Essential = (10)   Critical = (15)
Automatic failure results if any of the critical steps are omitted or performed incorrectly.

DETERMINE SCORE (divide points earned by total points possible, multiply results by 100)   _____ SCORE*

Evaluator's Name (print) _____ Signature _____

Comments _____

Name _____

Date _____ Score* _____

PROCEDURE 7-1   File Item(s) Alphabetically

PERFORMANCE OBJECTIVE—In a simulated situation, given the patient's file or other items, accurately file and store the file(s) and/or other items within acceptable time limit according to acceptable medical standards.

PROCEDURE STEPS	STEP PERFORMED	POINTS POSSIBLE	COMMENTS
EVALUATOR: Place check mark in space following each step performed satisfactorily			
NOTE TIME BEGAN _____			
1. Used rules for filing items alphabetically.	_____	10	
a. Double-checked spelling of name for accuracy when using cross-reference file	_____	15	
2. Determined appropriate storage file.	_____	10	
3. For new material, scanned guides for area nearest to letters of name(s) on items to file.	_____	10	
4. Placed folder in correct alphabetical order between two files.	_____	15	
a. Inserted new file *between* two other folders and *not* within another folder, where it could be lost	_____	15	
5. In filing material previously in file, scanned for the OUTguide.			
a. Removed OUTguide after removing file	_____	5	
b. Checked to be sure it was marking the space for the file just returned and not another	_____	5	
EVALUATOR: NOTE TIME COMPLETED _____			

ADD POINTS OF STEPS CHECKED   _____ EARNED

TOTAL POINTS POSSIBLE   85 POSSIBLE

Points assigned reflect importance of step to meeting objective: Important = (5)   Essential = (10)   Critical = (15)
Automatic failure results if any of the critical steps are omitted or performed incorrectly.

DETERMINE SCORE (divide points earned by total points possible, multiply results by 100)   _____ SCORE*

Evaluator's Name (print) _____ Signature _____

Comments _____

Name _____

Date _____ Score* _____

PROCEDURE 7-2   Pull File Folder from Alphabetic Files

PERFORMANCE OBJECTIVE—In a simulated situation, given the patient's name, accurately prepare the OUTguide and pull the file, replacing the file with the OUTguide within acceptable time limit according to accepted medical standards.

PROCEDURE STEPS	STEP PERFORMED	POINTS POSSIBLE	COMMENTS
EVALUATOR: Place check mark in space following each step performed satisfactorily			
NOTE TIME BEGAN _____			
1. Found name of patient in alphabetic file.	_____	15	
a. Double-checked the spelling of the name for accuracy	_____	15	
2. Completed OUTguide with date and name.	_____	5	
3. Pulled file(s) needed and replaced with OUTguide(s).	_____	5	
EVALUATOR: NOTE TIME COMPLETED _____			

ADD POINTS OF STEPS CHECKED   _____ EARNED
TOTAL POINTS POSSIBLE   40 POSSIBLE

Points assigned reflect importance of step to meeting objective: Important = (5)   Essential = (10)   Critical = (15)
Automatic failure results if any of the critical steps are omitted or performed incorrectly.

DETERMINE SCORE (divide points earned by total points possible, multiply results by 100)   _____ SCORE*

Evaluator's Name (print) _____ Signature _____

Comments _____

Name _____

Date _____ Score* _____

PROCEDURE 7-3   File Item(s) Numerically

PERFORMANCE OBJECTIVE—In a simulated situation, given the patient's file or other items, accurately file and store the file(s) and/or other items within acceptable time limit according to accepted medical standards.

PROCEDURE STEPS	STEP PERFORMED	POINTS POSSIBLE	COMMENTS
EVALUATOR: Place check mark in space following each step performed satisfactorily			
NOTE TIME BEGAN _____			
1. Used rules for numerical filing.	_____	15	
a. Double-checked spelling of name for accuracy using cross-reference file	_____	15	
2. Determined appropriate storage file.	_____	5	
3. Matched the first two or three numbers with those already in the file.	_____	15	
4. Matched remaining numbers with those in the file.	_____	15	
EVALUATOR: NOTE TIME COMPLETED _____			

ADD POINTS OF STEPS CHECKED   _____ EARNED

TOTAL POINTS POSSIBLE   35 POSSIBLE

Points assigned reflect importance of step to meeting objective: Important = (5)   Essential = (10)   Critical = (15)
Automatic failure results if any of the critical steps are omitted or performed incorrectly.

DETERMINE SCORE (divide points earned by total points possible, multiply results by 100)   _____ SCORE*

Evaluator's Name (print) _____ Signature _____

Comments _____

Name _____

Date _____ Score* _____

PROCEDURE 7-4   Pull File Folder from Numeric Files

PERFORMANCE OBJECTIVE—In a simulated situation, given the patient's name or account number, accurately prepare the OUTguide and pull the file, replacing the file with the OUTguide within acceptable time limit according to accepted medical standards.

PROCEDURE STEPS	STEP PERFORMED	POINTS POSSIBLE	COMMENTS
EVALUATOR: Place check mark in space following each step performed satisfactorily			
NOTE TIME BEGAN _____			
1. Found name of patient in card file and obtained account number.	_____	10	
a. Double-checked the spelling of name for accuracy	_____	10	
2. Completed OUTguide with date and name.	_____	5	
3. Located corresponding section of numeric file.	_____	10	
4. Scanned the files for the number.	_____	15	
5. Pulled requested file and replaced with prepared OUTguide.	_____	15	
EVALUATOR: NOTE TIME COMPLETED _____			

ADD POINTS OF STEPS CHECKED   _____ EARNED

TOTAL POINTS POSSIBLE   65 POSSIBLE

Points assigned reflect importance of step to meeting objective: Important = (5)   Essential = (10)   Critical = (15)
Automatic failure results if any of the critical steps are omitted or performed incorrectly.

DETERMINE SCORE (divide points earned by total points possible, multiply results by 100)   _____ SCORE*

Evaluator's Name (print) _____ Signature _____

Comments _____

Name _____

Date _____ Score* _____

PROCEDURE 8-1   Prepare Patient Ledger Card

PERFORMANCE OBJECTIVE—In a simulated medical office situation, prepare a patient ledger card following the steps in the procedure.

PROCEDURE STEPS	STEP PERFORMED	POINTS POSSIBLE	COMMENTS
EVALUATOR: Place check mark in space following each step performed satisfactorily			
NOTE TIME BEGAN _____			
1. Typed the name of patient, last name first.	_____	15	
2. Typed complete address with zip code.	_____	10	
3. Typed name and address of person responsible for charges if different from patient.	_____	5	
4. Typed telephone number of patient.	_____	10	
5. Typed name of insurance company.	_____	15	
6. Typed referring individual.	_____	5	
7. Typed balance due amount.	_____	10	
EVALUATOR: NOTE TIME COMPLETED _____			

ADD POINTS OF STEPS CHECKED   _____ EARNED
TOTAL POINTS POSSIBLE   70 POSSIBLE

Points assigned reflect importance of step to meeting objective: Important = (5)   Essential = (10)   Critical = (15)
Automatic failure results if any of the critical steps are omitted or performed incorrectly.

DETERMINE SCORE (divide points earned by total points possible, multiply results by 100)   _____ SCORE*

Evaluator's Name (print) _____ Signature _____

Comments _____

Name _____

Date _____ Score* _____

PROCEDURE 8-2   Record Charges and Credits

PERFORMANCE OBJECTIVE—In a simulated medical office situation, record charges and credits following the steps in the
procedure.

PROCEDURE STEPS	STEP PERFORMED	POINTS POSSIBLE	COMMENTS
EVALUATOR: Place check mark in space following each step performed satisfactorily			
NOTE TIME BEGAN _____			
1. Pulled patients' ledger cards.	_____	10	
2. Posted charges and credits on ledger cards.	_____	15	
a. Used small, neat figures	_____	5	
3. Checked each off on day sheet	_____	5	
4. Posted charges in debit column	_____	15	
a. Added balance and new debit for new balance	_____	10	
5. Posted payments in credit column	_____	15	
a. Subtracted payments from balance due	_____	10	
b. Showed credits in red	_____	5	

EVALUATOR: NOTE TIME COMPLETED _____

ADD POINTS OF STEPS CHECKED   _____ EARNED
TOTAL POINTS POSSIBLE   90 POSSIBLE

Points assigned reflect importance of step to meeting objective: Important = (5)   Essential = (10)   Critical = (15)
Automatic failure results if any of the critical steps are omitted or performed incorrectly.

DETERMINE SCORE (divide points earned by total points possible, multiply results by 100)   _____ SCORE*

Evaluator's Name (print) _____ Signature _____

Comments _____

Name _____

Date _____ Score* _____

PROCEDURE 8-3   Generate Itemized Statement

PERFORMANCE OBJECTIVE—In a simulated medical office situation, type itemized statement(s) with 100 percent accuracy
following the steps in the procedure.

PROCEDURE STEPS	STEP PERFORMED	POINTS POSSIBLE	COMMENTS
EVALUATOR: Place check mark in space following each step performed satisfactorily			
NOTE TIME BEGAN _____			
1. Stacked ledger cards beside typewriter.	_____	5	
2. Assembled statement forms and window envelopes.	_____	5	
3. Stamped ledger card on line below last entry with date stamp.	_____	5	
4. Typed name and complete address in area that shows in window of envelope.	_____	15	
5. Listed balance first under services.	_____	10	
6. Typed each service charge and payment for current month.	_____	15	
7. Folded and placed form in envelope	_____	5	
a. Address shown in window	_____	15	
b. Only one form in envelope	_____	15	
8. Fanned and exposed several envelope flaps.	_____	5	
9. Dampened flaps sufficiently.	_____	5	
10. Folded flaps of envelopes down to seal.	_____	10	
EVALUATOR: NOTE TIME COMPLETED _____			

ADD POINTS OF STEPS CHECKED   _____ EARNED
TOTAL POINTS POSSIBLE   110 POSSIBLE

Points assigned reflect importance of step to meeting objective: Important = (5)   Essential = (10)   Critical = (15)
Automatic failure results if any of the critical steps are omitted or performed incorrectly.

DETERMINE SCORE (divide points earned by total points possible, multiply results by 100)   _____ SCORE*

Evaluator's Name (print) _____ Signature _____

Comments _____

Name _____

Date _____ Score* _____

PROCEDURE 8-4   Compose Collection Letter

PERFORMANCE OBJECTIVE—In a simulated medical office situation, compose and type appropriate collection letters for assigned accounts to be collected following the procedure.

PROCEDURE STEPS	STEP PERFORMED	POINTS POSSIBLE	COMMENTS
EVALUATOR: Place check mark in space following each step performed satisfactorily			
NOTE TIME BEGAN _____			
1. Identified patients to whom an initial collection letter should be sent.	_____	10	
2. Composed a rough draft	_____	10	
a. First paragraph stated reason for letter	_____	10	
3. Second paragraph indicated expected response.	_____	10	
4. Reread rough draft	_____	5	
a. Had clear message	_____	10	
b. Contained correctly spelled words	_____	5	
c. Had correct punctuation	_____	5	
5. Typed letter according to standard form.	_____	5	
a. Proofread letter	_____	10	
b. Signed letter	_____	10	
6. Typed envelope.	_____	5	
7. Folded letter properly.	_____	5	
a. Sealed envelope	_____	5	
b. Stamped and mailed letter	_____	10	

EVALUATOR: NOTE TIME COMPLETED _____

ADD POINTS OF STEPS CHECKED   _____ EARNED
TOTAL POINTS POSSIBLE   115 POSSIBLE

Points assigned reflect importance of step to meeting objective: Important = (5)   Essential = (10)   Critical = (15)
Automatic failure results if any of the critical steps are omitted or performed incorrectly.

DETERMINE SCORE (divide points earned by total points possible, multiply results by 100)   _____ SCORE*

Evaluator's Name (print) _____ Signature _____

Comments _____

Name _____

Date _____ Score* _____

PROCEDURE 9-1   Complete a Claim Form

PERFORMANCE OBJECTIVE—Given access to all necessary equipment and information, follow the procedure to complete the HCFA-approved claim form without error within the instructor's prescribed time limit.

PROCEDURE STEPS	STEP PERFORMED	POINTS POSSIBLE	COMMENTS
EVALUATOR: Place check mark in space following each step performed satisfactorily			
NOTE TIME BEGAN _____			
1. Checked for a photocopy of the patient's insurance card.	_____	10	
2. Checked the chart to see if the patient signature was on file for release of information and assignment of benefits.	_____	15	
3. Explained procedure to obtain signature when not on file.	_____	10	
4. Using Figure 9–6 as an example, completed the HCFA claim form.			
a. Checked appropriate box at top of form	_____	5	
b. Entered name of patient	_____	10	
c. Entered birthdate using digits	_____	10	
d. Checked box for male or female			
5. Entered insured's name.	_____	5	
6. Entered patient's full address and telephone number.	_____	5	
7. Entered patient's relationship to insured.	_____	5	
8. Entered insured's full address and telephone number.	_____	5	
9. Entered patient's status.	_____	5	
10. Entered other insured's name, if applicable.	_____	—	
a. Other insured's policy or group number	_____	—	
b. Other insured's birthdate and box for male or female	_____	—	
c. Employer's name or school name	_____	—	
d. Insurance plan name or program name	_____	—	
11. Checked appropriate box regarding employment and/or accident.	_____	5	
12. Entered insured's policy number			
a. Insured's birthdate and box for male or female	_____	5	
b. Employer or school name	_____	5	
c. Insurance plan name or program name	_____	5	
d. Was there another health benefit plan?	_____	5	
13. Obtained signature or indicated "on file."	_____	15	

PROCEDURE 9-1   Complete a Claim Form—continued

PROCEDURE STEPS	STEP PERFORMED	POINTS POSSIBLE	COMMENTS
14. Obtained insured's or authorized signature.	_____	10	
15. Entered current illness date, accident, or pregnancy.	_____	10	
16. Entered date patient first treated for same or similar illness.	_____	5	
17. Entered dates unable to work or stated N/A.	_____	—	
18. Entered referring physician or other.	_____	5	
a. Physician's ID number	_____	5	
19. Entered hospital dates or stated N/A.	_____	—	
20. Left blank.	_____	—	
21. Completed outside lab as appropriate.	_____	—	
22. Entered ICN codes.	_____	15	
23. Completed Medicaid resubmission if applicable.	_____	—	
24. Entered prior authorization number.	_____	—	
25. Completed Section 24 A–E with dates, appropriate codes, and charges for services.	_____	15	
26. Entered physician's Social Security number or practice tax identification number.	_____	10	
27. Entered patient's account number if applicable.	_____	—	
28. Checked appropriate box for assignment.	_____	10	
29. Totaled charges.	_____	15	
30. Entered amount paid.	_____	15	
31. Entered balance due.	_____	15	
32. Obtained physician's signature and date.	_____	15	
33. Completed name and address where services given.	_____	5	
34. Completed physician's information.	_____	5	
35. Completed within time specified.	_____	15	

EVALUATOR: NOTE TIME COMPLETED _____

Note: Subtract 10 points each for steps 9, 16, 18, 19, 20, 23, and 26 if applicable and not entered.

ADD POINTS OF STEPS CHECKED   _____ EARNED
TOTAL POINTS POSSIBLE   295 POSSIBLE

Points assigned reflect importance of step to meeting objective: Important = (5)   Essential = (10)   Critical = (15)
Automatic failure results if any of the critical steps are omitted or performed incorrectly.

DETERMINE SCORE (divide points earned by total points possible, multiply results by 100)   _____ SCORE*

Evaluator's Name (print) _____ Signature _____

Comments _____

Name _____

Date _____ Score* _____

PROCEDURE 10-1   Prepare a Check

PERFORMANCE OBJECTIVE—Prepare a check following the steps of the procedure. The check must be dated, accurately identify the payer, have the correct numeric and written amount, and have appropriate signature. The register must accurately reflect the check.

PROCEDURE STEPS	STEP PERFORMED	POINTS POSSIBLE	COMMENTS
EVALUATOR: Place check mark in space following each step performed satisfactorily			
NOTE TIME BEGAN _____			
1. Filled out check register using black or blue ink.			
a. Check number	_____	5	
b. Date	_____	10	
c. Payee information	_____	10	
d. Amount	_____	15	
e. Previous balance	_____	10	
f. Entered new balance	_____	10	
2. Entered date on check.	_____	5	
3. Entered payee.	_____	15	
4. Entered numerically the amount of check.	_____	10	
5. Wrote out amount of check.			
a. Began as far left as possible	_____	10	
b. Wrote out amount correctly	_____	15	
c. Made straight line to fill space	_____	10	
6. Obtained signature; must agree with authorization card.	_____	15	
EVALUATOR: NOTE TIME COMPLETED _____			

ADD POINTS OF STEPS CHECKED   _____ EARNED

TOTAL POINTS POSSIBLE   140 POSSIBLE

Points assigned reflect importance of step to meeting objective: **Important** = (5)   **Essential** = (10)   **Critical** = (15)

Automatic failure results if any of the critical steps are omitted or performed incorrectly.

DETERMINE SCORE (divide points earned by total points possible, multiply results by 100)   _____ SCORE*

Evaluator's Name (print) _____ Signature _____

Comments _____

PERFORMANCE EVALUATION CHECKLIST

Name _____

Date _____ Score* _____

PROCEDURE 10-2   Prepare a Deposit Slip

PERFORMANCE OBJECTIVE—Prepare a bank deposit slip following the steps in the procedure. The slip will correctly reflect the currency, coin, and checks to be deposited, and be totaled accurately.

PROCEDURE STEPS	STEP PERFORMED	POINTS POSSIBLE	COMMENTS
EVALUATOR: Place check mark in space following each step performed satisfactorily			
NOTE TIME BEGAN _____			
1. Separated money to be deposited, by check, currency, and coin.	_____	5	
2. Listed currency.			
a. Sorted bills by denomination	_____	5	
b. Portrait side up	_____	5	
c. Highest denomination to lowest	_____	5	
d. Totaled currency accurately	_____	15	
e. Recorded accurately on deposit slip	_____	10	
3. Listed coin.			
a. Sorted by denomination	_____	5	
b. Totaled coin accurately	_____	15	
c. Recorded accurately on deposit slip	_____	10	
4. Listed checks.			
a. Checked for endorsement	_____	10	
b. Listed by number, maker, amount	_____	5	
c. Listed from largest to smallest amount	_____	5	
d. Listed money orders with MO and name	_____	5	
e. Accurately totaled and entered on slip	_____	15	
5. Accurately totaled currency, coin, and checks to be deposited.	_____	15	
6. Made copy of deposit slip for files.	_____	5	
7. Entered deposit total in checkbook.	_____	10	
8. Made deposit at bank and kept record for files.	_____	10	
EVALUATOR: NOTE TIME COMPLETED _____			

ADD POINTS OF STEPS CHECKED   _____ EARNED

TOTAL POINTS POSSIBLE   155 POSSIBLE

Points assigned reflect importance of step to meeting objective: Important = (5)   Essential = (10)   Critical = (15)
Automatic failure results if any of the critical steps are omitted or performed incorrectly.

DETERMINE SCORE (divide points earned by total points possible, multiply results by 100)   _____ SCORE*

Evaluator's Name (print) _____ Signature _____

Comments _____

Name _____

Date _____ Score* _____

PROCEDURE 10-3   Reconcile a Bank Statement

PERFORMANCE OBJECTIVE—Follow the steps in the procedure "Reconcile a Bank Statement;" after performing mathematical calculations, the checkbook and bank statement balance should agree.

PROCEDURE STEPS	STEP PERFORMED	POINTS POSSIBLE	COMMENTS
EVALUATOR: Place check mark in space following each step performed satisfactorily			
NOTE TIME BEGAN _____			
1. Compared the opening balance on the new statement with the closing balance on the previous statement.	_____	10	
2. Listed the bank balance in the appropriate space on the reconciliation worksheet.	_____	5	
3. Compared the check entries on the statement with the returned checks.	_____	10	
4. Determined if any outstanding checks.			
a. Marked stub or entry on register if check returned	_____	5	
b. Listed ones not checked on worksheet	_____	15	
c. Totaled outstanding checks	_____	10	
5. Subtracted from checkbook balance items such as withdrawals, automatic payments or service charges that appeared on the statement but not in the checkbook.	_____	15	
6. Added to checkbook any interest earned as indicated on statement.	_____	15	
7. Added to the bank statement balance any deposits not shown on the bank statement.	_____	15	
8. The balance in the checkbook and the bank statement agreed.	_____	15	
EVALUATOR: NOTE TIME COMPLETED _____			

ADD POINTS OF STEPS CHECKED   _____ EARNED
TOTAL POINTS POSSIBLE   115 POSSIBLE

Points assigned reflect importance of step to meeting objective: Important = (5)   Essential = (10)   Critical = (15)
Automatic failure results if any of the critical steps are omitted or performed incorrectly.

DETERMINE SCORE (divide points earned by total points possible, multiply results by 100)   _____ SCORE*

Evaluator's Name (print) _____ Signature _____

Comments _____

PERFORMANCE EVALUATION CHECKLIST   Name _____

Date _____ Score* _____

PROCEDURE 11-1   Handwashing

PERFORMANCE OBJECTIVE—Provided with liquid hand soap in a dispenser, cuticle stick, nail brush, paper towels, and a waste receptacle, the student will stand at a sink with hot and cold faucets and demonstrate each step in the handwashing procedure as specified in the procedure sheet.

PROCEDURE STEPS	STEP PERFORMED	POINTS POSSIBLE	COMMENTS
EVALUATOR: Place check mark in space following each step performed satisfactorily			
NOTE TIME BEGAN _____			
1. Removed jewelry.	_____	5	
2. a. Stood, not touching sink	_____	10	
b. Used paper towel to turn on faucets	_____	5	
c. Adjusted water temperature	_____	5	
d. Discarded paper towel	_____	5	
3. a. Wet hands	_____	10	
b. Dispensed 1 tsp soap into palm	_____	10	
c. Distributed soap into lather on both hands	_____	15	
d. Washed, in circular motion, for two minutes	_____	15	
4. a. Used nail brush/1 dozen circular motions	_____	5	
b. Used cuticle stick under nails	_____	5	
5. a. Rinsed thoroughly	_____	10	
b. Wet arms to elbow	_____	5	
c. Re-applied soap (1 tsp) to palm	_____	5	
d. Did not touch inside of sink or faucets	_____	10	
e. Used brush in one dozen circular motions to elbow	_____	5	
f. Rinsed thoroughly	_____	5	
6 a. Let water continue to run	_____	5	
b. Got paper towels	_____	5	
c. Dried hands and arms to elbow	_____	5	
d. Turned water off with paper towel	_____	5	
e. Discarded paper towel in proper receptacle			
EVALUATOR: NOTE TIME COMPLETED _____			

ADD POINTS OF STEPS CHECKED   _____ EARNED
TOTAL POINTS POSSIBLE   155 POSSIBLE

Points assigned reflect importance of step to meeting objective: Important = (5)   Essential = (10)   Critical = (15)
Automatic failure results if any of the critical steps are omitted or performed incorrectly.

DETERMINE SCORE (divide points earned by total points possible, multiply results by 100)   _____ SCORE*

Evaluator's Name (print) _____ Signature _____

Comments _____

Name _____

Date _____ Score* _____

PROCEDURE 11-2   Wrap Items for Autoclave

PERFORMANCE OBJECTIVE—Provided with several items to be autoclaved or sterilized, the student will wrap each in autoclave
paper in preparation for the sterilization process. Each item must be wrapped neatly and snugly but not too tightly. After the
paper wrapping procedure is demonstrated and checked, the paper should be removed and discarded. This procedure should be
performed with both paper and muslin wrap.

PROCEDURE STEPS	STEP PERFORMED	POINTS POSSIBLE	COMMENTS
EVALUATOR: Place check mark in space following each step performed satisfactorily			
NOTE TIME BEGAN _____			
Wrapping Items			
1. Washed hands.	_____	10	
a. Assembled all necessary items	_____	10	
b. Worked in a clean area	_____	5	
c. Allowed for sufficient work space	_____	5	
2. Checked items for flaws.	_____	15	
a. Checked items for proper functioning	_____	15	
b. Made sure items were sanitized before wrapping	_____	15	
3. Wrapped items in double thickness paper wrap.	_____	10	
a. Made sure of no opening	_____	10	
b. Sealed with autoclave tape	_____	5	
c. Wrapped items snugly	_____	10	
d. Did not wrap items too tight	_____	10	
4. Made tab with tape for ease in opening following sterilization.	_____	5	
5. Labeled contents.	_____	15	
a. Wrote date on package	_____	10	
b. Wrote your initials on package	_____	5	_____ EARNED
6. Returned all items to proper storage.	_____	5	160 POSSIBLE
Envelope Type			
Repeated steps 1–2	_____	65	
3. Placed item in envelope and	_____	15	
a. Sealed	_____	5	
b. Labeled contents	_____	15	
c. Dated label	_____	10	
d. Initialed label	_____	5	_____ EARNED
4. Returned items to proper storage.	_____	5	120 POSSIBLE

PROCEDURE 11-2   Wrap Items for Autoclave—continued

PROCEDURE STEPS	STEP PERFORMED	POINTS POSSIBLE	COMMENTS
Spinal needle(s), small items			
Repeated steps 1–2.	_____	65	
3. Placed cotton/gauze in bottom of glass test tube.	_____	10	
4. Wrapped autoclave tape around top of test tube to seal.	_____	15	
a. Made pull tab with tape	_____	5	
5. Labeled contents on piece of tape, secured to glass and	_____	15	
a. Dated label	_____	15	
b. Initialed	_____	5	
6. Returned items to storage.	_____	5	
			_____ EARNED
EVALUATOR: NOTE TIME COMPLETED _____			135 POSSIBLE

ADD POINTS OF STEPS CHECKED
TOTAL POINTS POSSIBLE

Points assigned reflect importance of step to meeting objective: Important = (5)   Essential = (10)   Critical = (15)
Automatic failure results if any of the critical steps are omitted or performed incorrectly.

DETERMINE SCORE (divide points earned by total points possible, multiply results by 100)   _____ SCORE*

Evaluator's Name (print) _____ Signature _____

Comments _____

Name _____

Date _____ Score* _____

PROCEDURE 12-1   Interview Patient to Complete Medical History Form

PERFORMANCE OBJECTIVE—Using copies of the medical history forms included in the textbook and a blue or black pen, obtain and record a medical history from a patient within a set time specified by the instructor.

PROCEDURE STEPS	STEP PERFORMED	POINTS POSSIBLE	COMMENTS
EVALUATOR: Place check mark in space following each step performed satisfactorily			
NOTE TIME BEGAN _____			
1. Assembled necessary items.	_____	15	
2. Courteously escorted patient to private area.	_____	5	
3. Sat opposite patient.	_____	5	
4. Explained procedure to patient and put them at ease.	_____	15	
5. Maintained eye contact with patient throughout procedure.	_____	10	
6. Asked questions clearly and distinctly.	_____	15	
7. Gave patient sufficient time to answer.	_____	10	
8. Recorded information neatly and accurately.	_____	15	
9. Avoided getting off subject.	_____	5	
10. Made necessary comments.	_____	5	
11. Highlighted in red ink when necessary (example: allergies).	_____	10	
12. Clearly stated patient's chief complaint.	_____	15	
13. Thanked patient for cooperation.	_____	5	
14. Explained next procedure to patient.	_____	5	
15. Made patient comfortable.	_____	5	
16. Placed patient's history form in chart.	_____	10	
17. Placed chart in appropriate area for physician.	_____	10	
EVALUATOR: NOTE TIME COMPLETED _____			

ADD POINTS OF STEPS CHECKED   _____ EARNED
TOTAL POINTS POSSIBLE   160 POSSIBLE

Points assigned reflect importance of step to meeting objective: Important = (5)   Essential = (10)   Critical = (15)
Automatic failure results if any of the critical steps are omitted or performed incorrectly.

DETERMINE SCORE (divide points earned by total points possible, multiply results by 100)   _____ SCORE*

Evaluator's Name (print) _____ Signature _____

Comments _____

Name _____

Date _____ Score* _____

PROCEDURE 12-2   Measure Height

PERFORMANCE OBJECTIVE—Demonstrate each step of the height measurement procedure to determine the precise height of five students who have been measured previously by the instructor. Measurements should be recorded and agree with instructor by ± ⅛ inch.

PROCEDURE STEPS	STEP PERFORMED	POINTS POSSIBLE	COMMENTS
EVALUATOR: Place check mark in space following each step performed satisfactorily			
NOTE TIME BEGAN _____			
1. Raised measuring bar higher than patient.	_____	15	
2. Aware of patient's safety.	_____	10	
3. Asked patient to remove shoes.	_____	5	
4. Placed paper towel on platform.	_____	5	
5. Helped patient onto scale.	_____	10	
6. Moved measuring bar slowly and carefully to rest on top of patient's head.	_____	10	
7. Gently compressed hair.	_____	15	
8. Read measurement correctly.	_____	15	
9. Told patient the reading.	_____	5	
10. Helped patient down from scale.	_____	10	
11. Asked patient to put shoes back on.	_____	5	
12. Placed measuring extension bar back.	_____	5	
13. Discarded paper towel.	_____	5	
14. Recorded measurement accurately on patient's chart.	_____	15	
EVALUATOR: NOTE TIME COMPLETED _____			

ADD POINTS OF STEPS CHECKED   _____ EARNED

TOTAL POINTS POSSIBLE   130 POSSIBLE

Points assigned reflect importance of step to meeting objective: Important = (5)   Essential = (10)   Critical = (15)
Automatic failure results if any of the critical steps are omitted or performed incorrectly.

DETERMINE SCORE (divide points earned by total points possible, multiply results by 100)   _____ SCORE*

Evaluator's Name (print) _____ Signature _____

Comments _____

DOCUMENTATION

Chart the procedure in the patient's medical record.

Date: _____

Charting: _____

_____

_____

_____

Student's Name: _____   **Physician's Initials:** __(____)__

Name _____

Date _____ Score* _____

PROCEDURE 12-3   Weigh Patient on Upright Scale

PERFORMANCE OBJECTIVE—Demonstrate each step of the procedure of weighing a patient on an upright scale and record; weight measurement should agree with instructor's by ± ¼ lb.

PROCEDURE STEPS	STEP PERFORMED	POINTS POSSIBLE	COMMENTS
EVALUATOR: Place check mark in space following each step performed satisfactorily			
NOTE TIME BEGAN _____			
1. Washed hands.	_____	5	
2. Balanced scales.	_____	15	
3. Asked patient to remove shoes.	_____	5	
4. Placed paper towel on scale.	_____	5	
5. Helped patient onto scale.	_____	5	
6. Asked patient to stand in center of platform.	_____	10	
7. Asked patient to stand still.	_____	10	
8. Adjusted balance.	_____	10	
9. Read weight accurately.	_____	15	
10. Told patient the reading.	_____	5	
11. Helped patient from scales.	_____	5	
12. Discarded paper towel.	_____	5	
13. Recorded weight accurately on patient's chart.	_____	15	
a. Noted what patient was wearing	_____	10	
14. Returned scales to balance at zero.	_____	5	

EVALUATOR: NOTE TIME COMPLETED _____

ADD POINTS OF STEPS CHECKED   _____ EARNED
TOTAL POINTS POSSIBLE   125 POSSIBLE

Points assigned reflect importance of step to meeting objective: Important = (5)   Essential = (10)   Critical = (15)
Automatic failure results if any of the critical steps are omitted or performed incorrectly.

DETERMINE SCORE (divide points earned by total points possible, multiply results by 100)   _____ SCORE*

Evaluator's Name (print) _____ Signature _____

Comments _____

DOCUMENTATION

Chart the procedure in the patient's medical record.

Date: _____

Charting: _____

_____

_____

_____

Student's Name: _____   Physician's Initials: __(___)__

PROCEDURE 12-4   Clean and Store Mercury Thermometers

PERFORMANCE OBJECTIVE—Given soiled mercury thermometers and access to all necessary equipment and supplies, clean, inspect, disinfect, and store the thermometers aseptically, in accordance with procedure technique and observing aseptic and safety precautions.

PROCEDURE STEPS	STEP PERFORMED	POINTS POSSIBLE	COMMENTS
EVALUATOR: Place check mark in space following each step performed satisfactorily. Check to see if oral and rectal are separated. Subtract 15 pts if not.			
NOTE TIME BEGAN _____			
1. Washed hands, assembled equipment, and put on gloves.	_____	15	
2. Took soiled thermometers to sink.	_____	—	
3. Applied soap or other cleanser to cotton ball and added water to make solution.	_____	10	
4. While holding thermometer by stem, rotated and wiped it from stem to bulb with soapy solution.	_____	5	
5. Discarded cotton ball in biohazardous waste container.	_____	5	
6. While holding by stem with bulb pointed downward, rinsed thermometer in cool running water.	_____	5	
7. Inspected for cleanliness and condition, discarded damaged thermometer in a sharps biohazardous waste container.	_____	15	
8. Grasped stem firmly between thumb and index finger.	_____	5	
9. Shook mercury down to 95.0°F or below.	_____	15	
10. Placed thermometers in gauze-lined container filled with disinfectant.	_____	10	
11. Using correct procedure, removed and discarded gloves.	_____	10	
12. Washed hands.	_____	5	
13. Noted time or set timer for at least 20 minutes.	_____	15	
14. After allowing time for disinfection, washed hands.	_____	5	
15. Rinsed, inspected, and placed clean thermometers in individual envelopes, individual dry holders, or storage container.	_____	15	

PROCEDURE STEPS	STEP PERFORMED	POINTS POSSIBLE	COMMENTS
16. Cleaned area and equipment. Returned thermometers to appropriate locations.	_____	5	
EVALUATOR: NOTE TIME COMPLETED _____			

ADD POINTS OF STEPS CHECKED   _____ EARNED
TOTAL POINTS POSSIBLE   140 POSSIBLE

Points assigned reflect importance of step to meeting objective: Important = (5)   Essential = (10)   Critical = (15)
Automatic failure results if any of the critical steps are omitted or performed incorrectly.

DETERMINE SCORE (divide points earned by total points possible, multiply results by 100)   _____ SCORE*

Evaluator's Name (print) _____ Signature _____

Comments _____

PROCEDURE 12-5   Measure Oral Temperature with Mercury Thermometer

PERFORMANCE OBJECTIVE—In a simulated or actual situation and given access to all necessary equipment and supplies, measure and record a patient's oral temperature. The procedure will be done within six minutes, following correct procedural technique and observing aseptic and safety precautions. The recorded findings must agree with the instructor's reading.

PROCEDURE STEPS	STEP PERFORMED	POINTS POSSIBLE	COMMENTS
EVALUATOR: Place check mark in space following each step performed satisfactorily			
NOTE TIME BEGAN _____			
1. Washed hands, assembled equipment, and put on gloves.	_____	15	
2. Identified patient.	_____	5	
3. Explained procedure.	_____	5	
4. Determined if patient had recently had a hot or cold drink or smoked.	_____	15	
5. Removed thermometer from holder or envelope. Avoided touching bulb end with fingers.	_____	5	
6. Inspected thermometer. Discarded a chipped or cracked thermometer in a sharps biohazardous waste container.	_____	15	
7. Read thermometer and shook down to 95°F or below if necessary.	_____	15	
8. Put plastic sheath on thermometer and ensured it is intact.	_____	10	
9. Placed bulb sublingually in patient's mouth.	_____	10	
10. Told patient how to maintain proper position of thermometer: to keep lips closed, breathe through nose, and avoid biting.	_____	5	
11. Left thermometer in position a minimum of three minutes.	_____	15	
12. Removed and read thermometer. Reinserted for one minute if less than 97°F.	_____	10	
13. Reread thermometer, if appropriate.	_____	—	
14. Holding by stem, pulled off plastic sheath and discarded in biohazardous waste container.	_____	5	
EVALUATOR: NOTE TIME COMPLETED _____			
Completed within six minutes	_____	15	
EVALUATOR: Read thermometer and record temperature: _____			

PROCEDURE STEPS	STEP PERFORMED	POINTS POSSIBLE	COMMENTS
15. Followed procedure for soiled thermometers.	_____	5	
16. Removed gloves and discarded in biohazardous waste container.	_____	5	
17. Washed hands.	_____	5	
18. Accurately noted temperature.	_____	15	
19. Recorded and signed procedure on patient's chart.	_____	10	

ADD POINTS OF STEPS CHECKED   _____ EARNED

TOTAL POINTS POSSIBLE   185 POSSIBLE

Points assigned reflect importance of step to meeting objective: Important = (5)   Essential = (10)   Critical = (15)

Automatic failure results if any of the critical steps are omitted or performed incorrectly.

DETERMINE SCORE (divide points earned by total points possible, multiply results by 100)   _____ SCORE*

Evaluator's Name (print) _____ Signature _____

Comments _____

DOCUMENTATION

Chart the procedure in the patient's medical record.

Date: _____

Charting: _____

_____

_____

_____

Student's Name: _____   Physician's Initials: __( )__

Name _____

Date _____ Score* _____

PROCEDURE 12-6   Measure Rectal Temperature with Mercury Thermometer

PERFORMANCE OBJECTIVE—In a simulated or actual situation and given access to all necessary equipment and supplies, measure and record a patient's rectal temperature within eight minutes, following correct procedural technique and observing aseptic and safety precautions. The recorded findings must agree with the instructor's reading.

PROCEDURE STEPS	STEP PERFORMED	POINTS POSSIBLE	COMMENTS
EVALUATOR: Place check mark in space following each step performed satisfactorily			
NOTE TIME BEGAN _____			
1. Washed hands, assembled equipment, and put on gloves.	_____	15	
2. Identified patient.	_____	5	
3. Explained procedure.	_____	5	
4. Placed a small amount of lubricant on a tissue.	_____	5	
5. Removed thermometer from holder or envelope.	_____	5	
6. Inspected thermometer. Discarded a chipped or cracked thermometer in a sharps biohazardous waste container.	_____	15	
7. Read thermometer and shook down to 95°F, or below.	_____	15	
8. Placed thermometer in plastic sheath. Checked that sheath is intact.	_____	15	
9. Rotated thermometer bulb in lubricant on tissue and placed in convenient location.	_____	5	
10. Instructed patient to remove appropriate clothing, assisting as needed.	_____	5	
11. Provided privacy.	_____	5	
12. Assisted adult patient onto examining table and covered with drape. Avoided overexposure.	_____	5	
13. Positioned patient on side. Ensured patient's comfort and safety.	_____	5	
14. Arranged drape to expose buttocks.	_____	5	
15. With one hand raised upper buttock to expose anus.	_____	5	
16. With other hand, carefully inserted lubricated thermometer into anal canal approximately 1½ ".	_____	5	
a. Did not force thermometer. Rotated if necessary to facilitate insertion	_____	10	
b. If opening was not apparent, requested patient to bear down slightly	_____	5	
17. Held thermometer in place for a minimum of three minutes.	_____	15	

PROCEDURE STEPS	STEP PERFORMED	POINTS POSSIBLE	COMMENTS
18. Withdrew thermometer. Carefully removed plastic sheath and discarded it in biohazardous waste container.	_____	10	
19. Read thermometer.	_____	5	
20. Reread to check temperature.	_____	5	
21. Placed thermometer on tissue.	_____	5	
EVALUATOR: NOTE TIME COMPLETED _____			
Completed within eight minutes	_____	15	
EVALUATOR: Read thermometer and record temperature: _____			
22. Removed any excess lubricant from anal area with tissue; wiped from front to back.	_____	5	
23. Assisted adult patient from examining table and instructed to redress.	_____	5	
24. Followed procedure for soiled thermometer.	_____	5	
25. Removed and discarded gloves in biohazardous waste container.	_____	5	
26. Accurately noted temperature.	_____	15	
27. Recorded and signed procedure on patient's chart.	_____	10	

ADD POINTS OF STEPS CHECKED   _____ EARNED

TOTAL POINTS POSSIBLE   235 POSSIBLE

Points assigned reflect importance of step to meeting objective: Important = (5)   Essential = (10)   Critical = (15)
Automatic failure results if any of the critical steps are omitted or performed incorrectly.

DETERMINE SCORE (divide points earned by total points possible, multiply results by 100)   _____ SCORE*

Evaluator's Name (print) _____ Signature _____

Comments _____

DOCUMENTATION

Chart the procedure in the patient's medical record.

Date: _____

Charting: _____

_____

_____

_____

Student's Name: _____   Physician's Initials: _(_____)_

Name _____

Date _____ Score* _____

PROCEDURE 12-7   Measure Axillary Temperature with Mercury Thermometer

PERFORMANCE OBJECTIVE—In a simulated or actual situation and given access to all necessary equipment and supplies, measure and record axillary temperature within 14 minutes, following correct procedural technique and observing aseptic and safety precautions. Recorded findings must agree with the instructor's reading.

PROCEDURE STEPS	STEP PERFORMED	POINTS POSSIBLE	COMMENTS
EVALUATOR: Place check mark in space following each step performed satisfactorily			
NOTE TIME BEGAN _____			
1. Washed hands, assembled equipment.	_____	5	
2. Identified patient.	_____	5	
3. Explained procedure.	_____	5	
4. Removed thermometer from holder or envelope.	_____	5	
5. Inspected thermometer. Discarded a chipped or cracked thermometer in a sharps biohazardous waste container.	_____	15	
6. Read thermometer and shook down to 95°F or below.	_____	15	
7. Placed thermometer on tissue or in envelope in convenient location.	_____	5	
8. Assisted patient, as necessary, to expose axilla, provided privacy.	_____	5	
9. Patted axillary space with tissue to remove perspiration.	_____	10	
10. Placed thermometer deep in the axillary space.	_____	10	
a. Bulb at top of axillary space	_____	5	
b. Stem projecting anteriorly or posteriorly	_____	5	
11. Instructed patient to hold arm tightly against body and to maintain position for a minimum of ten minutes.	_____	15	
12. Removed thermometer and wiped with tissue from stem to bulb.	_____	5	
13. Read and noted findings accurately.	_____	15	
14. Reread and checked recording.	_____	5	
EVALUATOR: NOTE TIME COMPLETED _____ Completed within fourteen minutes.		15	
EVALUATOR: Read thermometer and record temperature: _____			

PROCEDURE STEPS	STEP PERFORMED	POINTS POSSIBLE	COMMENTS
15. Helped patient replace clothing.	_____	5	
16. Followed procedure for soiled thermometer.	_____	5	.
17. Washed hands.	_____	5	
18. Recorded and signed procedure on patient's chart.	_____	10	

ADD POINTS OF STEPS CHECKED   _____ EARNED
TOTAL POINTS POSSIBLE   170   POSSIBLE

Points assigned reflect importance of step to meeting objective: Important = (5)   Essential = (10)   Critical = (15)
Automatic failure results if any of the critical steps are omitted or performed incorrectly.

DETERMINE SCORE (divide points earned by total points possible, multiply results by 100)   _____ SCORE*

Evaluator's Name (print) _____ Signature _____

Comments _____

DOCUMENTATION

Chart the procedure in the patient's medical record.

Date: _____

Charting: _____

_____

_____

_____

Student's Name: _____   Physician's Initials: __(____)__

PERFORMANCE EVALUATION CHECKLIST

Name _____

Date _____ Score* _____

PROCEDURE 12-8   Measure Oral Temperature with Disposable Plastic Thermometer

PERFORMANCE OBJECTIVE—In a simulated or actual situation and given access to all necessary equipment and supplies, measure and record oral temperature within four minutes, following correct procedural technique and observing aseptic and safety precautions. Recorded findings must agree with the instructor's reading.

PROCEDURE STEPS	STEP PERFORMED	POINTS POSSIBLE	COMMENTS
EVALUATOR: Place check mark in space following each step performed satisfactorily			
NOTE TIME BEGAN _____			
1. Washed hands, assembled equipment, put on gloves.	_____	5	
2. Identified patient.	_____	5	
3. Explained procedure.	_____	5	
4. Determined if patient had recently had a hot or cold drink or smoked.	_____	15	
5. Opened package by peeling back top of wrapper to expose handle end of thermometer.	_____	5	
6. Grasped handle and removed from wrapper without touching matrix section.	_____	15	
7. Inserted thermometer into patient's mouth as far back as possible into one of the heat pockets.	_____	10	
8. Instructed patient to press tongue down on thermometer and keep mouth closed.	_____	10	
9. Instructed patient to maintain position for sixty seconds; timed by watch.	_____	15	
10. Removed thermometer and waited ten seconds for dots to stabilize. Did not touch dots.	_____	15	
11. Read thermometer.	_____	—	
EVALUATOR: NOTE TIME COMPLETED _____			
Completed within four minutes.		15	
EVALUATOR: Read thermometer and record temperature: _____			
12. Discarded thermometer in biohazardous waste container.	_____	10	
13. Washed hands.	_____	5	
14. Accurately noted temperature.	_____	15	
15. Recorded and signed procedure on patient's chart.	_____	10	

ADD POINTS OF STEPS CHECKED   _____ EARNED

TOTAL POINTS POSSIBLE   155 POSSIBLE

Points assigned reflect importance of step to meeting objective: Important = (5)   Essential = (10)   Critical = (15)
Automatic failure results if any of the critical steps are omitted or performed incorrectly.

DETERMINE SCORE (divide points earned by total points possible, multiply results by 100)   _____ SCORE*

Evaluator's Name (print) _____ Signature _____

Comments _____

DOCUMENTATION

Chart the procedure in the patient's medical record.

Date: _____

Charting: _____

_____

_____

_____

Student's Name: _____   Physician's Initials: _(_____)_

Name _____

Date _____ Score* _____

PROCEDURE 12-9   Measure Oral Temperature Electronically

PERFORMANCE OBJECTIVE—In a simulated or actual situation and given access to all necessary equipment and supplies, measure the patient's temperature electronically. The temperature will be read and recorded in two minutes, following correct procedural technique and observing aseptic and safety precautions. Recorded findings must agree with instructor's reading.

PROCEDURE STEPS	STEP PERFORMED	POINTS POSSIBLE	COMMENTS
EVALUATOR: Place check mark in space following each step performed satisfactorily			
NOTE TIME BEGAN _____			
1. Washed hands, assembled equipment.	_____	5	
2. Identified patient.	_____	5	
3. Explained procedure.	_____	5	
4. Placed probe connector in receptacle of unit base and checked to make sure it was properly seated.	_____	10	
5. Holding it by the collar, removed appropriate probe from stored position.	_____	5	
6. Inserted probe firmly into probe cover to ensure that it was properly seated.	_____	5	
7. Inserted covered probe into mouth, and provided support.	_____	15	
8. Maintained covered probe in position until unit signals.	_____	10	
9. Removed probe; avoided touching cover.	_____	15	
10. Accurately read and noted temperature measurement.	_____	15	
11. Rechecked reading and recording.	_____	5	
12. Pressed the eject button and discarded used probe cover into biohazardous waste container.	_____	10	
13. Returned probe to stored position in unit. Thermometer display read zero and shut off.	_____	5	
14. Stored unit in charging stand.	_____	5	
15. Recorded and signed procedure on patient's chart.	_____	10	
EVALUATOR: NOTE TIME COMPLETED _____			
Completed within two minutes	_____	15	
EVALUATOR: Read thermometer and record temperature: _____			

ADD POINTS OF STEPS CHECKED   _____ EARNED
TOTAL POINTS POSSIBLE   140 POSSIBLE

Points assigned reflect importance of step to meeting objective: Important = (5)   Essential = (10)   Critical = (15)
Automatic failure results if any of the critical steps are omitted or performed incorrectly.

DETERMINE SCORE (divide points earned by total points possible, multiply results by 100)   _____ SCORE*

Evaluator's Name (print) _____ Signature _____

Comments _____

DOCUMENTATION

Chart the procedure in the patient's medical record.

Date: _____

Charting: _____

_____

_____

_____

Student's Name: _____   Physician's Initials: __(____)__

Name _____

Date _____ Score* _____

PROCEDURE 12-10   Measure Core Body Temperature
with an Infrared Tympanic Thermometer

PERFORMANCE OBJECTIVE—In a simulated or actual situation and given access to all necessary equipment and supplies, measure and record core temperature within three minutes, following correct procedural technique and observing aseptic and safety precautions. Recorded findings must agree with the instructor's reading.

PROCEDURE STEPS	STEP PERFORMED	POINTS POSSIBLE	COMMENTS
EVALUATOR: Place check mark in space following each step performed satisfactorily			
NOTE TIME BEGAN _____			
1. Washed hands, assembled equipment.	_____	5	
2. Identified patient.	_____	5	
3. Explained procedure.	_____	5	
4. Removed thermometer from base.	_____	5	
5. Attached a disposable probe cover to the earpiece.	_____	10	
6. Inserted covered probe into ear canal, sealing opening.	_____	15	
7. Pressed the scan button to activate the thermometer.	_____	5	
8. Withdrew the thermometer.	_____	—	
9. Observed the display window, noting the temperature.	_____	5	
10. Pressed the release button on the thermometer and ejected probe cover into a biohazardous waste container.	_____	5	
11. Accurately read and noted temperature.	_____	15	
12. Returned thermometer to base.	_____	5	
13. Recorded and signed procedure on patient's chart.	_____	10	
EVALUATOR: NOTE TIME COMPLETED _____			
Completed within three minutes.	_____	15	
EVALUATOR: Read thermometer and record temperature: _____			

ADD POINTS OF STEPS CHECKED   _____ EARNED
TOTAL POINTS POSSIBLE   105 POSSIBLE

Points assigned reflect importance of step to meeting objective: Important = (5)   Essential = (10)   Critical = (15)
Automatic failure results if any of the critical steps are omitted or performed incorrectly.

DETERMINE SCORE (divide points earned by total points possible, multiply results by 100)   _____ SCORE*

Evaluator's Name (print) _____ Signature _____

Comments _____

DOCUMENTATION

Chart the procedure in the patient's medical record.

Date: _____

Charting: _____

_____

_____

_____

Student's Name: _____   Physician's Initials: __( )__

Name _____

Date _____ Score* _____

PROCEDURE 12-11   Measure Radial Pulse

PERFORMANCE OBJECTIVE—In a simulated or actual situation and given access to all necessary equipment and supplies, within four minutes, assess and record the quality and measure and record the rate of a patient's radial pulse following correct procedural technique. Recorded rate findings must be within two beats per minute of instructor's measurement and agree as to rhythm and quality characteristics.

PROCEDURE STEPS	STEP PERFORMED	POINTS POSSIBLE	COMMENTS
EVALUATOR: Place check mark in space following each step performed satisfactorily			
NOTE TIME BEGAN _____			
1. Washed hands, assembled equipment.	_____	5	
2. Identified patient.	_____	5	
3. Explained procedure.	_____	5	
4. Determined patient's recent activity.	_____	10	
5. Had patient assume a comfortable position.	_____	5	
6. Located radial artery.	_____	15	
7. Observed quality of pulse before beginning to count.	_____	15	
8. Counted pulse.	_____	15	
a. Regular for 30 seconds—*or*—			
b. Irregular for one minute			
9. Accurately recorded pulse rate.	_____	15	
10. Described characteristics.	_____	15	
11. Recorded and signed procedure on patient's chart.	_____	10	
EVALUATOR: NOTE TIME COMPLETED _____			
Completed within four minutes.	_____	15	
EVALUATOR: Record pulse rate _____			
Characteristics _____			
_____			
_____			

ADD POINTS OF STEPS CHECKED   _____ EARNED
TOTAL POINTS POSSIBLE   130 POSSIBLE

Points assigned reflect importance of step to meeting objective: Important = (5)   Essential = (10)   Critical = (15)
Automatic failure results if any of the critical steps are omitted or performed incorrectly.

DETERMINE SCORE (divide points earned by total points possible, multiply results by 100)   _____ SCORE*

Evaluator's Name (print) _____ Signature _____

Comments _____

DOCUMENTATION

Chart the procedure in the patient's medical record.

Date: _____

Charting: _____

_____

_____

_____

Student's Name: _____   Physician's Initials: _( )_

Name _____

Date _____ Score* _____

PROCEDURE 12-12   Measure Apical Pulse

PERFORMANCE OBJECTIVE—In a simulated or actual situation and given access to all necessary equipment and supplies, within five minutes, locate the apex of the heart, assess and record the quality and measure and record the rate of a patient's apical pulse following correct technique and observing aseptic precautions. Recorded rate findings must be within one beat per minute of instructor's measurement and agree as to rhythm and quality characteristics.

PROCEDURE STEPS	STEP PERFORMED	POINTS POSSIBLE	COMMENTS
EVALUATOR: Place check mark in space following each step performed satisfactorily			
NOTE TIME BEGAN _____			
1. Washed hands, assembled equipment.	_____	5	
2. Prepared stethoscope by wiping earpieces and chestpiece with germicidal solution to prevent transfer of organisms.	_____	10	
3. Identified patient.	_____	5	
4. Explained procedure. If infant or small child, explained to parent.	_____	5	
5. Provided privacy and a gown or drape if indicated.	_____	5	
6. Uncovered left side of chest.	_____	10	
7. Placed earpieces in ears. Openings in tips should be forward, entering auditory canal: held chestpiece in hand.	_____	10	
8. Located apex.	_____	15	
9. Placed chestpiece of stethoscope at apex.	_____	5	
10. Determined quality of heart sounds.	_____	15	
11. Counted beats for a full minute.	_____	15	
12. Removed earpieces from ears.	_____	5	
13. Accurately noted rate of heart sounds.	_____	15	
14. Accurately noted quality of heart sounds.	_____	15	
15. Assisted patient as necessary to redress.	_____	—	
16. Wiped earpieces and chestpiece of stethoscope with disinfectant. Returned to storage.	_____	5	
17. Washed hands.	_____	5	
18. Recorded and signed procedure on patient's chart.	_____	10	
EVALUATOR: NOTE TIME COMPLETED _____			
Completed within five minutes.	_____	15	
EVALUATOR: Record rate _____			
Characteristics _____			

ADD POINTS OF STEPS CHECKED   _____ EARNED

TOTAL POINTS POSSIBLE   170 POSSIBLE

Points assigned reflect importance of step to meeting objective: Important = (5)   Essential = (10)   Critical = (15)
Automatic failure results if any of the critical steps are omitted or performed incorrectly.

DETERMINE SCORE (divide points earned by total points possible, multiply results by 100)   _____ SCORE*

Evaluator's Name (print) _____ Signature _____

Comments _____

DOCUMENTATION

Chart the procedure in the patient's medical record.

Date: _____

Charting: _____

_____

_____

_____

Student's Name: _____   **Physician's Initials:** __(____)__

Name _____

Date _____ Score* _____

PROCEDURE 12-13   Measure Respirations

PERFORMANCE OBJECTIVE—In a simulated or actual situation and given access to all necessary equipment and supplies, assess and record the quality and rate of a patient's respirations within three minutes, following correct procedural technique. Recorded rate findings must be within two breaths per minute of instructor's measurement and agree as to rhythm, sound, and depth quality characteristics.

PROCEDURE STEPS	STEP PERFORMED	POINTS POSSIBLE	COMMENTS
EVALUATOR: Place check mark in space following each step performed satisfactorily			
NOTE TIME BEGAN _____			
1. Washed hands, assembled equipment.	_____	5	
2. Identified patient.	_____	5	
3. Asked about recent activity level.	_____	10	
4. Avoided identifying respiration evaluation.	_____	10	
5. Placed patient in comfortable position.	_____	5	
6. Assumed pulse measurement position.	_____	10	
7. Assessed respiration quality.	_____	15	
8. Accurately counted respirations for thirty seconds.	_____	15	
9. Accurately noted rate.	_____	15	
10. Recorded characteristics.	_____	15	
11. Recorded and signed procedure on patient's chart.	_____	10	
EVALUATOR: NOTE TIME COMPLETED _____			
Completed within three minutes.	_____	15	
EVALUATOR: Record rate _____			
Characteristics _____			
_____			

ADD POINTS OF STEPS CHECKED   _____ EARNED
TOTAL POINTS POSSIBLE   130 POSSIBLE

Points assigned reflect importance of step to meeting objective: Important = (5)   Essential = (10)   Critical = (15)
Automatic failure results if any of the critical steps are omitted or performed incorrectly.

DETERMINE SCORE (divide points earned by total points possible, multiply results by 100)   _____ SCORE*

Evaluator's Name (print) _____ Signature _____

Comments _____

DOCUMENTATION

Chart the procedure in the patient's medical record.

Date: _____

Charting: _____

_____

_____

_____

Student's Name: _____   Physician's Initials: __(____)__

PROCEDURE 12-14   Measure Blood Pressure

PERFORMANCE OBJECTIVE—In a simulated or actual situation and given access to all necessary equipment and supplies, within
a four-minute period of time, measure palpatory and auscultatory blood pressure and record findings, following correct
procedural technique and observing safety and aseptic precautions. Recorded rate findings must be within 4 mmHg of
instructor's measurement using teaching stethoscope.

PROCEDURE STEPS	STEP PERFORMED	POINTS POSSIBLE	COMMENTS
EVALUATOR: Place check mark in space following each step performed satisfactorily			
NOTE TIME BEGAN _____			
1. Washed hands.	_____	5	
2. Assembled equipment.	_____	5	
3. Cleaned earpieces and head of stethoscope with antiseptic.	_____	5	
4. Identified patient.	_____	5	
5. Explained procedure.	_____	5	
6. Placed a mercury manometer on a flat, level surface near patient. Put aneroid type within easy reach.	_____	5	
7. Placed patient in a relaxed and comfortable sitting or lying position.	_____	5	
8. a. Positioned arm, palm up	_____	5	
b. Clothing appropriately managed	_____	10	
9. a. Opened valve, deflated bladder completely	_____	5	
b. Located center of bladder; assured adequate cuff size	_____	15	
c. Applied cuff to upper arm, bladder centered over brachial artery; 1″ to 2″ above elbow	_____	15	
d. Attached tubing if disconnected	_____	—	
10. Assured manometer in proper view.	_____	5	
11. Closed valve with one hand.	_____	5	
12. Positioned other hand to palpate radial pulse.	_____	5	
13. Observing manometer, rapidly inflated cuff to 30 mm above level where radial pulse disappears.	_____	10	
14. Opened valve, slowly releasing air until radial pulse was detected.	_____	10	
15. Observed mercury or dial reading.	_____	10	
16. Deflated cuff rapidly and completely. Squeezed cuff with hands to empty **air.**	_____	5	
17. Positioned earpieces of stethoscope in ears with openings entering ear canal; held head of scope in one hand.	_____	5	
18. Palpated brachial artery at medial antecubital space with fingertips.	_____	15	
19. Placed head of stethoscope directly over palpated pulse.	_____	5	
20. Closed valve on bulb and rapidly inflated cuff to 30 mm above palpated systolic pressure.	_____	10	

PROCEDURE 12-14   Measure Blood Pressure—continued

PROCEDURE STEPS	STEP PERFORMED	POINTS POSSIBLE	COMMENTS
21. Opened valve, slowly deflating cuff.	_____	10	
22. With eyes at level of descending meniscus or directly in line with dial, noted reading at which systolic pressure heard.	_____	10	
23. Allowed pressure to lower steadily.	_____	5	
24. Continued to release pressure until all sound disappears.	_____	5	
25. Released remaining air. Squeezed cuff between hands.	_____	5	
26. Recorded accurate systolic and whichever diastolic instructed to read.	_____	15	
27. Reevaluated if indicated after a minimum of fifteen seconds.	_____	—	
28. Removed stethoscope from ears.	_____	—	
29. Removed cuff from patient's arm.	_____	—	
EVALUATOR: NOTE TIME COMPLETED _____			
Completed within four minutes.	_____	15	
EVALUATOR: Record B/P _____			
30. Assisted patient with clothing, if necessary.	_____	—	
31. Cleaned tips and head of stethoscope with alcohol to disinfect.	_____	10	
32. Folded cuff properly and placed with manometer and stethoscope in storage.	_____	5	
33. Washed hands.	_____	5	
34. Recorded and signed procedure on patient's chart.	_____	10	

ADD POINTS OF STEPS CHECKED   _____ EARNED
TOTAL POINTS POSSIBLE   265 POSSIBLE

Points assigned reflect importance of step to meeting objective: Important = (5)   Essential = (10)   Critical = (15)
Automatic failure results if any of the critical steps are omitted or performed incorrectly.

DETERMINE SCORE (divide points earned by total points possible, multiply results by 100)   _____ SCORE*

Evaluator's Name (print) _____ Signature _____

Comments _____

DOCUMENTATION

Chart the procedure in the patient's medical record.

Date: _____

Charting: _____

_____

_____

_____

Student's Name: _____   Physician's Initials: __(___)__

Name _____

Date _____ Score* _____

PROCEDURE 13-1   Irrigate the Eye

PERFORMANCE OBJECTIVE—Provided with a mannequin and all equipment required for eye irrigation, demonstrate the steps of the procedure in proper order.

PROCEDURE STEPS	STEP PERFORMED	POINTS POSSIBLE	COMMENTS
EVALUATOR: Place check mark in space following each step performed satisfactorily			
NOTE TIME BEGAN _____			
1. Assembled necessary items.	_____	10	
2. Washed hands and put on gloves.	_____	15	
3. Prepared solution.	_____	10	
4. Identified patient, called by name.	_____	5	
5. Explained procedure to patient.	_____	5	
6. Positioned patient comfortably.	_____	5	
7. Draped patient.	_____	5	
8. Asked patient to turn head to side then back.	_____	10	
9. Placed emesis basin against head to catch solution, gave tissues.	_____	10	
10. Wiped eye with gauze square from bridge of nose out.	_____	10	
11. Filled bulb syringe with solution.	_____	10	
12. Held eye open with thumb and index finger.	_____	15	
13. Released solution over eye gently from inner canthus to outer canthus.	_____	15	
14. Used sterile gauze square to blot area dry.	_____	5	
15. Attended to patient's comfort.	_____	5	
16. Removed gloves and washed hands.	_____	10	
17. Provided patient education.	_____	5	
18. Recorded procedure in patient's chart.	_____	10	
19. Initialed procedure.	_____	5	
20. Noted observations during procedure.	_____	5	
21. Washed items and returned to storage.	_____	5	
EVALUATOR: NOTE TIME COMPLETED _____			

ADD POINTS OF STEPS CHECKED   _____ EARNED
TOTAL POINTS POSSIBLE   175 POSSIBLE

Points assigned reflect importance of step to meeting objective: Important = (5)   Essential = (10)   Critical = (15)
Automatic failure results if any of the critical steps are omitted or performed incorrectly.

DETERMINE SCORE (divide points earned by total points possible, multiply results by 100)   _____ SCORE*

Evaluator's Name (print) _____ Signature _____

Comments _____

DOCUMENTATION

Chart the procedure in the patient's medical record.

Date: _____

Charting: _____

_____

_____

_____

Student's Name: _____   Physician's Initials: _(___)_

Name _____

Date _____ Score* _____

PROCEDURE 13-2   Irrigate the Ear

PERFORMANCE OBJECTIVE—Provided with anatomical model of the ear and all equipment required for ear irrigation, demonstrate the steps of the procedure in proper order.

PROCEDURE STEPS	STEP PERFORMED	POINTS POSSIBLE	COMMENTS
EVALUATOR: Place check mark in space following each step performed satisfactorily			
NOTE TIME BEGAN _____			
1. Washed hands and put on gloves.	_____	10	
2. Assembled necessary items.	_____	15	
3. Prepared solution between 100°F and 105°F as directed by the physician.	_____	15	
4. a. Identified patient, called by name	_____	10	
b. Explained procedure to patient	_____	5	
5. Viewed affected area with otoscope.	_____	10	
6. Asked patient to turn head to side and back.	_____	10	
7. Placed ear basin under ear.	_____	5	
8. Placed towel over patient's shoulder.	_____	5	
9. Used gauze square to wipe ear.	_____	5	
10. Filled syringe with solution.	_____	10	
11. Pulled auricle up and back for adult or down and back for child.	_____	15	
12. Placed tip of syringe into side of ear canal.	_____	5	
13. Irrigated ear with solution to desired results.	_____	15	
14. Used gauze square to wipe excess solution from outside of patient's ear.	_____	5	
15. Instructed patient to tilt head to allow drainage, give tissues.	_____	5	
16. Inspected ear canal with otoscope to determine results of irrigation. Repeat irrigation PRN.	_____	5	
17. Provided patient education.	_____	5	
18. a. Recorded procedure in patient's chart	_____	10	
b. Initialed chart	_____	5	
c. Wrote observations	_____	5	

PROCEDURE 13-2 Irrigate the Ear—continued

PROCEDURE STEPS	STEP PERFORMED	POINTS POSSIBLE	COMMENTS
19. Washed equipment.	_____	5	
20. Removed gloves and washed hands.	_____	5	
21. Returned equipment to proper storage area.	_____	5	

EVALUATOR: NOTE TIME COMPLETED _____

ADD POINTS OF STEPS CHECKED _____ EARNED

TOTAL POINTS POSSIBLE 190 POSSIBLE

Points assigned reflect importance of step to meeting objective: Important = (5) Essential = (10) Critical = (15)
Automatic failure results if any of the critical steps are omitted or performed incorrectly.

DETERMINE SCORE (divide points earned by total points possible, multiply results by 100) _____ SCORE*

Evaluator's Name (print) _____ Signature _____

Comments _____

DOCUMENTATION

Chart the procedure in the patient's medical record.

Date: _____

Charting: _____

_____

_____

_____

Student's Name: _____   Physician's Initials: __(____)__

Name _____

Date _____ Score* _____

PROCEDURE 13-3   Instill Eardrops

PERFORMANCE OBJECTIVE—Provided with a mannequin or anatomical model of the ear and all necessary equipment, demonstrate each step of the procedure for instilling eardrops in proper order.

PROCEDURE STEPS	STEP PERFORMED	POINTS POSSIBLE	COMMENTS
EVALUATOR: Place check mark in space following each step performed satisfactorily			
NOTE TIME BEGAN _____			
1. Verified medication ordered.	_____	15	
a. Assembled items	_____	5	
2. Washed hands and put on gloves.	_____	10	
3. Called patient by name.	_____	10	
a. Explained procedure	_____	10	
4. Opened medication container/drew up ordered amount in dropper.	_____	15	
5. Positioned patient/tilt head to instill left for right ear (right for left).	_____	10	
6. Asked for assistance if necessary.	_____	5	
7. Gave patient tissues.	_____	5	
8. Instilled drops in ear (without touching ear tissues).	_____	15	
9. Advised patient to remain in position for drops to settle in ear.	_____	10	
10. Provided patient education.	_____	5	
11. Repeated for other ear if ordered.	_____	10	
12. Closed medication container without touching outside of the container.	_____	15	
13. Removed gloves and washed hands.	_____	10	
14. Recorded procedure on patient's chart.	_____	5	
a. Noted observations	_____	5	
b. Initialed	_____	10	
15. Returned items to proper storage area.	_____	5	
EVALUATOR: NOTE TIME COMPLETED _____			

ADD POINTS OF STEPS CHECKED   _____ EARNED
TOTAL POINTS POSSIBLE   175 POSSIBLE

Points assigned reflect importance of step to meeting objective: Important = (5)   Essential = (10)   Critical = (15)
Automatic failure results if any of the critical steps are omitted or performed incorrectly.

DETERMINE SCORE (divide points earned by total points possible, multiply results by 100)   _____ SCORE*

Evaluator's Name (print) _____ Signature _____

Comments _____

DOCUMENTATION

Chart the procedure in the patient's medical record.

Date: _____

Charting: _____

_____

_____

_____

Student's Name: _____   Physician's Initials: __(__)__

Name _____

Date _____ Score* _____

PROCEDURE 13-4   Instill Eyedrops

PERFORMANCE OBJECTIVE—Provided with a mannequin or anatomical model of the eye and all necessary equipment, demonstrate each step of the procedure for instilling eyedrops in proper order.

PROCEDURE STEPS	STEP PERFORMED	POINTS POSSIBLE	COMMENTS
EVALUATOR: Place check mark in space following each step performed satisfactorily			
NOTE TIME BEGAN _____			
1. Verified medication ordered.	_____	15	
a. Assembled items	_____	5	
2. Washed hands and put on gloves.	_____	10	
3. Called patient by name.	_____	10	
a. Explained procedure	_____	10	
4. Opened medication container/drew up ordered amount in dropper.	_____	15	
5. Positioned patient/asked for assistance if necessary.	_____	10	
6. Used gauze to touch area just under eyelid to form pocket.	_____	10	
7. Instilled drops into pocket of eye without touching tissues.	_____	15	
8. Asked patient to blink to distribute medication.	_____	15	
a. Repeated for other eye	_____	10	
9. Advised patient not to rub eyes.	_____	10	
10. Offered patient tissues to blot excess medication gently.	_____	5	
11. Provided patient education.	_____	5	
12. Closed medication container without touching cap to the outside of the container.	_____	10	
13. Removed gloves and washed hands.	_____	5	
14. Recorded procedure on patient's chart.	_____	10	
a. Noted observations	_____	5	
b. Initialed	_____	5	
15. Returned items to proper storage area.	_____	5	
EVALUATOR: NOTE TIME COMPLETED _____			

ADD POINTS OF STEPS CHECKED   _____ EARNED
TOTAL POINTS POSSIBLE   185 POSSIBLE

Points assigned reflect importance of step to meeting objective: Important = (5)   Essential = (10)   Critical = (15)
Automatic failure results if any of the critical steps are omitted or performed incorrectly.

DETERMINE SCORE (divide points earned by total points possible, multiply results by 100)   _____ SCORE*

Evaluator's Name (print) _____ Signature _____

Comments _____

DOCUMENTATION

Chart the procedure in the patient's medical record.

Date: _____

Charting: _____

_____

_____

_____

Student's Name: _____   **Physician's Initials:** _(   )_

PERFORMANCE EVALUATION CHECKLIST   Name _____

                                       Date _____ Score* _____

PROCEDURE 13-5   Screen Visual Acuity with Snellen Chart

PERFORMANCE OBJECTIVE—Measure the visual acuity of a patient by demonstrating each step of the vision screening procedure using the Snellen chart; record the results accurately on the patient's chart.

PROCEDURE STEPS	STEP PERFORMED	POINTS POSSIBLE	COMMENTS
EVALUATOR: Place check mark in space following each step performed satisfactorily			
NOTE TIME BEGAN _____			
1. Identified patient.	_____	10	
2. Explained the procedure to the patient.	_____	10	
3. Instructed patient to stand 20 feet from chart.	_____	10	
a. Adjusted eye chart to patient's eye level	_____	10	
4. Told patient to keep both eyes open.	_____	10	
a. Instructed patient to keep corrective lenses on/in during the first part of the screening	_____	10	
5. Instructed patient to read lines as you point to them.	_____	5	
6. Asked patient to read chart with both eyes.	_____	5	
7. Recorded smallest line patient could read (without making a mistake).	_____	15	
8. Asked patient to cover left eye.	_____	10	
a. Instructed patient to leave both eyes open	_____	10	
b. Recorded smallest line patient could read (without making a mistake)	_____	15	
9. Asked patient to cover right eye.	_____	10	
a. Instructed patient to leave both eyes open	_____	10	
10. Recorded smallest line patient could read (without making a mistake).	_____	15	
11. Recorded observations of patient during screening.	_____	5	
EVALUATOR: NOTE TIME COMPLETED _____			

ADD POINTS OF STEPS CHECKED   _____ EARNED
TOTAL POINTS POSSIBLE   160 POSSIBLE

Points assigned reflect importance of step to meeting objective: Important = (5)   Essential = (10)   Critical = (15)
Automatic failure results if any of the critical steps are omitted or performed incorrectly.

DETERMINE SCORE (divide points earned by total points possible, multiply results by 100)   _____ SCORE*

Evaluator's Name (print) _____ Signature _____

Comments _____

DOCUMENTATION

Chart the procedure in the patient's medical record.

Date: _____

Charting: _____

_____

_____

_____

Student's Name: _____   Physician's Initials: __(____)__

Name _____

Date _____ Score* _____

PROCEDURE 13-6   Screen Visual Acuity with Jaeger System

PERFORMANCE OBJECTIVE—Determine the near distance visual acuity of a patient using the Jaeger near vision acuity chart by demonstrating each step of the visual acuity procedure; record results accurately in patient's chart.

PROCEDURE STEPS	STEP PERFORMED	POINTS POSSIBLE	COMMENTS
EVALUATOR: Place check mark in space following each step performed satisfactorily			
NOTE TIME BEGAN _____			
1. Identified patient.	_____	10	
2. Positioned patient for procedure.	_____	10	
3. Instructed patient to hold Jaeger chart between 14″ and 16″ from eyes.	_____	15	
4. Instructed patient to read various paragraphs/both eyes open first without corrective lenses.	_____	10	
a. With corrective lenses	_____	10	
5. Instructed patient to cover left eye and read.	_____	10	
6. Instructed patient to cover right eye and read.	_____	10	
7. Observed patient during procedure.	_____	5	
8. Listened to remarks made by patient during procedure.	_____	5	
9. Recorded results on patient's chart listing the smallest print patient could read (without making a mistake).	_____	15	
10. Initialed patient's chart.	_____	5	
11. Thanked patient for cooperation.	_____	5	
12. Answered patient's questions.	_____	5	
13. Returned Jaeger chart to proper storage.	_____	5	
EVALUATOR: NOTE TIME COMPLETED _____			

ADD POINTS OF STEPS CHECKED   _____ EARNED

TOTAL POINTS POSSIBLE   120 POSSIBLE

Points assigned reflect importance of step to meeting objective: Important = (5)   Essential = (10)   Critical = (15)
Automatic failure results if any of the critical steps are omitted or performed incorrectly.

DETERMINE SCORE (divide points earned by total points possible, multiply results by 100)   _____ SCORE*

Evaluator's Name (print) _____ Signature _____

Comments _____

DOCUMENTATION

Chart the procedure in the patient's medical record.

Date: _____

Charting: _____

_____

_____

_____

Student's Name: _____   Physician's Initials: __(____)__

Name _____

Date _____ Score* _____

PROCEDURE 13-7   Determine Color Vision Acuity by Ishihara Method

PERFORMANCE OBJECTIVE—In a well-lighted area, determine the color vision acuity of a patient using the Ishihara method demonstrating each step of the procedure and accurately recording the results in the patient's chart.

PROCEDURE STEPS	STEP PERFORMED	POINTS POSSIBLE	COMMENTS
EVALUATOR: Place check mark in space following each step performed satisfactorily			
NOTE TIME BEGAN _____			
1. Identified patient.	_____	10	
a. Explained procedure to patient	_____	10	
2. Obtained chart from back of Ishihara book.	_____	10	
a. Worked in well-lighted area	_____	10	
3. Instructed patient to wear corrective lenses during procedure.	_____	10	
4. Asked patient to read plates with both eyes.	_____	10	
5. Instructed patient to trace the letters/numbers, etc. with finger.	_____	5	
6. Asked patient to cover left eye.	_____	5	
a. Repeated steps 3–5	_____	25	
7. Asked patient to cover right eye.	_____	5	
a. Repeated steps 3–5	_____	25	
8. Recorded any difficulty/complaints on patient's chart.	_____	5	
9. Compared answers of patient with Ishihara chart.	_____	10	
10. Recorded frames patient missed.	_____	10	
11. Recorded what patient reports.	_____	5	
12. Initialed procedure on patient's chart.	_____	5	

EVALUATOR: NOTE TIME COMPLETED _____

ADD POINTS OF STEPS CHECKED   _____ EARNED
TOTAL POINTS POSSIBLE   160 POSSIBLE

Points assigned reflect importance of step to meeting objective: Important = (5)   Essential = (10)   Critical = (15)
Automatic failure results if any of the critical steps are omitted or performed incorrectly.

DETERMINE SCORE (divide points earned by total points possible, multiply results by 100)   _____ SCORE*

Evaluator's Name (print) _____ Signature _____

Comments _____

DOCUMENTATION

Chart the procedure in the patient's medical record.

Date: _____

Charting: _____

_____

_____

_____

Student's Name: _____   Physician's Initials: __(____)__

Name _____

Date _____ Score* _____

PROCEDURE 13-8   Assist Patient to Horizontal Recumbent Position

PERFORMANCE OBJECTIVE—Assist patient to assume the horizontal recumbent position while providing for safety and privacy according to the standards identified in the procedure.

PROCEDURE STEPS	STEP PERFORMED	POINTS POSSIBLE	COMMENTS
EVALUATOR: Place check mark in space following each step performed satisfactorily			
NOTE TIME BEGAN _____			
1. Checked examination room for cleanliness.	_____	5	
a. Provided clean table paper	_____	5	
b. Provided clean pillow cover	_____	5	
2. Identified patient.	_____	15	
3. Instructed patient to remove appropriate clothing.	_____	10	
a. Instructed patient where to put belongings	_____	5	
4. Instructed patient in putting on gown.	_____	5	
5. Assisted patient as necessary.	_____	5	
6. Instructed patient to sit on side of exam table.	_____	5	
7. Instructed patient to lie flat on table with legs together.	_____	15	
8. Pulled out extension of table for leg support.	_____	5	
9. Provided pillow under patient's head.	_____	5	
10. Asked patient to put arms at side or crossed over chest.	_____	5	
11. Placed drape sheet over patient.	_____	5	
12. Assisted with examination as necessary.	_____	5	
13. Assisted patient from table as necessary.	_____	5	
14. Cleaned up examination room as needed.	_____	5	
a. Replaced supplies as needed (Gloves PRN)	_____	5	
EVALUATOR: NOTE TIME COMPLETED _____			

ADD POINTS OF STEPS CHECKED   _____ EARNED

TOTAL POINTS POSSIBLE   115 POSSIBLE

Points assigned reflect importance of step to meeting objective: Important = (5)   Essential = (10)   Critical = (15)
Automatic failure results if any of the critical steps are omitted or performed incorrectly.

DETERMINE SCORE (divide points earned by total points possible, multiply results by 100)   _____ SCORE*

Evaluator's Name (print) _____ Signature _____

Comments _____

Name _____

Date _____ Score* _____

PROCEDURE 13-9   Assist Patient to Prone Position

PERFORMANCE OBJECTIVE—Assist patient to assume the prone position while providing for safety and privacy according to the standards identified in the procedure.

PROCEDURE STEPS	STEP PERFORMED	POINTS POSSIBLE	COMMENTS
EVALUATOR: Place check mark in space following each step performed satisfactorily			
NOTE TIME BEGAN _____			
1. Checked examination room for cleanliness.	_____	5	
a. Provided clean table paper	_____	5	
b. Provided clean pillow cover	_____	5	
2. Identified patient.	_____	15	
3. Instructed patient to remove appropriate clothing.	_____	10	
a. Instructed patient where to put belongings	_____	5	
4. Instructed patient in putting on gown.	_____	5	
5. Assisted patient as necessary.	_____	5	
6. Instructed patient to sit on side of exam table.	_____	5	
7. Instructed patient to lie flat on table with legs together.	_____	10	
8. Pulled out extension of table for leg support.	_____	5	
9. Placed drape sheet over patient.	_____	5	
10. Asked patient to turn toward you onto her stomach.	_____	15	
a. Cautioned patient to stay in center of table to avoid falling	_____	5	
11. Instructed patient to turn her head to one side.	_____	5	
12. Instructed patient to flex arms at elbows with her hands at side or under head.	_____	5	
13. Adjusted drape sheet evenly and loosely on all sides.	_____	5	
14. Assisted with examination as necessary.	_____	5	
15. Instructed patient to turn on back.	_____	5	
a. Reminded her to stay in center of table	_____	5	
16. Assisted patient in sitting up.	_____	5	
17. Advised patient to regain balance before standing.	_____	5	

PROCEDURE STEPS	STEP PERFORMED	POINTS POSSIBLE	COMMENTS
18. Assisted patient from table as necessary.	_____	5	
19. Cleaned up examination room as needed.	_____	5	
a. Replaced supplies as needed (Gloves PRN)	_____	5	
EVALUATOR: NOTE TIME COMPLETED _____			

ADD POINTS OF STEPS CHECKED   _____ EARNED

TOTAL POINTS POSSIBLE   155 POSSIBLE

Points assigned reflect importance of step to meeting objective: Important = (5)   Essential = (10)   Critical = (15)
Automatic failure results if any of the critical steps are omitted or performed incorrectly.

DETERMINE SCORE (divide points earned by total points possible, multiply results by 100)   _____ SCORE*

Evaluator's Name (print) _____ Signature _____

Comments _____

Name _____

Date _____ Score* _____

PROCEDURE 13-10   Assist Patient to Sims' Position

PERFORMANCE OBJECTIVE—Assist patient to assume the Sims' position while providing for safety and privacy according to the standards identified in the procedure.

PROCEDURE STEPS	STEP PERFORMED	POINTS POSSIBLE	COMMENTS
EVALUATOR: Place check mark in space following each step performed satisfactorily			
NOTE TIME BEGAN _____			
1. Checked examination room for cleanliness.	_____	5	
a. Provided clean table paper	_____	5	
b. Provided clean pillow cover	_____	5	
2. Identified patient.	_____	15	
3. Instructed patient to remove appropriate clothing.	_____	10	
a. Instructed patient where to put belongings	_____	5	
4. Instructed patient in putting on gown.	_____	5	
5. Assisted patient as necessary.	_____	5	
6. Instructed patient to sit on side of exam table.	_____	5	
7. Instructed patient to lie on left side.	_____	10	
8. Provided pillow under patient's head.	_____	5	
9. Asked patient to put left arm and shoulder behind body.	_____	5	
10. Asked patient to flex right arm with hand toward head.	_____	5	
11. Asked patient to flex left leg slightly.	_____	5	
12. Asked patient to move buttocks near side of table.	_____	5	
13. Instruct patient to flex right leg sharply toward chest.	_____	15	
14. Placed fenestrated drape sheet over patient.	_____	5	
15. Assisted with examination as necessary.	_____	5	
16. Assisted patient from table as necessary.	_____	5	
17. Cleaned up examination room as needed.	_____	5	
a. Replaced supplies as needed (Gloves PRN)	_____	5	
EVALUATOR: NOTE TIME COMPLETED _____			

ADD POINTS OF STEPS CHECKED   _____ EARNED

TOTAL POINTS POSSIBLE   135 POSSIBLE

Points assigned reflect importance of step to meeting objective: Important = (5)   Essential = (10)   Critical = (15)
Automatic failure results if any of the critical steps are omitted or performed incorrectly.

DETERMINE SCORE (divide points earned by total points possible, multiply results by 100)   _____ SCORE*

Evaluator's Name (print) _____ Signature _____

Comments _____

PROCEDURE 13-11   Assist Patient to Knee-Chest Position

PERFORMANCE OBJECTIVE—Assist patient to assume the knee-chest position while providing for safety and privacy according to the standards identified in the procedure.

PROCEDURE STEPS	STEP PERFORMED	POINTS POSSIBLE	COMMENTS
EVALUATOR: Place check mark in space following each step performed satisfactorily			
NOTE TIME BEGAN _____			
1. Checked examination room for cleanliness.	_____	5	
a. Provided clean table paper	_____	5	
b. Provided clean pillow cover	_____	5	
2. Prepared examination equipment on tray.	_____	5	
3. Identified patient.	_____	15	
4. Instructed patient to remove appropriate clothing.	_____	15	
a. Instructed patient where to put belongings	_____	5	
5. Instructed patient in putting on gown.	_____	5	
6. Assisted patient as necessary.	_____	5	
7. Instructed patient to sit on side of exam table.	_____	5	
8. Instructed patient to lie down on table.	_____	5	
9. Placed drape sheet over patient.	_____	5	
10. Instructed patient to turn toward you onto stomach.	_____	5	
a. Guided patient to center of table	_____	5	
11. Instructed patient to get on hands and knees.	_____	10	
12. Instructed patient to flex arms and fold under head.	_____	5	
13. Asked patient to separate knees slightly and keep thighs at right angle to table.	_____	15	
14. Adjusted drape sheet as needed.	_____	5	
15. Called physician to begin exam.	_____	5	
16. Assisted with examination as necessary.	_____	5	
17. Instructed patient to lie flat on stomach.	_____	5	
a. Assisted patient to turn over on back	_____	5	

PROCEDURE 13-11 Assist Patient to Knee-Chest Position—continued

PROCEDURE STEPS	STEP PERFORMED	POINTS POSSIBLE	COMMENTS
18. Assisted patient to sit up.	_____	5	
19. Assisted patient from table as necessary.	_____	5	
20. Cleaned up examination room as needed.	_____	5	
a. Replaced supplies as needed (Gloves PRN)	_____	5	

EVALUATOR: NOTE TIME COMPLETED _____

ADD POINTS OF STEPS CHECKED   _____ EARNED
TOTAL POINTS POSSIBLE   165 POSSIBLE

Points assigned reflect importance of step to meeting objective: Important = (5) Essential = (10) Critical = (15)
Automatic failure results if any of the critical steps are omitted or performed incorrectly.

DETERMINE SCORE (divide points earned by total points possible, multiply results by 100)   _____ SCORE*

Evaluator's Name (print) _____ Signature _____

Comments _____

Name _____

Date _____ Score* _____

PROCEDURE 13-12 Assist Patient to Semi-Fowler's Position

PERFORMANCE OBJECTIVE—Assist patient to assume the semi-Fowler's position while providing for safety and privacy according to the standards identified in the procedure.

PROCEDURE STEPS	STEP PERFORMED	POINTS POSSIBLE	COMMENTS
EVALUATOR: Place check mark in space following each step performed satisfactorily			
NOTE TIME BEGAN _____			
1. Checked examination room for cleanliness.	_____	5	
a. Provided clean table paper	_____	5	
b. Provided clean pillow cover	_____	5	
2. Identified patient.	_____	15	
3. Instructed patient to remove appropriate clothing.	_____	15	
a. Instructed patient where to put belongings	_____	5	
4. Instructed patient in putting on gown.	_____	5	
5. Assisted patient as necessary.	_____	5	
6. Instructed patient to sit at end of exam table.	_____	10	
a. Asked patient to scoot back toward center of table	_____	10	
7. Raised head of table to desired height—45° angle for semi-Fowler's (90° angle for Fowler's)	_____	15	
8. Instructed patient to lie flat on table with legs together.	_____	5	
9. Asked patient to lean back for comfort.	_____	5	
10. Pulled out extension of table for leg support.	_____	5	
11. Placed drape sheet over patient.	_____	5	
12. Assisted patient as necessary.	_____	5	
13. Assisted patient in sitting up.	_____	5	
14. Advised patient to regain balance before standing.	_____	5	
15. Assisted patient from table as necessary.	_____	5	
16. Cleaned up examination room as needed.	_____	5	
a. Replaced supplies as needed (Gloves PRN)	_____	5	
EVALUATOR: NOTE TIME COMPLETED _____			

ADD POINTS OF STEPS CHECKED   _____ EARNED

TOTAL POINTS POSSIBLE   145 POSSIBLE

Points assigned reflect importance of step to meeting objective: Important = (5)   Essential = (10)   Critical = (15)
Automatic failure results if any of the critical steps are omitted or performed incorrectly.

DETERMINE SCORE (divide points earned by total points possible, multiply results by 100)   _____ SCORE*

Evaluator's Name (print) _____ Signature _____

Comments _____

Name _____

Date _____ Score* _____

PROCEDURE 13-13   Assist Patient to Lithotomy Position

PERFORMANCE OBJECTIVE—Assist patient to assume the lithotomy position while providing for safety and privacy according to the standards identified in the procedure.

PROCEDURE STEPS	STEP PERFORMED	POINTS POSSIBLE	COMMENTS
EVALUATOR: Place check mark in space following each step performed satisfactorily			
NOTE TIME BEGAN _____			
1. Checked examination room for cleanliness.	_____	5	
a. Provided clean table paper	_____	5	
b. Provided clean pillow cover	_____	5	
2. Assembled necessary equipment.	_____	5	
3. Identified patient.	_____	15	
4. Instructed patient to remove appropriate clothing.	_____	10	
a. Instructed patient where to put belongings	_____	5	
5. Instructed patient in putting on gown.	_____	5	
6. Assisted patient as necessary.	_____	5	
7. Instructed patient to sit at end of exam table.	_____	10	
8. Instructed patient to lie back on table.	_____	10	
9. Pulled out extension of table for leg support.	_____	5	
10. Positioned stirrups away from table.	_____	5	
a. Adjusted height of stirrups	_____	5	
b. Secured stirrups in place	_____	5	
11. Asked patient to move buttocks toward end of table.	_____	10	
a. Placed the back of your hand at end of table to guide patient	_____	5	
b. Assisted patient's feet into stirrups	_____	15	
12. Pushed table extension in.	_____	5	
a. Positioned examination stool for physician	_____	5	
b. Positioned examination light for physician	_____	5	
13. Placed drape sheet over patient.	_____	5	
14. Assisted with examination as necessary.	_____	5	

PROCEDURE 13-13   Assist Patient to Lithotomy Position—continued

PROCEDURE STEPS	STEP PERFORMED	POINTS POSSIBLE	COMMENTS
15. Assisted patient from table as necessary.	_____	5	
16. Cleaned up examination room as needed.	_____	5	
a. Replaced supplies as needed (Gloves PRN)	_____	5	

EVALUATOR: NOTE TIME COMPLETED _____

ADD POINTS OF STEPS CHECKED   _____ EARNED
TOTAL POINTS POSSIBLE   170 POSSIBLE

Points assigned reflect importance of step to meeting objective: Important = (5)   Essential = (10)   Critical = (15)
Automatic failure results if any of the critical steps are omitted or performed incorrectly.

DETERMINE SCORE (divide points earned by total points possible, multiply results by 100)   _____ SCORE*

Evaluator's Name (print) _____ Signature _____

Comments _____

Name _____

Date _____ Score* _____

PROCEDURE 13-14   Assist with a Gynecological Examination and Pap Test

PERFORMANCE OBJECTIVE—Demonstrate each of the steps required in assisting with he gynecological (GYN) examination and Pap test.

PROCEDURE STEPS	STEP PERFORMED	POINTS POSSIBLE	COMMENTS
EVALUATOR: Place check mark in space following each step performed satisfactorily			
NOTE TIME BEGAN _____			
1. Stated purpose of procedure.	_____	10	
2. Washed hands.	_____	5	
3. Assembled all needed items on Mayo table.	_____	10	
4. Asked patient to empty her bladder.	_____	5	
(Instructed patient to leave urine specimen if ordered by physician).	_____	—	
5. Printed patient's name in pencil on frosted end of slide(s).	_____	10	
6. Explained procedure to patient.	_____	5	
7. Gave gown/drape sheet to patient and instructed her how to put it on.	_____	10	
a. Assisted patient PRN	_____	5	
b. Instructed patient to sit at end of table when ready and left door unlocked	_____	5	
8. Assisted patient to horizontal recumbent position.	_____	10	
9. Assisted patient into lithotomy position and draped.	_____	15	
10. Encouraged patient to breathe slowly and deeply through the mouth during exam.	_____	10	
11. Put on gloves.	_____	5	
12. Warmed vaginal speculum with warm water.	_____	5	
13. Handed speculum and spatula to physician.	_____	10	
14. Held slide for physician to apply smear.	_____	10	
15. Marked smear(s) accordingly.	_____	15	
16. Applied fixative or placed in alcohol-ether solution bottle.	_____	10	
17. Placed lubricant on physician's fingers for bimanual exam.	_____	5	
18. Discarded disposables in biohazardous container.	_____	10	
19. Removed gloves and washed hands.	_____	5	

PROCEDURE 13-14 Assist with a Gynecological Examination and Pap Test—continued

PROCEDURE STEPS	STEP PERFORMED	POINTS POSSIBLE	COMMENTS
20. Helped patient to sit up.	_____	5	
a. Pushed foot rest in	_____	5	
21. Helped patient down from exam table.	_____	5	
22. Returned items to proper storage area.	_____	5	
a. If metal speculum was used—placed in cool water to soak	_____	5	
23. Regloved PRN.	_____	5	
24. Instructed patient to dress.	_____	5	
25. Placed Pap smear slide(s) with completed request form in lab pick-up area.	_____	10	

EVALUATOR: NOTE TIME COMPLETED _____

ADD POINTS OF STEPS CHECKED   _____ EARNED
TOTAL POINTS POSSIBLE   220 POSSIBLE

Points assigned reflect importance of step to meeting objective: Important = (5)   Essential = (10)   Critical = (15)
Automatic failure results if any of the critical steps are omitted or performed incorrectly.

DETERMINE SCORE (divide points earned by total points possible, multiply results by 100)   _____ SCORE*

Evaluator's Name (print) _____ Signature _____

Comments _____

DOCUMENTATION

Chart the procedure in the patient's medical record.

Date: _____

Charting: _____

_____

_____

_____

Student's Name: _____   Physician's Initials: __(____)__

Name _____

Date _____ Score* _____

PROCEDURE 13-15 Measure Recumbent Length of Infant

PERFORMANCE OBJECTIVE—Demonstrate each step required in measuring the recumbent length of an infant and record; measurement should agree with instructor's by ± ⅛ inch.

PROCEDURE STEPS	STEP PERFORMED	POINTS POSSIBLE	COMMENTS
EVALUATOR: Place check mark in space following each step performed satisfactorily			
NOTE TIME BEGAN _____			
1. Washed hands.	_____	15	
2. Asked parent to place infant on exam table and explained procedure.	_____	5	
3. Instructed parent to remove shoes, socks/booties from infant.	_____	5	
4. Moved infant to end of table so that infant's head was at the zero mark of the ruler.	_____	15	
5. Asked parent to hold infant's head against the end of the table.	_____	15	
6. Straightened (gently) infant's back and legs to line up along ruler.	_____	10	
7. Placed infant's heels against footboard.	_____	10	
8. Read length of infant in inches or centimeters from ruler accurately.	_____	15	
9. Returned infant to parent.	_____	5	
10. Recorded measurement on			
a. Growth chart	_____	10	
b. Patient's chart	_____	10	
c. Parent's booklet	_____	5	
d. Initialed all	_____	5	
EVALUATOR: NOTE TIME COMPLETED _____			

ADD POINTS OF STEPS CHECKED   _____ EARNED
TOTAL POINTS POSSIBLE   125 POSSIBLE

Points assigned reflect importance of step to meeting objective: Important = (5)   Essential = (10)   Critical = (15)
Automatic failure results if any of the critical steps are omitted or performed incorrectly.

DETERMINE SCORE (divide points earned by total points possible, multiply results by 100)   _____ SCORE*

Evaluator's Name (print) _____ Signature _____

Comments _____

DOCUMENTATION

Chart the procedure in the patient's medical record.

Date: _____

Charting: _____

_____

_____

_____

Student's Name: _____   Physician's Initials: __(____)__

PERFORMANCE EVALUATION CHECKLIST   Name _____

Date _____ Score* _____

PROCEDURE 13-17   Weigh Infant

PERFORMANCE OBJECTIVE—Demonstrate each step of the procedure of weighing infants and record; weight must agree with instructor's by ± ⅛ lb.

PROCEDURE STEPS	STEP PERFORMED	POINTS POSSIBLE	COMMENTS
EVALUATOR: Place check mark in space following each step performed satisfactorily			
NOTE TIME BEGAN _____			
1. Washed hands.	_____	15	
2. Asked parent to remove infant's clothes.	_____	5	
3. Placed towel on scale.	_____	5	
4. Balanced scale at zero with towel in place.	_____	15	
5. Placed infant gently on scale.	_____	5	
6. Held hand over infant—not touching.	_____	5	
7. Talked to infant in quiet tone.	_____	5	
8. Kept diaper over genital area.	_____	5	
9. Slid weight easily.	_____	10	
10. Returned infant to parent.	_____	5	
11. Read weight accurately.	_____	15	
12. Removed towel from scale.	_____	5	
13. Placed towel in proper receptacle.	_____	5	
14. Balanced scale at zero.	_____	10	
15. Recorded weight accurately on:			
a. Growth chart	_____	15	
b. Patient's chart	_____	15	
c. Parent's booklet	_____	5	
d. Initialed all	_____	5	
EVALUATOR: NOTE TIME COMPLETED _____			

ADD POINTS OF STEPS CHECKED   _____ EARNED
TOTAL POINTS POSSIBLE   150 POSSIBLE

Points assigned reflect importance of step to meeting objective: Important = (5)   Essential = (10)   Critical = (15)
Automatic failure results if any of the critical steps are omitted or performed incorrectly.

DETERMINE SCORE (divide points earned by total points possible, multiply results by 100)   _____ SCORE*

Evaluator's Name (print) _____ Signature _____

Comments _____

411

DOCUMENTATION

Chart the procedure in the patient's medical record.

Date: _____

Charting: _____

_____

_____

_____

Student's Name: _____   Physician's Initials: __(____)__

Name _____

Date _____ Score* _____

PROCEDURE 13-18   Measure Head Circumference

PERFORMANCE OBJECTIVE—Demonstrate each step of the procedure for measuring head circumference of infants and record; measurement must agree with instructor's by ± ½ inch or 0.1 cm.

PROCEDURE STEPS	STEP PERFORMED	POINTS POSSIBLE	COMMENTS
EVALUATOR: Place check mark in space following each step performed satisfactorily			
NOTE TIME BEGAN _____			
1. Washed hands.	_____	15	
2. Talked to infant.	_____	5	
3. Asked parent for assistance.	_____	5	
4. Used thumb to hold tape measure at zero mark against forehead over the eyebrows.	_____	15	
5. Brought tape measure around infant's head over the ears to meet in front.	_____	15	
6. Pulled tape measure snugly to compress hair.	_____	10	
7. Read measurement to nearest 0.1 cm or 0.5 inch.	_____	15	
8. Recorded measurement accurately on:			
a. Growth chart	_____	15	
b. Patient's chart	_____	15	
c. Parent's booklet	_____	5	
d. Initialed all	_____	5	
EVALUATOR: NOTE TIME COMPLETED _____			

ADD POINTS OF STEPS CHECKED   _____ EARNED
TOTAL POINTS POSSIBLE   120 POSSIBLE

Points assigned reflect importance of step to meeting objective: Important = (5)   Essential = (10)   Critical = (15)
Automatic failure results if any of the critical steps are omitted or performed incorrectly.

DETERMINE SCORE (divide points earned by total points possible, multiply results by 100)   _____ SCORE*

Evaluator's Name (print) _____ Signature _____

Comments _____

DOCUMENTATION

Chart the procedure in the patient's medical record.

Date: _____

Charting: _____

_____

_____

_____

Student's Name: _____   Physician's Initials: ___(_____)___

Name _____

Date _____ Score* _____

PROCEDURE 13-19   Measure Infant's Chest

PERFORMANCE OBJECTIVE—Provided with a lifelike clinical infant doll and a flexible tape measure, demonstrate each step required in obtaining the chest measurement and record; the chest measurement must agree with instructor's by ± ⅛ inch (0.3 cm).

PROCEDURE STEPS	STEP PERFORMED	POINTS POSSIBLE	COMMENTS
EVALUATOR: Place check mark in space following each step performed satisfactorily			
NOTE TIME BEGAN _____			
1. Washed hands.	_____	15	
2. Talked to infant/gained cooperation.	_____	5	
3. Asked parent for assistance.	_____	5	
4. Held tape at zero with thumb at mid-sternal area of chest.	_____	15	
5. Brought tape around child's back to meet in front at zero mark under axillary region.	_____	15	
6. Made tape snug against chest.	_____	10	
7. Read measurement to nearest 0.1 cm or ½ inch.	_____	15	
8. Recorded measurement accurately on:			
a. Patient's chart	_____	15	
b. Parent's booklet	_____	15	
c. Initialed both	_____	5	
EVALUATOR: NOTE TIME COMPLETED _____			

ADD POINTS OF STEPS CHECKED   _____ EARNED

TOTAL POINTS POSSIBLE   115 POSSIBLE

Points assigned reflect importance of step to meeting objective: Important = (5)   Essential = (10)   Critical = (15)
Automatic failure results if any of the critical steps are omitted or performed incorrectly.

DETERMINE SCORE (divide points earned by total points possible, multiply results by 100)   _____ SCORE*

Evaluator's Name (print) _____ Signature _____

Comments _____

DOCUMENTATION

Chart the procedure in the patient's medical record.

Date: _____

Charting: _____

_____

_____

_____

Student's Name: _____   Physician's Initials: __(____)__

Name _____

Date _____ Score* _____

PROCEDURE 13-20   Assist with Sigmoidoscopy

PERFORMANCE OBJECTIVE—Demonstrate each of the steps required in assisting with the sigmoidoscopy procedure.

PROCEDURE STEPS	STEP PERFORMED	POINTS POSSIBLE	COMMENTS
EVALUATOR: Place check mark in space following each step performed satisfactorily			
NOTE TIME BEGAN _____			
1. Stated purpose of procedure.	_____	10	
2. Explained procedure to patient.	_____	5	
3. Asked patient to empty bladder.	_____	10	
4. Assembled all needed items on Mayo table at end of exam table.	_____	10	
a. Completed lab request form for biopsy if requested; labeled container	_____	10	
5. Checked light source.	_____	5	
6. Instructed patient to disrobe from waist down.	_____	5	
a. Assisted patient to sit at end of exam table	_____	5	
b. Covered patient with drape	_____	5	
7. Assisted patient with knee-chest or Sims' position just before exam.	_____	15	
8. Applied approximately two tablespoons of lubricant on gauze square for physician to use during exam.	_____	5	
9. Plugged in light source of sigmoidoscope.	_____	5	
a. Secured air inflation tubing	_____	5	
10. Washed hands and put on gloves.	_____	10	
11. Handed sigmoidoscope to physician.	_____	10	
a. Assisted as needed	_____	5	
12. Cleaned patient's anal area with tissues.	_____	5	
13. Removed gloves and washed hands.	_____	5	
14. Assisted patient to resting prone position.	_____	5	
15. Assisted patient to sitting position.	_____	5	
a. Then from table to dress	_____	5	
16. Regloved.	_____	5	
17. Cleaned up exam area.	_____	5	
a. Placed used instruments in basin of detergent solution to soak	_____	5	

PROCEDURE STEPS	STEP PERFORMED	POINTS POSSIBLE	COMMENTS
18. Removed gloves and washed hands.	_____	5	
19. Scheduled patient for further appointment(s).	_____	5	
20. Recorded procedure on patient's chart.	_____	5	
a. Initialed	_____	5	
21. Cleaned exam room; readied instruments for autoclave (regloved as necessary).	_____	5	

EVALUATOR: NOTE TIME COMPLETED _____

ADD POINTS OF STEPS CHECKED   _____ EARNED

TOTAL POINTS POSSIBLE   185 POSSIBLE

Points assigned reflect importance of step to meeting objective: Important = (5)   Essential = (10)   Critical = (15)

Automatic failure results if any of the critical steps are omitted or performed incorrectly.

DETERMINE SCORE (divide points earned by total points possible, multiply results by 100)   _____ SCORE*

Evaluator's Name (print) _____ Signature _____

Comments _____

DOCUMENTATION

Chart the procedure in the patient's medical record.

Date: _____

Charting: _____

_____

_____

_____

Student's Name: _____   Physician's Initials: __( )__

Name _____

Date _____ Score* _____

PROCEDURE 13-21   Administer Disposable Cleansing Enema

PERFORMANCE OBJECTIVE—Demonstrate each of the steps required in administering a cleansing enema.

PROCEDURE STEPS	STEP PERFORMED	POINTS POSSIBLE	COMMENTS
EVALUATOR: Place check mark in space following each step performed satisfactorily			
NOTE TIME BEGAN _____			
1. Identified patient.	_____	5	
a. Explained procedure to patient	_____	5	
2. Instructed patient to disrobe from waist down.	_____	5	
a. Provided drape sheet	_____	5	
b. Assisted patient onto exam table	_____	5	
3. Helped patient into Sims' position:	_____	10	
a. Instructed patient to lie on left side	_____	10	
b. Asked patient to bring right knee up to waist level	_____	15	
c. Adjusted drape sheet over patient	_____	5	
4. Washed hands.	_____	5	
a. Put on gloves	_____	5	
5. Removed protective covering from tip of enema container.	_____	10	
a. Applied small amount of lubricant to the tip	_____	5	
6. Separated buttocks to expose anus.	_____	10	
7. Inserted tip of bottle into anus.	_____	10	
a. Advised patient to breathe deeply and slowly through the mouth	_____	5	
8. Expressed entire contents into the anus.	_____	15	
a. Advised patient to retain contents for as long as possible	_____	15	
9. Withdrew enema tip slowly.	_____	5	
a. Provided tissues to patient	_____	5	
b. Disposed of used tissues in biohazardous container	_____	5	
10. Directed patient to restroom.	_____	5	
a. Asked patient to show results before flushing	_____	15	
11. Reported results to physician.	_____	10	

PROCEDURE STEPS	STEP PERFORMED	POINTS POSSIBLE	COMMENTS
12. Cleaned room	_____	5	
a. Discarded disposables in appropriate waste containers	_____	5	
13. Removed gloves	_____	10	
a. Washed hands	_____	10	
14. Initialed chart.	_____	5	

EVALUATOR: NOTE TIME COMPLETED _____

ADD POINTS OF STEPS CHECKED _____ EARNED
TOTAL POINTS POSSIBLE   225 POSSIBLE

Points assigned reflect importance of step to meeting objective: Important = (5)   Essential = (10)   Critical = (15)
Automatic failure results if any of the critical steps are omitted or performed incorrectly.

DETERMINE SCORE (divide points earned by total points possible, multiply results by 100) _____ SCORE*

Evaluator's Name (print) _____ Signature _____

Comments _____

DOCUMENTATION

Chart the procedure in the patient's medical record.

Date: _____

Charting: _____

_____

_____

_____

Student's Name: _____   Physician's Initials: _(____)_

Name _____

Date _____ Score* _____

PROCEDURE 14-1   Use a Microscope

PERFORMANCE OBJECTIVE—Provided with all necessary equipment and supplies, demonstrate the use of the microscope following the steps in the procedure with the instructor observing each step.

PROCEDURE STEPS	STEP PERFORMED	POINTS POSSIBLE	COMMENTS
EVALUATOR: Place check mark in space following each step performed satisfactorily			
NOTE TIME BEGAN _____			
1. Washed hands and put on gloves.	_____	5	
2. Assembled necessary equipment.	_____	5	
3. Labeled specimen on frosted end of slide with pencil.	_____	10	
4. Cleaned ocular lens with lens cleaning tissue.	_____	10	
5. Plugged light source into electrical outlet.	_____	15	
6. Turned light source on.	_____	10	
7. Placed specimen slide on stage with frosted side up between clips.	_____	10	
8. Secured slide over opening of stage.	_____	5	
9. Raised substage carefully.	_____	5	
10. Turned revolving nosepiece to 1pf (10X).	_____	5	
11. Began to focus until specimen was in view.	_____	10	
12. Turned fine adjustment until specimen was seen in detail.	_____	10	
13. Adjusted substage diaphragm lever for proper lighting.	_____	5	
14. Turned revolving nosepiece to intermediate (40X).	_____	5	
15. Adjusted fine focus for detail in viewing specimen.	_____	10	
16. Use hpf:			
a. Use cover slide	_____	10	
b. Clean lens after use	_____	5	
c. Adjust diaphragm lever	_____	5	
17. Identified specimen.	_____	5	
18. Turned light off.	_____	5	
19. Cleaned microscopic stage.	_____	5	
20. Disposed of clean slide(s).	_____	5	
21. Removed gloves and washed hands.	_____	5	

PROCEDURE STEPS	STEP PERFORMED	POINTS POSSIBLE	COMMENTS
22. Recorded findings of microscopic examination on chart	_____	15	
a. Initialed	_____	5	
EVALUATOR: NOTE TIME COMPLETED _____			

ADD POINTS OF STEPS CHECKED   _____ EARNED

TOTAL POINTS POSSIBLE   185 POSSIBLE

Points assigned reflect importance of step to meeting objective: Important = (5)   Essential = (10)   Critical = (15)
Automatic failure results if any of the critical steps are omitted or performed incorrectly.

DETERMINE SCORE (divide points earned by total points possible, multiply results by 100)   _____ SCORE*

Evaluator's Name (print) _____ Signature _____

Comments _____

Name _____

Date _____ Score* _____

PROCEDURE 14-2   Puncture Skin with Sterile Lancet

PERFORMANCE OBJECTIVE—Demonstrate skin puncture procedure following all steps to obtain capillary blood for test(s) specified by physician/instructor.

PROCEDURE STEPS	STEP PERFORMED	POINTS POSSIBLE	COMMENTS
EVALUATOR: Place check mark in space following each step performed satisfactorily			
NOTE TIME BEGAN _____			
1. Identified patient.	_____	5	
2. Explained procedure to patient.	_____	5	
3. Inspected patient's finger and selected puncture site.	_____	5	
4. Washed hands and put on gloves.	_____	5	
5. Assembled needed items next to patient.	_____	5	
6. Cleaned site with alcohol pad.	_____	5	
7. Allowed site to air dry.	_____	5	
8. Removed sterile lancet from package without contaminating it.	_____	10	
9. Secured puncture site between thumb and great finger.	_____	5	
10. Held lancet pointed downward between thumb and great finger of other hand.	_____	5	
11. Punctured site with a quick, firm, steady down-and-up motion.	_____	10	
a. Approximately 2mm deep	_____	5	
b. Control entry and exit of lancet to avoid ripping skin	_____	5	
12. Discarded first drop of blood by blotting with gauze square.	_____	10	
13. Applied gentle pressure on either side of puncture site to obtain desired amount of blood.	_____	15	
14. Wiped site with cotton ball/gauze square.	_____	10	
15. Asked patient to apply gentle pressure with gauze square over site to control bleeding.	_____	10	
16. Checked site and attended to patient.	_____	5	
17. Discarded disposables in proper receptacles.	_____	5	

PROCEDURE 14-2   Puncture Skin with Sterile Lancet—continued

PROCEDURE STEPS	STEP PERFORMED	POINTS POSSIBLE	COMMENTS
18. Removed gloves.	_____	5	
19. Washed hands.	_____	5	

EVALUATOR: NOTE TIME COMPLETED _____

ADD POINTS OF STEPS CHECKED   _____ EARNED

TOTAL POINTS POSSIBLE   140 POSSIBLE

Points assigned reflect importance of step to meeting objective: Important = (5)   Essential = (10)   Critical = (15)
Automatic failure results if any of the critical steps are omitted or performed incorrectly.

DETERMINE SCORE (divide points earned by total points possible, multiply results by 100)   _____ SCORE*

Evaluator's Name (print) _____ Signature _____

Comments _____

DOCUMENTATION

Chart the procedure in the patient's medical record.

Date: _____

Charting: _____

_____

_____

_____

Student's Name: _____   Physician's Initials: __(___)__

PERFORMANCE EVALUATION CHECKLIST

Name _____

Date _____ Score* _____

PROCEDURE 14-3   Obtain Blood for PKU Test

PERFORMANCE OBJECTIVE—Demonstrate the steps of the procedure for obtaining a blood specimen for determination of phenylketonuria level in the blood.

PROCEDURE STEPS	STEP PERFORMED	POINTS POSSIBLE	COMMENTS
EVALUATOR: Place check mark in space following each step performed satisfactorily			
NOTE TIME BEGAN _____			
1. Identified patient.	_____	5	
2. Explained procedure to patient.	_____	5	
3. Washed hands.	_____	5	
a. Put on gloves	_____	5	
4. Assembled all needed items.	_____	10	
5. Explained procedure to parent of patient.	_____	5	
6. Asked all necessary information.	_____	10	
7. Completed form.	_____	10	
8. Asked assistance of parent.	_____	5	
9. Performed skin puncture adequately.	_____	10	
10. Wiped first drop of blood from site.	_____	5	
11. Secured site between great finger and thumb.	_____	5	
12. Applied gentle pressure to produce large drop of blood.	_____	10	
13. Applied blood to the circles on the back of the form, saturating each circle completely.	_____	15	
14. Repeated steps 11 and 12 until all circles have been saturated.	_____	15	
15. Wiped puncture site with dry gauze square.	_____	5	
a. Asked patient to hold gently	_____	5	
b. Placed small round bandage over area	_____	5	
16. Placed completed PKU test form in protective paper envelope.	_____	10	
a. Then, into addressed envelope to health dept.	_____	10	
17. Discarded used items properly.	_____	5	
18. Removed gloves.	_____	5	
a. Washed hands	_____	5	

PROCEDURE STEPS	STEP PERFORMED	POINTS POSSIBLE	COMMENTS
19. Returned items to proper storage.	_____	5	
20. Recorded procedure on patient's chart.	_____	10	
a. Initialed	_____	5	

EVALUATOR: NOTE TIME COMPLETED _____

ADD POINTS OF STEPS CHECKED   _____ EARNED
TOTAL POINTS POSSIBLE   190 POSSIBLE

Points assigned reflect importance of step to meeting objective: Important = (5)   Essential = (10)   Critical = (15)
Automatic failure results if any of the critical steps are omitted or performed incorrectly.

DETERMINE SCORE (divide points earned by total points possible, multiply results by 100)   _____ SCORE*

Evaluator's Name (print) _____ Signature _____

Comments _____

DOCUMENTATION

Chart the procedure in the patient's medical record.

Date: _____

Charting: _____

_____

_____

_____

Student's Name: _____   Physician's Initials: __(____)__

Name _____

Date _____ Score* _____

PROCEDURE 14-4   Determine Hematocrit (Hct) Using Microhematocrit Centrifuge

PERFORMANCE OBJECTIVE—Demonstrate the steps of the procedure for determining hematocrit (Hct) readings using the microhematocrit centrifuge.

PROCEDURE STEPS	STEP PERFORMED	POINTS POSSIBLE	COMMENTS
EVALUATOR: Place check mark in space following each step performed satisfactorily			
NOTE TIME BEGAN _____			
1. Identified patient.	_____	5	
2. Explained procedure to patient.	_____	5	
3. Washed hands.	_____	5	
a. Put on gloves	_____	5	
4. Assembled necessary items.	_____	5	
5. Followed desired skin puncture procedure.	_____	5	
6. Held microhematocrit tube horizontally. (There should be no bubbles in tube. Subtract points if bubbles are present.)	_____	10	
7. Filled tube(s) to line.	_____	15	
8. Wiped puncture site with cotton ball.	_____	5	
9. Wiped outside end of glass tube while holding horizontally.	_____	5	
10. Placed carefully into clay tray to seal end of tube.	_____	10	
11. Instructed patient to hold dry gauze over site gently.	_____	5	
a. Make sure bleeding has stopped	_____	5	
12. Secured sealed end of tube against rubber padding of centrifuge.	_____	10	
13. Balanced centrifuge.	_____	10	
14. Noted number of placed tube in centrifuge.	_____	10	
15. Closed inside cover and locked by turning clockwise.	_____	10	
16. Closed and locked outside cover.	_____	10	
17. Listened for click to assure locking.	_____	5	
18. Turned timer switch past desired time and then to three minutes to set automatic timer.	_____	5	
19. Waited until completely stopped to unlock cover.	_____	15	
20. Placed bottom line of packed red cells up to buffy coat against calibrated chart (in centrifuge).	_____	15	
21. Used magnifying glass to read results.	_____	10	
22. Reclosed cover of centrifuge.	_____	5	

PROCEDURE STEPS	STEP PERFORMED	POINTS POSSIBLE	COMMENTS
23. Discarded used items in proper receptacle.	_____	5	
24. Removed gloves.	_____	5	
a. Washed hands	_____	5	
25. Returned items to proper storage.	_____	5	
26. Recorded reading in patient's chart as percentage	_____	15	
a. Initialed	_____	5	
EVALUATOR: NOTE TIME COMPLETED _____			

ADD POINTS OF STEPS CHECKED   _____ EARNED

TOTAL POINTS POSSIBLE   230 POSSIBLE

Points assigned reflect importance of step to meeting objective: Important = (5)   Essential = (10)   Critical = (15)
Automatic failure results if any of the critical steps are omitted or performed incorrectly.

DETERMINE SCORE (divide points earned by total points possible, multiply results by 100)   _____ SCORE*

Evaluator's Name (print) _____ Signature _____

Comments _____

DOCUMENTATION

Chart the procedure in the patient's medical record.

Date: _____

Charting: _____

_____

_____

_____

Student's Name: _____   Physician's Initials: __(____)__

Name _____

Date _____ Score* _____

PROCEDURE 14-5   Hemoglobin (Hb) Determination Using the Hemoglobinometer

PERFORMANCE OBJECTIVE—Demonstrate the steps of the procedure for determining hemoglobin (Hb) using the hemoglobinometer.

PROCEDURE STEPS	STEP PERFORMED	POINTS POSSIBLE	COMMENTS
EVALUATOR: Place check mark in space following each step performed satisfactorily			
NOTE TIME BEGAN _____			
1. Identified patient.	_____	5	
2. Washed hands.	_____	5	
a. Put on gloves	_____	5	
3. Assembled all necessary items.	_____	5	
4. Checked batteries and light bulb in hemoglobinometer.	_____	10	
5. Explained procedure to patient.	_____	5	
6. Followed desired skin puncture procedure.	_____	15	
7. Pulled glass chamber out of hemoglobinometer and fixed lower part of slide so that it was slightly offset.	_____	5	
8. Placed large drop of blood directly onto offset glass chamber.	_____	10	
9. Gave patient dry gauze to place over site gently.	_____	5	
10. Mixed blood on slide with hemolysis applicator.	_____	15	
11. Pushed chamber into clip and into slot on left side of hemoglobinometer.	_____	10	
12. Held hemoglobinometer in left hand at eye level.	_____	10	
13. Depressed light button on bottom of instrument.	_____	10	
14. Looked into hemoglobinometer to view green field.	_____	10	
15. Slid button on right of meter to match green field.	_____	15	
16. Left sliding scale lever where fields match.	_____	5	
17. Read hemoglobin level at top of calibrator scale.	_____	15	
18. Recorded reading on patient's chart.	_____	10	
a. Initialed	_____	5	
19. Washed chambers, rinsed, dried and returned to hemoglobinometer	_____	5	

PROCEDURE STEPS	STEP PERFORMED	POINTS POSSIBLE	COMMENTS
20. Removed gloves.	_____	5	
a. Washed hands.	_____	5	
21. Discarded disposable items.	_____	5	
22. Returned items to proper storage.	_____	5	

EVALUATOR: NOTE TIME COMPLETED _____

ADD POINTS OF STEPS CHECKED   _____ EARNED
TOTAL POINTS POSSIBLE   200 POSSIBLE

Points assigned reflect importance of step to meeting objective: Important = (5)   Essential = (10)   Critical = (15)
Automatic failure results if any of the critical steps are omitted or performed incorrectly.

DETERMINE SCORE (divide points earned by total points possible, multiply results by 100)   _____ SCORE*

Evaluator's Name (print) _____ Signature _____

Comments _____

DOCUMENTATION

Chart the procedure in the patient's medical record.

Date: _____

Charting: _____

_____

_____

_____

Student's Name: _____   Physician's Initials: _(____)_

Name _____

Date _____ Score* _____

PROCEDURE 14-6   Screen Blood Sugar (Glucose) Level

PERFORMANCE OBJECTIVE—Demonstrate the steps required in the procedure for determining blood glucose level.

PROCEDURE STEPS	STEP PERFORMED	POINTS POSSIBLE	COMMENTS
EVALUATOR: Place check mark in space following each step performed satisfactorily			
NOTE TIME BEGAN _____			
1. Identified patient.	_____	10	
2. Washed hands.	_____	5	
a. Put on gloves	_____	5	
3. Assembled all necessary items.	_____	5	
4. Calibrated instrument to be used (dextrometer).	_____	15	
5. Explained procedure to patient.	_____	5	
6. Followed desired skin puncture procedure.	_____	10	
7. Removed reagent strip from bottle without contaminating it.	_____	5	
8. Closed bottle.	_____	5	
9. Applied large drop of blood onto entire chemically treated surface of reagent strip.	_____	15	
10. Began timing immediately.	_____	15	
11. Wiped puncture site with cotton ball.	_____	5	
12. Gave patient dry gauze square to hold over site.	_____	5	
13. Blotted reagent strip after timing precisely.	_____	10	
14. Moved strip to clean area of tissue and blotted again.	_____	10	
15. Read strip by matching with color chart to determine glucose level of blood.	_____	15	
16. Recorded reading in patient's chart.	_____	15	
a. Initialed	_____	5	
17. Discarded used items.	_____	5	
18. Removed gloves.	_____	5	
a. Washed hands	_____	5	
19. Returned items to proper storage area.	_____	5	
EVALUATOR: NOTE TIME COMPLETED _____			

ADD POINTS OF STEPS CHECKED   _____ EARNED
TOTAL POINTS POSSIBLE   180 POSSIBLE

Points assigned reflect importance of step to meeting objective: Important = (5)   Essential = (10)   Critical = (15)
Automatic failure results if any of the critical steps are omitted or performed incorrectly.

DETERMINE SCORE (divide points earned by total points possible, multiply results by 100)   _____ SCORE*

Evaluator's Name (print) _____ Signature _____

Comments _____

431

DOCUMENTATION

Chart the procedure in the patient's medical record.

Date: _____

Charting: _____

_____

_____

_____

Student's Name: _____   Physician's Initials: _(___)_

432

Name _____

Date _____ Score* _____

PROCEDURE 14-7   Making a Blood Smear

PERFORMANCE OBJECTIVE—Demonstrate the steps required to make an adequate blood smear for a differential white blood cell count.

PROCEDURE STEPS	STEP PERFORMED	POINTS POSSIBLE	COMMENTS
EVALUATOR: Place check mark in space following each step performed satisfactorily			
NOTE TIME BEGAN _____			
1. Identified patient.	_____	10	
2. Explained procedure to patient.	_____	5	
3. Completed lab request form.	_____	5	
4. Printed patient's name on frosted end of slide(s).	_____	10	
5. Assembled necessary items near patient.	_____	5	
6. Washed hands.	_____	5	
a. Put on gloves	_____	5	
7. Performed desired method of obtaining blood specimen.	_____	10	
8. Placed a small drop of blood on end of slide	_____	5	
a. ¼″ from frosted end	_____	10	
b. Approximately ⅛″ in diameter	_____	10	
9. Held corners of frosted end of glass slide down on flat surface.	_____	10	
a. Held second slide at 45° angle	_____	10	
10. Rested spreader slide against frosted slide.	_____	10	
a. Moved slide back carefully into the blood	_____	10	
b. Allowed blood to flow to edge of slide	_____	15	
c. Moved angled slide toward frosted end quickly and gently	_____	15	
d. Made feathered edge	_____	15	
11. Allowed smear to air dry/fan dry.	_____	5	
12. Placed blood smear in lab container.	_____	5	
a. Attached lab request form	_____	5	

PROCEDURE 14-7   Making a Blood Smear—continued

PROCEDURE STEPS	STEP PERFORMED	POINTS POSSIBLE	COMMENTS
13. Removed gloves.	_____	5	
a. Washed hands	_____	5	
14. Discarded waste in appropriate containers.	_____	5	
15. Initialed procedure in patient's chart.	_____	5	

EVALUATOR: NOTE TIME COMPLETED _____

ADD POINTS OF STEPS CHECKED   _____ EARNED

TOTAL POINTS POSSIBLE   200 POSSIBLE

Points assigned reflect importance of step to meeting objective: Important = (5)   Essential = (10)   Critical = (15)

Automatic failure results if any of the critical steps are omitted or performed incorrectly.

DETERMINE SCORE (divide points earned by total points possible, multiply results by 100)   _____ SCORE*

Evaluator's Name (print) _____ Signature _____

Comments _____

DOCUMENTATION

Chart the procedure in the patient's medical record.

Date: _____

Charting: _____

_____

_____

_____

Student's Name: _____   Physician's Initials: _( )_

Name _____

Date _____ Score* _____

PROCEDURE 14-8   Obtain Venous Blood with Butterfly Needle Method

PERFORMANCE OBJECTIVE—Demonstrate the steps necessary for obtaining blood specimens using the butterfly needle method.

PROCEDURE STEPS	STEP PERFORMED	POINTS POSSIBLE	COMMENTS
EVALUATOR: Place check mark in space following each step performed satisfactorily			
NOTE TIME BEGAN _____			
1. Identified patient.	_____	5	
2. Explained procedure to patient.	_____	5	
3. Completed lab request form.	_____	5	
4. Assembled necessary items near patient.	_____	5	
5. Attached butterfly needle to syringe.	_____	10	
6. Put on gloves.	_____	5	
7. Palpated vein.	_____	5	
a. Cleaned skin with alcohol	_____	5	
b. Dried excess alcohol with cottonball	_____	5	
8. Applied tourniquet properly.	_____	10	
9. Asked patient to make fist and hold.	_____	10	
10. Removed needle guard.	_____	5	
a. Pushed air out of syringe	_____	5	
b. Quickly inserted needle into vein	_____	5	
c. Pulled back on plunger slowly	_____	10	
d. Obtained sufficient amount of blood	_____	15	
e. Removed tourniquet	_____	5	
f. Withdrew needle quickly	_____	5	
11. Filled appropriate blood tubes.	_____	15	
a. Filled in correct order	_____	15	
12. Applied gentle pressure to site with cottonball.	_____	5	
a. Advised patient to hold arm slightly upward	_____	5	
13. Applied bandaid to puncture site.	_____	5	
a. Asked if patient is allergic to adhesive	_____	5	
14. Placed used needle in biohazard sharps container.	_____	5	
15. Placed used disposables in biohazard bag.	_____	5	
16. Removed gloves and placed in biohazard bag.	_____	5	
17. Washed hands.	_____	5	

PROCEDURE STEPS	STEP PERFORMED	POINTS POSSIBLE	COMMENTS
18. Recorded procedure in patient's chart.	_____	5	
a. Initialed	_____	5	
EVALUATOR: NOTE TIME COMPLETED _____			

ADD POINTS OF STEPS CHECKED   _____ EARNED

TOTAL POINTS POSSIBLE   200 POSSIBLE

Points assigned reflect importance of step to meeting objective: Important = (5)   Essential = (10)   Critical = (15)

Automatic failure results if any of the critical steps are omitted or performed incorrectly.

DETERMINE SCORE (divide points earned by total points possible, multiply results by 100)   _____ SCORE*

Evaluator's Name (print) _____ Signature _____

Comments _____

DOCUMENTATION

Chart the procedure in the patient's medical record.

Date: _____

Charting: _____

_____

_____

_____

Student's Name: _____   Physician's Initials: __(   )__

Name _____

Date _____ Score* _____

PROCEDURE 14-9   Obtain Venous Blood with Sterile Needle and Syringe

PERFORMANCE OBJECTIVE—Demonstrate the steps necessary for obtaining venous blood using the sterile needle and syringe
method.

PROCEDURE STEPS	STEP PERFORMED	POINTS POSSIBLE	COMMENTS
EVALUATOR: Place check mark in space following each step performed satisfactorily			
NOTE TIME BEGAN _____			
1. Identified patient.	_____	10	
2. Washed hands.	_____	5	
a. Put on gloves	_____	5	
3. Assembled necessary items near patient.	_____	5	
4. Completed lab request form.	_____	5	
a. Labeled specimen tube(s)	_____	5	
5. Explained procedure to patient.	_____	5	
a. Asked patient for preferred venipuncture site	_____	5	
6. Positioned patient appropriately.	_____	5	
7. Secured needle into syringe.	_____	10	
a. Pushed in plunger to expel air from barrel	_____	10	
8. Applied tourniquet to patient's upper arm.	_____	5	
a. Placed 3″ above elbow	_____	10	
9. Cleansed site lightly with alcohol/cottonball.	_____	5	
a. Allowed alcohol to air dry/dried with cottonball	_____	5	
10. Asked patient to clench fist to make vein stand up.	_____	5	
11. Took needle guard off.	_____	5	
a. Pointed bevel of needle up	_____	10	
b. Inserted needle tip into vein with quick and steady motion	_____	10	
c. Inserted needle into vein at 15° angle	_____	10	
d. Held skin taut for easier insertion	_____	5	
e. Inserted needle between ¼″ and ½″	_____	15	
12. Held barrel of syringe in one hand.	_____	5	
a. Pulled plunger back with other hand	_____	5	
b. Pulled plunger slowly/steadily	_____	5	
c. Allowed sufficient blood collection for specimen tube(s)	_____	15	
d. Asked patient to release clenched fist slowly	_____	5	
e. Released tourniquet within one minute	_____	10	
f. Pulled needle out in same path as inserted	_____	5	

PROCEDURE STEPS	STEP PERFORMED	POINTS POSSIBLE	COMMENTS
g. Placed cottonball/gauze square over site	_____	5	
13. Instructed patient to apply gentle pressure to site and elevate arm slightly.	_____	5	
14. Filled specimen tube(s) quickly.	_____	10	
a. Angled flow of blood to run down side of tube	_____	10	
b. Filled tubes in correct order of draw	_____	15	
c. Made blood smears as needed	_____	5	
15. Stood red-stoppered tubes vertically.	_____	5	
a. Did not shake tubes/mixed additives carefully	_____	5	
16. Deposited needle/syringe in sharps container.	_____	5	
17. Assembled specimen tubes/lab form together in biobag.	_____	5	
18. Attended to patient's needs.	_____	5	
a. Applied bandage	_____	5	
19. Discarded disposables in proper containers.	_____	5	
20. Removed gloves/placed in biobag.	_____	5	
a. Washed hands	_____	5	
21. Returned items to proper storage.	_____	5	
22. Recorded procedure in patient's chart.	_____	10	
a. Initialed	_____	5	

EVALUATOR: NOTE TIME COMPLETED _____

ADD POINTS OF STEPS CHECKED   _____ EARNED
TOTAL POINTS POSSIBLE   320 POSSIBLE

Points assigned reflect importance of step to meeting objective: Important = (5)   Essential = (10)   Critical = (15)
Automatic failure results if any of the critical steps are omitted or performed incorrectly.

DETERMINE SCORE (divide points earned by total points possible, multiply results by 100)   _____ SCORE*

Evaluator's Name (print) _____ Signature _____

Comments _____

DOCUMENTATION

Chart the procedure in the patient's medical record.

Date: _____

Charting: _____

_____

_____

_____

Student's Name: _____   Physician's Initials: ___( )___

Name _____

Date _____ Score* _____

PROCEDURE 14-10   Obtain Venous Blood with Vacuum Tube

PERFORMANCE OBJECTIVE—Demonstrate the steps necessary for obtaining venous blood using the vacuum tube method.

PROCEDURE STEPS	STEP PERFORMED	POINTS POSSIBLE	COMMENTS
EVALUATOR: Place check mark in space following each step performed satisfactorily			
NOTE TIME BEGAN _____			
1. Identified patient.	_____	10	
2. Washed hands.	_____	5	
3. Assembled necessary items near patient.	_____	5	
4. Completed lab request form.	_____	5	
a. Labeled specimen tube(s)	_____	5	
5. Explained procedure to patient.	_____	5	
a. Asked patient for preferred venipuncture site	_____	5	
6. Positioned patient appropriately.	_____	5	
7. Put on gloves.	_____	5	
8. Secured needle into adapter.	_____	10	
9. Applied tourniquet to patient's upper arm.	_____	5	
a. Placed 3″ above elbow	_____	10	
10. Cleansed site lightly with alcohol/cottonball.	_____	5	
a. Allowed alcohol to air dry/dried with cottonball	_____	5	
11. Asked patient to clench fist to make vein stand up.	_____	5	
12. Took needle guard off.	_____	5	
a. Pointed bevel of needle up	_____	10	
b. Inserted needle tip into vein with quick and steady motion	_____	10	
c. Inserted needle into vein at 15° angle	_____	10	
d. Held skin taut for easier insertion	_____	5	
e. Inserted needle between ¼″ and ½″	_____	15	
13. Held adapter with one hand.	_____	5	
a. Placed index and great fingers of other hand on either side of protruding edges of adapter	_____	5	
b. Pushed vacuum tube completely into adapter with thumb	_____	10	
c. Allowed needle to puncture rubber stopper	_____	15	
d. Asked patient to release clenched fist slowly	_____	5	
e. Released tourniquet within one minute	_____	10	
f. Pulled filled tube out by holding it between			

PROCEDURE 14-10   Obtain Venous Blood with Vacuum Tube—continued

PROCEDURE STEPS	STEP PERFORMED	POINTS POSSIBLE	COMMENTS
thumb and great finger and pushed against adapter with index finger	_____	5	
g. Filled required number of tubes in correct order	_____	10	
h. Pulled needle out in same path as inserted	_____	5	
i. Placed cottonball/gauze square over site	_____	5	
14. Instructed patient to apply gentle pressure to site and elevate arm slightly.	_____	5	
15. Stood red-stoppered tubes vertically.	_____	5	
a. Did not shake tubes/mixed additives carefully	_____	5	
b. Made blood smear if ordered	_____	5	
16. Deposited needle/syringe in sharps container.	_____	5	
17. Assembled specimen tubes/lab form together in biobag.	_____	5	
18. Attended to patient's needs.	_____	5	
a. Applied bandage	_____	5	
19. Discarded disposables in proper containers.	_____	5	
20. Removed gloves/placed in biobag.	_____	5	
a. Washed hands	_____	5	
21. Returned items to proper storage.	_____	5	
22. Recorded procedure in patient's chart.	_____	5	
a. Initialed	_____	5	

EVALUATOR: NOTE TIME COMPLETED _____

ADD POINTS OF STEPS CHECKED   _____ EARNED
TOTAL POINTS POSSIBLE   290 POSSIBLE

Points assigned reflect importance of step to meeting objective: Important = (5)   Essential = (10)   Critical = (15)
Automatic failure results if any of the critical steps are omitted or performed incorrectly.

DETERMINE SCORE (divide points earned by total points possible, multiply results by 100)   _____ SCORE*

Evaluator's Name (print) _____ Signature _____

Comments _____

DOCUMENTATION

Chart the procedure in the patient's medical record.

Date: _____

Charting: _____
_____
_____
_____

Student's Name: _____   Physician's Initials: __( )__

Name _____

Date _____ Score* _____

PROCEDURE 14-11   Catheterize Urinary Bladder

PERFORMANCE OBJECTIVE—Demonstrate all required steps to perform a urinary bladder catheterization.

PROCEDURE STEPS	STEP PERFORMED	POINTS POSSIBLE	COMMENTS
EVALUATOR: Place check mark in space following each step performed satisfactorily			
NOTE TIME BEGAN _____			
1. Identify patient.	_____	5	
2. Placed catheter kit on Mayo table next to patient.	_____	5	
3. Explained procedure to patient.	_____	5	
4. a. Adjusted lamp	_____	5	
b. Turned lamp on	_____	5	
5. Asked patient to lie back on table.	_____	5	
a. Assisted patient into dorsal recumbent position	_____	10	
b. Assisted patient in positioning her feet in stirrups	_____	10	
6. Draped patient with sheet.	_____	5	
a. Exposed only external genitalia	_____	5	
7. Pulled out foot rest.	_____	5	
8. Opened outer wrapping of sterile kit.	_____	5	
9. Placed sterile towel between patient's knees.	_____	5	
10. Placed sterile plastic sheet under patient's buttocks.	_____	5	
11. Placed catheter kit on foot rest.	_____	5	
12. Asked patient to keep knees apart.	_____	5	
13. Washed and dried hands.	_____	5	
14. Put on sterile latex gloves.	_____	5	
15. Poured antiseptic solution over cotton balls in medicine cups.	_____	10	
16. Opened urine specimen container.	_____	5	
17. Applied sterile lubricant to one of the gauze squares.	_____	5	
18. Spread labia and wiped genitalia with each of the three antiseptic soaked cotton balls.	_____	10	
a. Used front to back motion	_____	10	
b. Discarded onto Mayo table	_____	5	
19. Placed tip of catheter in lubricant and other end of catheter into basin.	_____	5	
20. Held catheter about four inches from lubricated end.	_____	5	
21. Inserted lubricated tip of catheter into urinary meatus gently.	_____	15	
22. Instructed patient to breathe slowly and deeply.	_____	5	
23. Stopped urine flow by closing metal clamps attached to tubing.	_____	10	
24. Positioned end of tube into urine specimen container.	_____	10	

PROCEDURE 14-11   Catheterize Urinary Bladder—continued

PROCEDURE STEPS	STEP PERFORMED	POINTS POSSIBLE	COMMENTS
25. Released clamp to collect specimen.	_____	10	
26. Allowed remainder of urine flow to collect in basin.	_____	5	
a. Measured amount of urine—both specimen and basin	_____	15	
27. Withdrew catheter tube gently.	_____	5	
28. Dried area with sterile gauze squares or cotton balls.	_____	5	
29. Secured lid onto urine specimen container.	_____	5	
30. Placed reusable items in cold water to soak.	_____	5	
31. Removed items from foot rest.	_____	5	
32. Cleaned exam table.	_____	5	
33. Discarded gloves and other disposables.	_____	5	
34. Washed hands.	_____	5	
35. Turned lamp off and returned to usual position.	_____	5	
36. Assisted patient in sitting up or relaxing in a horizontal recumbent position.	_____	5	
37. Labeled specimen (completed request form and attached).	_____	5	
38. Assisted patient from exam table.	_____	5	
39. Recorded procedure and measured amount of urine.	_____	5	
a. Observations and comments	_____	5	
b. Initialed	_____	5	

EVALUATOR: NOTE TIME COMPLETED _____

ADD POINTS OF STEPS CHECKED   _____ EARNED

TOTAL POINTS POSSIBLE   300 POSSIBLE

Points assigned reflect importance of step to meeting objective: Important = (5)   Essential = (10)   Critical = (15)
Automatic failure results if any of the critical steps are omitted or performed incorrectly.

DETERMINE SCORE (divide points earned by total points possible, multiply results by 100)   _____ SCORE*

Evaluator's Name (print) _____ Signature _____

Comments _____

DOCUMENTATION

Chart the procedure in the patient's medical record.

Date: _____

Charting: _____

_____

_____

_____

Student's Name: _____   Physician's Initials: __(___)__

PERFORMANCE EVALUATION CHECKLIST

Name _____

Date _____ Score* _____

PROCEDURE 14-12   Test Urine with Multistix® 10   SG

PERFORMANCE OBJECTIVE—Demonstrate the steps required to perform the procedure for using Multistix® 10 SG.

PROCEDURE STEPS	STEP PERFORMED	POINTS POSSIBLE	COMMENTS
EVALUATOR: Place check mark in space following each step performed satisfactorily			
NOTE TIME BEGAN _____			
1. Washed hands.	_____	5	
a. Put on gloves	_____	5	
2. Assembled all needed items.	_____	5	
3. Stirred urine with tongue depressor.	_____	10	
4. Removed cap from bottle.	_____	5	
5. Took reagent strip out without touching test paper end.	_____	5	
6. Placed cap back on bottle securely.	_____	5	
7. Reviewed times given for reading each test on bottle.	_____	5	
8. Dipped test paper end of reagent strip into urine specimen.	_____	5	
9. Removed strip by touching its edge against inside of container to remove excess urine.	_____	5	
10. Began timing test immediately.	_____	15	
11. Placed reagent strip next to color chart.	_____	10	
12. Read each test section at proper time.	_____	15	
13. Discarded disposables in proper receptacle.	_____	5	
14. Returned items to proper storage.	_____	5	
15. Removed gloves.	_____	5	
a. Washed hands	_____	5	
16. Recorded results of each test section on patient's chart.	_____	15	
EVALUATOR: NOTE TIME COMPLETED _____			

ADD POINTS OF STEPS CHECKED   _____ EARNED
TOTAL POINTS POSSIBLE   130 POSSIBLE

Points assigned reflect importance of step to meeting objective: Important = (5)   Essential = (10)   Critical = (15)
Automatic failure results if any of the critical steps are omitted or performed incorrectly.

DETERMINE SCORE (divide points earned by total points possible, multiply results by 100)   _____ SCORE*

Evaluator's Name (print) _____ Signature _____

Comments _____

DOCUMENTATION

Chart the procedure in the patient's medical record.

Date: _____

Charting: _____

_____

_____

_____

Student's Name: _____   Physician's Initials: __(____)__

Name _____

Date _____ Score* _____

PROCEDURE 14-13   Determine Glucose Content of Urine with Clinitest Tablet

PERFORMANCE OBJECTIVE—Demonstrate the steps in the procedure for using Clinitest tablets to determine the glucose content of urine.

PROCEDURE STEPS	STEP PERFORMED	POINTS POSSIBLE	COMMENTS
EVALUATOR: Place check mark in space following each step performed satisfactorily			
NOTE TIME BEGAN _____			
1. Washed hands.	_____	5	
a. Put on gloves	_____	5	
2. Assembled needed items.	_____	5	
3. Stirred urine with tongue depressor.	_____	5	
4. Filled dropper halfway with urine.	_____	5	
5. Held test tube near top between thumb and index finger.	_____	5	
6. Released five drops of urine into test tube.	_____	10	
7. Rinsed dropper.	_____	5	
8. Half filled dropper with water.	_____	10	
9. Released ten drops water into test tube.	_____	10	
10. Mixed gently.	_____	5	
11. Set test tube in rack.	_____	5	
12. Opened bottle.	_____	5	
13. Shook out one Clinitest tablet into bottle cap.	_____	10	
14. Dropped one tablet into test tube from cap.	_____	10	
15. Recapped bottle.	_____	5	
16. Watched reaction of tablet and urine-water mixture.	_____	15	
17. Began 15 second timing immediately when boiling stopped.	_____	15	
18. Held test tube at top.	_____	10	
19. Tilted test tube back and forth to mix contents.	_____	10	
20. Compared color of contents to color chart to read results.	_____	15	
21. Recorded results as % of milligrams/deciliter on patient's chart.	_____	15	
a. Initialed	_____	5	
22. Rinsed test tube with cold water.	_____	5	
23. Washed and dried test tube and dropper.	_____	5	

PROCEDURE 14-13   Determine Glucose Content of Urine with Clinitest Tablet—continued

PROCEDURE STEPS	STEP PERFORMED	POINTS POSSIBLE	COMMENTS
24. Discarded disposables in proper receptacle.	_____	5	
25. Removed gloves.	_____	5	
a. Washed hands	_____	5	
26. Returned items to proper storage.	_____	5	
EVALUATOR: NOTE TIME COMPLETED _____			

ADD POINTS OF STEPS CHECKED   _____ EARNED

TOTAL POINTS POSSIBLE   220 POSSIBLE

Points assigned reflect importance of step to meeting objective: Important = (5)   Essential = (10)   Critical = (15)

Automatic failure results if any of the critical steps are omitted or performed incorrectly.

DETERMINE SCORE (divide points earned by total points possible, multiply results by 100)   _____ SCORE*

Evaluator's Name (print) _____ Signature _____

Comments _____

DOCUMENTATION

Chart the procedure in the patient's medical record.

Date: _____

Charting: _____

_____

_____

_____

Student's Name: _____   Physician's Initials: __(_____)__

Name _____

Date _____ Score* _____

PROCEDURE 14-14   Obtain Urine Sediment for Microscopic Examination

PERFORMANCE OBJECTIVE—Demonstrate all steps required in the procedure for obtaining urine sediment for microscopic examination.

PROCEDURE STEPS	STEP PERFORMED	POINTS POSSIBLE	COMMENTS
EVALUATOR: Place check mark in space following each step performed satisfactorily			
NOTE TIME BEGAN _____			
1. Washed hands.	_____	5	
a. Put on gloves	_____	5	
2. Assembled all needed items near patient.	_____	5	
a. Explained procedure	_____	5	
3. Identified patient.	_____	5	
4. Performed skin puncture.	_____	5	
5. Filled RBC unopette pipette and reservoir:	_____	10	
a. Punctured diaphragm of reservoir	_____	10	
b. Removed shield from pipette assembly with a twist	_____	5	
c. Held pipette almost horizontally to touch tip of pipette to sample	_____	5	
d. Wiped excess sample from pipette	_____	5	
e. Squeezed reservoir slightly	_____	5	
f. Covered opening of overflow chamber with index finger and seated pipette securely in reservoir neck	_____	5	
g. Released pressure on reservoir	_____	5	
h. Squeezed reservoir gently 2 to 3 times to rinse capillary bore	_____	5	
i. Placed index finger over upper opening and gently inverted several times to mix well	_____	5	
6. Converted to dropper assembly:			
a. Withdrew pipette from reservoir and reseated securely in reverse position	_____	5	
b. Inverted reservoir and gently squeezed sides to discard first 3 to 4 drops	_____	5	
7. Positioned cover glass onto hemocytometer.	_____	5	
8. Placed tip of pipette almost touching the "V" on the slide's chamber.	_____	10	
9. Released moderate drop of solution onto both sides of chamber.	_____	10	
10. Waited 2 to 3 minutes for cells to settle.	_____	5	
11. Placed slide on microscope stage.	_____	5	
a. Turned light on	_____	5	

PROCEDURE STEPS	STEP PERFORMED	POINTS POSSIBLE	COMMENTS
22. Removed gloves.	_____	5	
a. Washed hands	_____	5	
23. Returned items to proper storage.	_____	5	

EVALUATOR: NOTE TIME COMPLETED _____

ADD POINTS OF STEPS CHECKED   _____ EARNED

TOTAL POINTS POSSIBLE   195 POSSIBLE

Points assigned reflect importance of step to meeting objective: Important = (5)   Essential = (10)   Critical = (15)

Automatic failure results if any of the critical steps are omitted or performed incorrectly.

DETERMINE SCORE (divide points earned by total points possible, multiply results by 100)   _____ SCORE*

Evaluator's Name (print) _____ Signature _____

Comments _____

DOCUMENTATION

Chart the procedure in the patient's medical record.

Date: _____

Charting: _____

_____

_____

_____

Student's Name: _____   Physician's Initials: _( )_

Name _____

Date _____ Score* _____

PROCEDURE 14-15   Instruct Patient to Collect Sputum Specimen

PERFORMANCE OBJECTIVE—Demonstrate all steps required in the procedure for instructing a patient in the collection of a sputum specimen for analysis.

PROCEDURE STEPS	STEP PERFORMED	POINTS POSSIBLE	COMMENTS
EVALUATOR: Place check mark in space following each step performed satisfactorily			
NOTE TIME BEGAN _____			
1. Assembled items next to patient.	_____	10	
2. Wrote patient's name on specimen cup label.	_____	10	
3. Completed lab request form.	_____	5	
4. Explained physician's orders to patient.	_____	10	
a. Wrote instructions out/gave printed instructions to patient	_____	15	
5. Instructed patient to:			
a. Expel only those secretions of first AM coughing episode into center of cup	_____	15	
b. Fill cup one-half full	_____	10	
c. Seal with cover	_____	5	
d. Write time and date on label and request form	_____	10	
e. Take to lab/medical office as soon as possible	_____	10	
f. Secure lab request form to specimen container with tape or rubber band	_____	5	
g. Refrigerate if she/he cannot take within two hours	_____	10	
6. Record what instructions were given to patient.	_____	5	
a. Initialed	_____	5	
EVALUATOR: NOTE TIME COMPLETED _____			

ADD POINTS OF STEPS CHECKED   _____ EARNED
TOTAL POINTS POSSIBLE   125 POSSIBLE

Points assigned reflect importance of step to meeting objective: Important = (5)   Essential = (10)   Critical = (15)
Automatic failure results if any of the critical steps are omitted or performed incorrectly.

DETERMINE SCORE (divide points earned by total points possible, multiply results by 100)   _____ SCORE*

Evaluator's Name (print) _____ Signature _____

Comments _____

DOCUMENTATION

Chart the procedure in the patient's medical record.

Date: _____

Charting: _____

_____

_____

_____

Student's Name: _____   Physician's Initials: __( )__

Name _____

Date _____ Score* _____

PROCEDURE 14-16   Instruct Patient to Collect a Stool Specimen

PERFORMANCE OBJECTIVE—Demonstrate the steps required in the procedure for instructing a patient in the collection of an adequate stool specimen for laboratory analysis.

PROCEDURE STEPS	STEP PERFORMED	POINTS POSSIBLE	COMMENTS
EVALUATOR: Place check mark in space following each step performed satisfactorily			
NOTE TIME BEGAN _____			
1. Assembled items next to patient.	_____	10	
2. Identified patient.	_____	10	
3. Explained physician's orders.	_____	10	
4. Gave printed instructions or wrote out.	_____	10	
5. Wrote information on label of specimen cups and lab request form.	_____	5	
6. Instructed patient to:			
a. Obtain small amount of stool from next bowel movement with tongue depressor	_____	15	
b. Place specimen in container	_____	10	
c. Secure cup with cover	_____	5	
d. Write date and time of specimen on label	_____	5	
e. Write time and date on request form and attach request form to specimen container	_____	5	
f. Take to lab/medical office as soon as possible	_____	10	
g. Refrigerate specimen if she/he cannot take within two hours	_____	10	
7. Explained when report would be available.	_____	5	
8. Recorded that instructions were given on patient's chart.	_____	15	
a. Initialed	_____	5	

EVALUATOR: NOTE TIME COMPLETED _____

ADD POINTS OF STEPS CHECKED _____ EARNED

TOTAL POINTS POSSIBLE 130 POSSIBLE

Points assigned reflect importance of step to meeting objective: Important = (5)   Essential = (10)   Critical = (15)
Automatic failure results if any of the critical steps are omitted or performed incorrectly.

DETERMINE SCORE (divide points earned by total points possible, multiply results by 100) _____ SCORE*

Evaluator's Name (print) _____ Signature _____

Comments _____

DOCUMENTATION

Chart the procedure in the patient's medical record.

Date: _____

Charting: _____

_____

_____

_____

Student's Name: _____   **Physician's Initials:** __(____)__

Name _____

Date _____ Score* _____

PROCEDURE 14-17   Perform a Hemoccult® Sensa® Test

PERFORMANCE OBJECTIVE—Demonstrate each step required in the Hemoccult® Sensa® testing procedure.

PROCEDURE STEPS	STEP PERFORMED	POINTS POSSIBLE	COMMENTS
EVALUATOR: Place check mark in space following each step performed satisfactorily			
NOTE TIME BEGAN _____			
1. Washed hands.	_____	5	
2. Put on gloves.	_____	5	
3. Assembled items needed for testing on counter.	_____	10	
4. Opened test slide of Hemoccult paper slide.	_____	10	
5. Removed cap from bottle of developer.	_____	5	
6. Placed 2 drops of developer on each of three sections:			
a. A	_____	15	
b. B	_____	15	
c. Control	_____	15	
7. Began timing immediately for 60 seconds.	_____	15	
8. Watched closely for any change of color at 30 seconds.	_____	5	
9. Compared test with control and read results after 60-second time period.	_____	15	
10. Recorded results on patient's chart.	_____	15	
a. Initialed	_____	5	
11. Discarded disposables.	_____	5	
12. Returned items to proper storage.	_____	5	
13. Removed gloves.	_____	5	
a. Washed hands	_____	5	

EVALUATOR: NOTE TIME COMPLETED _____

ADD POINTS OF STEPS CHECKED   _____ EARNED

TOTAL POINTS POSSIBLE   155 POSSIBLE

Points assigned reflect importance of step to meeting objective: Important = (5)   Essential = (10)   Critical = (15)

Automatic failure results if any of the critical steps are omitted or performed incorrectly.

DETERMINE SCORE (divide points earned by total points possible, multiply results by 100)   _____ SCORE*

Evaluator's Name (print) _____ Signature _____

Comments _____

DOCUMENTATION

Chart the procedure in the patient's medical record.

Date: _____

Charting: _____

_____

_____

_____

Student's Name: _____   Physician's Initials: __(____)__

Name _____

Date _____ Score* _____

PROCEDURE 14-18   Prepare Bacteriological Smear

PERFORMANCE OBJECTIVE—Demonstrate the steps of the procedure for preparing a bacteriological smear for microscopic analysis.

PROCEDURE STEPS	STEP PERFORMED	POINTS POSSIBLE	COMMENTS
EVALUATOR: Place check mark in space following each step performed satisfactorily			
NOTE TIME BEGAN _____			
1. Assembled all needed items.	_____	10	
2. Penciled patient's name on frosted end of glass slide.	_____	10	
3. Completed lab request form.	_____	5	
4. Washed hands.	_____	5	
a. Put on gloves	_____	5	
5. Prepared smear(s):	_____	5	
a. Held slide with thumb and great finger	_____	5	
b. Rolled swab containing specimen evenly over two-thirds of slide	_____	15	
6. Lit bunsen burner.	_____	5	
a. Adjusted flame	_____	5	
7. Held frosted part of slide with forceps or thumb and index finger.	_____	5	
8. Passed smear (side up) of slide through blue flame two or three times.	_____	15	
9. Turned burner off.	_____	5	
10. Placed heat-fixed smear on staining rack or Placed on stage of microscope for observation.	_____	10	
11. Discarded used disposables in proper receptacle.	_____	5	
12. Returned items to proper storage.	_____	5	
13. Removed gloves.	_____	5	
a. Washed hands	_____	5	
14. Recorded procedure on patient's chart	_____	5	
a. Initialed	_____	5	

EVALUATOR: NOTE TIME COMPLETED _____

ADD POINTS OF STEPS CHECKED   _____ EARNED
TOTAL POINTS POSSIBLE   135 POSSIBLE

Points assigned reflect importance of step to meeting objective: Important = (5)   Essential = (10)   Critical = (15)
Automatic failure results if any of the critical steps are omitted or performed incorrectly.

DETERMINE SCORE (divide points earned by total points possible, multiply results by 100)   _____ SCORE*

Evaluator's Name (print) _____ Signature _____

Comments _____

DOCUMENTATION

Chart the procedure in the patient's medical record.

Date: _____

Charting: _____

_____

_____

_____

Student's Name: _____   Physician's Initials: __(____)__

Name _____

Date _____ Score* _____

PROCEDURE 14-19   Obtain a Throat Culture

PERFORMANCE OBJECTIVE—Demonstrate the steps required to perform the procedure for obtaining a throat culture.

PROCEDURE STEPS	STEP PERFORMED	POINTS POSSIBLE	COMMENTS
EVALUATOR: Place check mark in space following each step performed satisfactorily			
NOTE TIME BEGAN _____			
1. Identified patient.	_____	5	
2. Washed hands.	_____	10	
a. Put on gloves	_____	5	
b. Assembled needed items near patient	_____	5	
3. Labeled culture plate.	_____	5	
a. Completed lab request form if required	_____	10	
4. Explained procedure to patient.	_____	5	
5. Assisted patient into comfortable position.	_____	5	
a. Asked for assistance if child.	_____	5	
6. Opened sterile swab.	_____	5	
7. Asked patient to open mouth wide.	_____	5	
8. Examined patient's throat visually with light.	_____	10	
9. Depressed tongue with sterile tongue depressor.	_____	15	
10. Asked patient to say "ahh."	_____	15	
11. Inserted sterile swab to back of throat.	_____	5	
12. Rolled swab over area to obtain specimen.	_____	15	
13. Removed swab and depressor from patient's mouth.	_____	10	
14. Attended to patient; offered tissue.	_____	10	
15. Applied specimen to agar of petri dish in pattern.	_____	15	
16. Placed lid on dish.	_____	5	
a. Secured with tape	_____	5	
17. Discarded disposables in proper receptacle.	_____	5	
18. Placed culture dish in incubator bottom up or Attached request form and sent to lab.	_____	5	
19. Removed gloves.	_____	5	
a. Washed hands	_____	5	

PROCEDURE 14-19   Obtain a Throat Culture—continued

PROCEDURE STEPS	STEP PERFORMED	POINTS POSSIBLE	COMMENTS
20. Recorded procedure in patient's chart.	_____	5	
a. Initialed	_____	5	

EVALUATOR: NOTE TIME COMPLETED _____

ADD POINTS OF STEPS CHECKED   _____ EARNED
TOTAL POINTS POSSIBLE   200 POSSIBLE

Points assigned reflect importance of step to meeting objective: Important = (5)   Essential = (10)   Critical = (15)
Automatic failure results if any of the critical steps are omitted or performed incorrectly.

DETERMINE SCORE (divide points earned by total points possible, multiply results by 100)   _____ SCORE*

Evaluator's Name (print) _____ Signature _____

Comments _____

DOCUMENTATION

Chart the procedure in the patient's medical record.

Date: _____

Charting: _____

_____

_____

_____

Student's Name: _____   Physician's Initials: __(_____)__

PERFORMANCE EVALUATION CHECKLIST

Name _____

Date _____ Score* _____

PROCEDURE 14-20   Prepare Gram Stain

PERFORMANCE OBJECTIVE—Demonstrate the steps of the procedure for preparing a Gram stain.

PROCEDURE STEPS	STEP PERFORMED	POINTS POSSIBLE	COMMENTS
EVALUATOR: Place check mark in space following each step performed satisfactorily			
NOTE TIME BEGAN _____			
1. Assembled all needed items on counter.	_____	10	
2. Washed hands.	_____	5	
a. Put apron/gloves on	_____	5	
3. Placed heat-fixed slide on staining rack.	_____	5	
4. Opened crystal violet dye.	_____	5	
5. Filled dropper.	_____	5	
6. Applied over entire specimen area of slide.	_____	10	
7. Timed for sixty seconds.	_____	10	
8. Held frosted end with forceps.	_____	5	
9. Tipped slide to allow stain to run off into tray.	_____	5	
10. Washed slide with water from top to bottom.	_____	10	
11. Placed slide flat on rack.	_____	5	
12. Filled dropper with Gram's iodine.	_____	10	
13. Applied over entire specimen area.	_____	10	
14. Tipped slide to allow stain to run off.	_____	5	
15. Refilled dropper with Gram's iodine.	_____	10	
16. Applied to entire specimen area.	_____	10	
a. Timed for sixty seconds	_____	5	
17. Tipped slide to allow stain to run off.	_____	5	
18. Washed slide with water.	_____	10	
19. Applied alcohol/acetone with dropper until purple color in excess runoff was gone.	_____	15	
20. Washed with water immediately.	_____	10	
21. Applied Safranin solution with dropper.	_____	10	
22. Immediately washed with water.	_____	10	
23. Held slide by frosted end.	_____	5	
24. Wiped excess solution from underneath.	_____	5	

PROCEDURE STEPS	STEP PERFORMED	POINTS POSSIBLE	COMMENTS
25. Held slide on its side and tapped onto paper towel to remove excess.	_____	5	
26. Allowed slide to air dry or Blotted slide carefully between two paper towels.	_____	5	
27. Applied small drop of immersion oil to specimen.	_____	5	
a. Placed cover glass on slide	_____	5	
28. Placed slide on stage of microscope to view.	_____	5	
a. Turned light source on to view	_____	5	
29. Discarded disposables in proper receptacle.	_____	5	
30. Washed used items.	_____	5	
31. Returned items to proper storage.	_____	5	
a. Replaced caps on bottles immediately after use	_____	5	
32. Removed gloves.	_____	5	
a. Washed hands	_____	5	
33. Recorded procedure and results on patient's chart.	_____	5	
a. Initialed	_____	15	

EVALUATOR: NOTE TIME COMPLETED _____

ADD POINTS OF STEPS CHECKED   _____ EARNED

TOTAL POINTS POSSIBLE   280 POSSIBLE

Points assigned reflect importance of step to meeting objective: Important = (5) Essential = (10) Critical = (15)
Automatic failure results if any of the critical steps are omitted or performed incorrectly.

DETERMINE SCORE (divide points earned by total points possible, multiply results by 100)   _____ SCORE*

Evaluator's Name (print) _____ Signature _____

Comments _____

DOCUMENTATION

Chart the procedure in the patient's medical record.

Date: _____

Charting: _____

_____

_____

_____

Student's Name: _____   Physician's Initials: __(__)__

PROCEDURE 15-1   Perform a Scratch Test

PERFORMANCE OBJECTIVE—Demonstrate each of the steps required in the scratch test procedure.

PROCEDURE STEPS	STEP PERFORMED	POINTS POSSIBLE	COMMENTS
EVALUATOR: Place check mark in space following each step performed satisfactorily			
NOTE TIME BEGAN _____			
1. Identified patient.	_____	10	
2. Assembled all needed items next to patient.	_____	10	
3. Washed hands.	_____	5	
4. Put on gloves.	_____	5	
5. Explained procedure to patient.	_____	5	
6. Assisted patient into comfortable position.	_____	5	
7. Prepared test site with alcohol pad.	_____	5	
a. Allowed to air dry	_____	5	
8. Marked site(s) with initials or number of extract in pen.	_____	10	
a. Spaced adequately (about 1½″ to 2″ between each)	_____	10	
9. Applied small drop of extract onto site.	_____	10	
a. Repeated for each extract ordered	_____	10	
10. Removed sterile needle or lancet without contaminating it.	_____	15	
a. Made one-eighth inch scratch in surface of skin at site.	_____	15	
11. Began timing for 20 minutes.	_____	15	
12. Checked each site as soon as 20-minute period was up.	_____	15	
a. Cleaned each site with alcohol pad	_____	10	
b. Did not wash off extract identification	_____	15	
13. Washed hands.	_____	5	
14. Compared reaction sites with package insert drawing or measured reaction sites in centimeters.	_____	15	
15. Recorded test results on patient's chart.	_____	15	
a. Initialed	_____	5	
b. Attended to patient	_____	5	
16. Discarded disposables in proper receptacle.	_____	5	

PROCEDURE STEPS	STEP PERFORMED	POINTS POSSIBLE	COMMENTS
17. Returned items to proper storage area.	_____	5	
18. Removed gloves.	_____	5	
a. Washed hands	_____	5	

EVALUATOR: NOTE TIME COMPLETED _____

ADD POINTS OF STEPS CHECKED   _____ EARNED

TOTAL POINTS POSSIBLE   240 POSSIBLE

Points assigned reflect importance of step to meeting objective: Important = (5) Essential = (10) Critical = (15)
Automatic failure results if any of the critical steps are omitted or performed incorrectly.

DETERMINE SCORE (divide points earned by total points possible, multiply results by 100)   _____ SCORE*

Evaluator's Name (print) _____ Signature _____

Comments _____

DOCUMENTATION

Chart the procedure in the patient's medical record.

Date: _____

Charting: _____

_____

_____

_____

Student's Name: _____   Physician's Initials: ___(   )___

Name _____

Date _____ Score* _____

PROCEDURE 15-2   Apply a Patch Test

PERFORMANCE OBJECTIVE—Demonstrate each of the steps required in carrying out the skin patch test, including the 48 hour recheck.

PROCEDURE STEPS	STEP PERFORMED	POINTS POSSIBLE	COMMENTS
EVALUATOR: Place check mark in space following each step performed satisfactorily			
NOTE TIME BEGAN _____			
1. Identified patient.	_____	10	
2. Assembled items next to patient.	_____	10	
3. Washed hands.	_____	5	
4. Put on gloves.	_____	5	
5. Explained procedure to patient.	_____	5	
6. Assisted patient into comfortable sitting position.	_____	5	
7. Cleaned test site with alcohol pad.	_____	5	
a. Allowed to air dry	_____	5	
8. Applied substance to test site.	_____	10	
9. Secured substance to test site with non-allergic tape.	_____	15	
10. Recorded date, time, substance, and area tested on patient's chart.	_____	15	
a. Initialed	_____	5	
11. Scheduled patient to return in 48 hours for check.	_____	5	
12. Instructed patient to keep test area clean and dry.	_____	10	
13. Removed gloves.	_____	5	
a. Washed hands	_____	5	
When patient returned after 48 hours:			
14. Washed hands.	_____	5	
a. Put on gloves	_____	5	
15. Removed patch.	_____	5	
16. Read results of test.	_____	15	
17. Removed gloves.	_____	5	
a. Washed hands	_____	5	

PROCEDURE 15-2   Apply a Patch Test—continued

PROCEDURE STEPS	STEP PERFORMED	POINTS POSSIBLE	COMMENTS
Recorded results on patient's chart.	_____	5	
a. Initialed	_____	5	
EVALUATOR: NOTE TIME COMPLETED _____			

ADD POINTS OF STEPS CHECKED   _____ EARNED
TOTAL POINTS POSSIBLE   170 POSSIBLE

Points assigned reflect importance of step to meeting objective: Important = (5)   Essential = (10)   Critical = (15)
Automatic failure results if any of the critical steps are omitted or performed incorrectly.

DETERMINE SCORE (divide points earned by total points possible, multiply results by 100)   _____ SCORE*

Evaluator's Name (print) _____ Signature _____

Comments _____

DOCUMENTATION

Chart the procedure in the patient's medical record.

Date: _____

Charting: _____

_____

_____

_____

Student's Name: _____   Physician's Initials: __(   )__

Name _____

Date _____ Score* _____

PROCEDURE 15-3   Obtain a Standard 12-Lead Electrocardiogram

PERFORMANCE OBJECTIVE—Demonstrate each of the steps required in obtaining a standard 12-lead ECG reading.

PROCEDURE STEPS	STEP PERFORMED	POINTS POSSIBLE	COMMENTS
EVALUATOR: Place check mark in space following each step performed satisfactorily			
NOTE TIME BEGAN _____			
1. Identified patient.	_____	5	
2. Plugged in ECG machine to electrical outlet, away from known electrical interference.	_____	5	
3. Assembled electrodes.	_____	5	
a. Attached to straps	_____	5	
b. Applied electrolyte pads	_____	5	
4. Turned machine on.	_____	5	
5. Washed hands.	_____	5	
6. Asked patient to disrobe from waist up and remove clothing from lower legs.	_____	5	
7. Explained procedure to patient.	_____	5	
8. Assisted patient to table.	_____	5	
a. Asked patient to lie down.	_____	5	
b. Covered patient with drape sheet.	_____	5	
c. Pulled out foot rest.	_____	5	
d. Adjusted pillow under patient's head.	_____	5	
Note: For computerized electrocardiographs:			
a. Applied limb and chest lead wires by clipping to disposable electrodes.	_____	15	
b. Pressed "auto" to run complete 12-lead recording.	_____	10	
c. Removed patient cable and proceeded with step 28.	_____	5	
9. Placed chest strap with hard plastic end under left side of patient's back.	_____	5	
a. Weighed end at patient's right side.	_____	5	
10. Placed upper limb electrodes on outer fleshy area of upper arms.	_____	10	
a. Pointed connectors of electrodes toward shoulders.	_____	5	
b. Moved straps one space tighter than relaxed.	_____	5	
11. Placed lower limb electrodes on inner fleshy area of lower legs.	_____	5	
a. Pointed connectors toward upper part of body	_____	5	

PROCEDURE STEPS	STEP PERFORMED	POINTS POSSIBLE	COMMENTS
12. Connected lead wire tips to electrodes, all pointing downward.	_____	5	
13. Placed power cord directed away from patient.	_____	5	
14. Placed chest electrode under chest strap.	_____	5	
a. Placed electrolyte side up	_____	5	
15. Turned lead selector switch to STD.	_____	5	
a. Adjusted stylus to center of graph paper.	_____	5	
16. Moved record switch to 25 mm/second position.	_____	10	
a. Ran for a few seconds to adjust centering	_____	5	
b. Made standardization mark correctly	_____	5	
c. Turned off	_____	5	
17. Turned lead selector switch to Lead I.	_____	15	
a. Ran 8″–12″ of tracing.	_____	15	
b. Proceeded to run 8″–12″ of Leads II and III.	_____	15	
18. Ran 4″–6″ of leads aVR, aVL and aVF.	_____	15	
19. Paused between leads to allow machine to adjust automatically.	_____	5	
20. Made standardization mark at the beginning of each lead.	_____	5	
21. Marked each lead appropriately with correct code marking.	_____	15	
22. Placed chest electrode in proper positions, V1–V6.	_____	15	
a. Standardized each lead	_____	5	
b. Ran 4″–6″ of each	_____	5	
c. Marked each lead correctly	_____	15	
d. Turned switch to AMP off when changing electrode position	_____	5	
e. Paused a few seconds between leads to allow stylus to adjust	_____	5	
23. Turned lead selector switch back to STD slowly.	_____	5	
a. Ran tracing out until only baseline appears	_____	5	
24. Turned machine off.	_____	5	
25. Tore tracing from machine.	_____	5	
a. Marked immediately with patient's name, age, date	_____	10	
b. Initialed	_____	5	
26. Rolled or loosely overlapped tracing and secured with paper clip.	_____	5	
27. Removed tips of lead wires from limb electrodes.	_____	5	
a. Removed chest electrode and strap	_____	5	
b. Removed limb straps from patient	_____	5	

PROCEDURE STEPS	STEP PERFORMED	POINTS POSSIBLE	COMMENTS
c. Instructed patient to wash areas well	_____	5	
28. Removed electrolyte from areas with warmed towel; dried area.	_____	5	
a. Discarded in proper receptacle	_____	5	
29. Assisted patient to sitting position.	_____	5	
a. Assisted patient down from table	_____	5	
b. Assisted to dress PRN	_____	5	
30. Changed table paper and pillow cover.	_____	5	
a. Discarded disposables	_____	5	
31. Washed hands.	_____	5	
32. Placed tracing in patient's chart.	_____	5	
a. Initialed ECG order in chart	_____	5	
b. Placed tracing in appropriate area for physician to read or Mounted tracing/placed in patient's chart for physician to read.	_____	5	
33. Recorded any unusual findings or observations on patient's chart.	_____	10	

EVALUATOR: NOTE TIME COMPLETED _____

ADD POINTS OF STEPS CHECKED   _____ EARNED
TOTAL POINTS POSSIBLE   455 POSSIBLE Steps 1–33
                                                                                      140 *Steps 1–8; 28–33

Points assigned reflect importance of step to meeting objective: Important = (5)   Essential = (10)   Critical = (15)
Automatic failure results if any of the critical steps are omitted or performed incorrectly.

DETERMINE SCORE (divide points earned by total points possible, multiply results by 100)   _____ SCORE*

Evaluator's Name (print) _____ Signature _____

Comments _____

DOCUMENTATION

Chart the procedure in the patient's medical record.

Date: _____

Charting: _____

_____

_____

_____

Student's Name: _____   Physician's Initials: __(   )__

Name _____

Date _____ Score* _____

PROCEDURE 15-4   Holter Monitoring

PERFORMANCE OBJECTIVE—Demonstrate the steps of the procedure for hooking up a patient for the Holter monitor.

PROCEDURE STEPS	STEP PERFORMED	POINTS POSSIBLE	COMMENTS
EVALUATOR: Place check mark in space following each step performed satisfactorily			
NOTE TIME BEGAN _____			
1. Identified patient.	_____	5	
2. Explained procedure to patient.	_____	5	
3. Asked patient to remove clothing from the waist up.	_____	5	
4. Provided drape sheet.	_____	5	
5. Assisted patient to end of exam table.	_____	5	
6. Washed hands.	_____	5	
7. Assembled equipment and supplies near patient.	_____	5	
8. Tested Holter monitor for proper function.	_____	15	
9. Used shaving cream and razor to remove excess hair from patient's chest.	_____	10	
10. Rinsed, dried, and used alcohol on electrode sites.	_____	5	
11. Rubbed each site vigorously with gauze squares.	_____	10	
12. Applied electrodes/lead wires.	_____	15	
a. Made good contact	_____	15	
b. Secured electrodes with tape	_____	10	
13. Placed belt with recorder around patient's waist.	_____	10	
a. Advised patient in care of recorder	_____	10	
14. Assisted patient in dressing.	_____	5	
15. Instructed patient to perform routine activities.	_____	5	
a. Advised not to bathe in tub or shower	_____	10	
16. Recorded date and time monitor began on patient's chart.	_____	15	
a. Recorded in patient's diary	_____	10	
17. Instructed patient to record symptoms in diary.	_____	10	
18. Gave patient return appointment time in 24 hours.	_____	10	
19. When patient returned:			
a. Assisted patient in disrobing	_____	5	
b. Removed electrodes and wires	_____	5	

PROCEDURE 15-4   Holter Monitoring—continued

PROCEDURE STEPS	STEP PERFORMED	POINTS POSSIBLE	COMMENTS
c. Placed cassette in computerized ECG for printout of tracing	_____	15	
d. Placed diary and recording of ECG in patient's chart	_____	10	
e. Initialed	_____	5	
EVALUATOR: NOTE TIME COMPLETED _____			

ADD POINTS OF STEPS CHECKED   _____ EARNED

TOTAL POINTS POSSIBLE   240 POSSIBLE

Points assigned reflect importance of step to meeting objective: Important = (5)   Essential = (10)   Critical = (15)

Automatic failure results if any of the critical steps are omitted or performed incorrectly.

DETERMINE SCORE (divide points earned by total points possible, multiply results by 100)   _____ SCORE*

Evaluator's Name (print) _____ Signature _____

Comments _____

DOCUMENTATION

Chart the procedure in the patient's medical record.

Date: _____

Charting: _____

_____

_____

_____

Student's Name: _____   Physician's Initials: __(____)__

Name _____

Date _____ Score* _____

PROCEDURE 16-1   Prepare Skin for Minor Surgery

PERFORMANCE OBJECTIVE—Demonstrate each of the steps required in the skin prep procedure for minor surgery.

PROCEDURE STEPS	STEP PERFORMED	POINTS POSSIBLE	COMMENTS
EVALUATOR: Place check mark in space following each step performed satisfactorily			
NOTE TIME BEGAN _____			
1. Washed hands.	_____	5	
2. Assembled all necessary items.	_____	10	
3. Identified patient.	_____	5	
a. Explained procedure to patient	_____	5	
4. Asked patient to remove necessary clothing.	_____	5	
a. Instructed patient where to put clothing	_____	5	
b. Assisted patient as necessary	_____	5	
5. Positioned patient appropriately.	_____	5	
a. Draped patient appropriately	_____	5	
6. Positioned Mayo table over patient near surgical site.	_____	5	
7. Positioned gooseneck lamp over site.	_____	5	
8. Placed gauze squares in soapy solution.	_____	10	
a. Used one at a time to soap area to be shaved.	_____	10	
b. Discarded each in basin after use	_____	10	
9. Used scissors to clip hair as necessary.	_____	10	
10. Shaved hair placing razor at 30° angle.	_____	10	
a. Held skin taut while shaving	_____	10	
b. Shaved in direction hair grows	_____	15	
c. Wiped hair and soap from razor with tissues	_____	10	
d. Swished razor through soapy water	_____	5	
e. Shook excess water from razor	_____	5	
f. Repeated steps 10 a through e as necessary	_____	15	
11. Removed all soap and hair from site with sterile gauze and water.	_____	10	
a. Dried area with sterile gauze squares	_____	5	
12. Applied antiseptic solution to site with sterile gauze.	_____	15	
a. Applied in a circular motion from center outward	_____	10	

PROCEDURE STEPS	STEP PERFORMED	POINTS POSSIBLE	COMMENTS
13. Covered skin prep area with sterile drape sheet.	_____	10	
a. Instructed patient not to touch site/tray	_____	5	
14. Discarded disposable items in proper container.	_____	5	
15. Returned reusable items to proper storage.	_____	5	
16. Removed gloves and discarded properly.	_____	5	
17. Washed hands.	_____	5	
18. Initialed procedure completed.	_____	5	
19. Attended to patient comfort.	_____	5	

EVALUATOR: NOTE TIME COMPLETED _____

ADD POINTS OF STEPS CHECKED   _____ EARNED
TOTAL POINTS POSSIBLE   255 POSSIBLE

Points assigned reflect importance of step to meeting objective: Important = (5)   Essential = (10)   Critical = (15)
Automatic failure results if any of the critical steps are omitted or performed incorrectly.

DETERMINE SCORE (divide points earned by total points possible, multiply results by 100)   _____ SCORE*

Evaluator's Name (print) _____ Signature _____

Comments _____

DOCUMENTATION

Chart the procedure in the patient's medical record.

Date: _____

Charting: _____

_____

_____

_____

Student's Name: _____   Physician's Initials: __(_____)__

Name _____

Date _____ Score* _____

PROCEDURE 16-2   Put on Sterile Gloves

PERFORMANCE OBJECTIVE—Demonstrate the correct method of putting on sterile gloves.

PROCEDURE STEPS	STEP PERFORMED	POINTS POSSIBLE	COMMENTS
EVALUATOR: Place check mark in space following each step performed satisfactorily			
NOTE TIME BEGAN _____			
1. Selected appropriate size gloves.	_____	10	
2. Removed jewelry.	_____	5	
3. Performed surgical scrub.	_____	10	
a. Used nail brush	_____	5	
b. Thoroughly dried hands	_____	5	
4. Opened sterile gloves without contaminating them.	_____	15	
a. Placed package on counter with cuffs of gloves toward body	_____	10	
5. Grasped cuff with finger and thumb of non-dominant hand.	_____	10	
a. Inserted dominant hand in glove	_____	10	
b. Pulled glove onto dominant hand by pulling cuff with non-dominant hand	_____	10	
6. Placed gloved fingers under cuff of other glove.	_____	15	
a. Inserted hand into glove	_____	10	
b. Pushed up on folded cuff	_____	10	
7. Placed gloved fingers under each cuff to smooth gloves over wrists	_____	15	
a. Checked gloves for tears and holes.	_____	10	
8. Kept hands above waist level.	_____	10	
a. Did not touch anything other than sterile items.	_____	10	
9. Removed gloves by pulling outside cuff with thumb and fingers.	_____	10	
a. Pulled gloves off inside out	_____	5	
b. Did not touch contaminated side	_____	5	

PROCEDURE STEPS	STEP PERFORMED	POINTS POSSIBLE	COMMENTS
10. Placed gloves in biohazard bag.	_____	5	
EVALUATOR: NOTE TIME COMPLETED _____			

ADD POINTS OF STEPS CHECKED   _____ EARNED

TOTAL POINTS POSSIBLE   195 POSSIBLE

Points assigned reflect importance of step to meeting objective: Important = (5)   Essential = (10)   Critical = (15)
Automatic failure results if any of the critical steps are omitted or performed incorrectly.

DETERMINE SCORE (divide points earned by total points possible, multiply results by 100)   _____ SCORE*

Evaluator's Name (print) _____ Signature _____

Comments _____

PROCEDURE 16-3   Assist with Minor Surgery

PERFORMANCE OBJECTIVE—Demonstrate each of the steps required in assisting with minor surgery.

PROCEDURE STEPS	STEP PERFORMED	POINTS POSSIBLE	COMMENTS
EVALUATOR: Place check mark in space following each step performed satisfactorily			
NOTE TIME BEGAN _____			
1. Identified patient.	_____	10	
2. Washed hands.	_____	5	
3. Assembled appropriate items on Mayo tray (sterile packs).	_____	15	
a. Positioned next to treatment table	_____	10	
b. Checked expiration dates of items	_____	10	
4. Explained procedure to patient.	_____	5	
a. Obtained signature on consent form	_____	5	
b. Advised patient to empty bladder	_____	5	
c. Took vital signs and recorded	_____	5	
d. Instructed patient to disrobe as indicated for procedure	_____	10	
e. Advised where to put belongings	_____	5	
5. Assisted patient to treatment table.	_____	5	
a. Positioned patient	_____	10	
6. Performed skin prep procedure.	_____	10	
7. Draped patient appropriately.	_____	5	
8. Placed sterile towel on Mayo tray.	_____	5	
a. Put sterile gloves on	_____	10	
b. Opened sterile items at tabs	_____	10	
c. Placed items in order of use	_____	10	
d. Covered with sterile towel	_____	10	
e. Removed gloves	_____	5	
f. Washed hands	_____	5	
9. When physician was ready to begin:			
a. Removed cover	_____	5	
b. Handed physician sterile gloves	_____	5	
c. Wiped top of vial with alcohol	_____	5	
d. Held anesthetic vial for doctor	_____	5	
10. Washed hands and regloved to assist.	_____	10	
a. Mopped with sterile gauze	_____	15	
b. Handed sterile items to physician PRN	_____	15	

PROCEDURE STEPS	STEP PERFORMED	POINTS POSSIBLE	COMMENTS
c. Opened specimen container for biopsy	_____	15	
d. Clipped suture PRN	_____	10	
11. Cleaned and bandaged surgery site.	_____	5	
a. Asked patient if allergic to adhesive	_____	5	
12. Removed gloves.	_____	5	
a. Washed hands	_____	5	
13. Assisted patient to sitting position.	_____	5	
a. And then from table	_____	5	
14. Provided patient education.	_____	5	
a. Care of site	_____	5	
b. Return visit appointment given	_____	5	
15. Regloved to clean up room.	_____	5	
a. Discarded disposables in biohazardous waste container	_____	5	
b. Rinsed instruments in cool water and placed in detergent solution to soak	_____	5	
16. Removed gloves.	_____	5	
a. Washed hands	_____	5	
17. Restocked room	_____	5	

EVALUATOR: NOTE TIME COMPLETED _____

ADD POINTS OF STEPS CHECKED   _____ EARNED
TOTAL POINTS POSSIBLE   330 POSSIBLE

Points assigned reflect importance of step to meeting objective: Important = (5)   Essential = (10)   Critical = (15)
Automatic failure results if any of the critical steps are omitted or performed incorrectly.

DETERMINE SCORE (divide points earned by total points possible, multiply results by 100)   _____ SCORE*

Evaluator's Name (print) _____ Signature _____

Comments _____

DOCUMENTATION

Chart the procedure in the patient's medical record.

Date: _____

Charting: _____

_____

_____

_____

Student's Name: _____   Physician's Initials: __(____)__

Name _____

Date _____ Score* _____

PROCEDURE 16-4 Assisting with Suturing a Laceration

PERFORMANCE OBJECTIVE—Demonstrate each of the steps required in the procedure to assist with suturing a laceration.

PROCEDURE STEPS	STEP PERFORMED	POINTS POSSIBLE	COMMENTS
EVALUATOR: Place check mark in space following each step performed satisfactorily			
NOTE TIME BEGAN _____			
1. Washed hands.	_____	5	
2. Assembled all necessary items.	_____	10	
3. Identified patient.	_____	5	
a. Explained procedure to patient	_____	5	
b. Advised patient to empty bladder	_____	5	
4. Took and recorded patient's vital signs.	_____	5	
5. Asked/assisted patient in removing clothing.	_____	5	
a. Explained where to store clothing	_____	5	
6. Positioned patient appropriately.	_____	10	
7. Performed skin prep of site.	_____	15	
8. Draped patient appropriately.	_____	10	
9. Assembled unsterile items on Mayo tray.	_____	10	
10. Answered patient's questions.	_____	5	
11. Opened sterile pack on Mayo tray.	_____	5	
a. Handled sterile towel from underneath	_____	10	
b. Dropped sterile items on sterile field as appropriate	_____	15	
12. Put PPE and sterile gloves on.	_____	15	
13. Arranged sterile items in order of use.	_____	15	
a. Covered sterile field with sterile towel	_____	5	
14. Removed gloves.	_____	5	
a. Washed hands.	_____	5	
Assisting physician with actual procedure:			
15. Removed cover from set-up.	_____	5	
16. Handed sterile gloves to physician.	_____	10	
17. Held vial of anesthetic for physician.	_____	5	
a. Wiped top of vial with alcohol pad	_____	5	
18. Washed hands.	_____	5	
a. Put on sterile gloves	_____	15	
19. Handed sterile items to physician as needed.	_____	15	
20. Mopped excess blood from site/sterile gauze.	_____	15	
21. Clipped sutures as directed by physician.	_____	15	

PROCEDURE 16-4   Assisting with Suturing a Laceration—continued

PROCEDURE STEPS	STEP PERFORMED	POINTS POSSIBLE	COMMENTS
22. Assisted with cleaning site.	_____	15	
a. Bandaged site appropriately	_____	10	
b. Asked if patient has adhesive allergy	_____	10	
c. Regloved as necessary	_____	5	
d. Disposed of soiled items in biohazardous bag	_____	5	
e. Washed hands	_____	5	
23. Administered tetanus toxoid as directed by physician.	_____	5	
24. Assisted patient in sitting.	_____	5	
a. Assisted patient in dressing	_____	5	
b. Assisted patient from exam table	_____	5	
25. Instructed patient in caring for suture site.	_____	5	
26. Provided return appointment.	_____	10	
27. Put on gloves to clean up room.	_____	5	
a. Placed disposables in biobag/sharps	_____	10	
b. Rinsed instruments in cool water	_____	5	
c. Placed instruments in detergent solution	_____	5	
28. Removed gloves/PPE.	_____	5	
a. Placed soiled disposables in biobag	_____	5	
b. Washed hands	_____	5	
29. Restocked treatment room.	_____	5	
30. Recorded procedure in patient's chart.	_____	5	
a. Initialed	_____	5	

EVALUATOR: NOTE TIME COMPLETED _____

ADD POINTS OF STEPS CHECKED   _____ EARNED
TOTAL POINTS POSSIBLE   400 POSSIBLE

Points assigned reflect importance of step to meeting objective: Important = (5)   Essential = (10)   Critical = (15)
Automatic failure results if any of the critical steps are omitted or performed incorrectly.

DETERMINE SCORE (divide points earned by total points possible, multiply results by 100)   _____ SCORE*

Evaluator's Name (print) _____ Signature _____

Comments _____

DOCUMENTATION

Chart the procedure in the patient's medical record.

Date: _____

Charting: _____

_____

_____

_____

Student's Name: _____   Physician's Initials: __(____)__

Name _____

Date _____ Score* _____

PROCEDURE 16-5   Remove Sutures

PERFORMANCE OBJECTIVE—Demonstrate the steps required in removing sutures.

PROCEDURE STEPS	STEP PERFORMED	POINTS POSSIBLE	COMMENTS
EVALUATOR: Place check mark in space following each step performed satisfactorily			
NOTE TIME BEGAN _____			
1. Identified patient.	_____	5	
2. Washed hands.	_____	5	
3. Placed Mayo tray next to treatment table.	_____	5	
a. Assembled items on tray	_____	5	
4. Asked about condition of suture site.	_____	5	
a. If laceration/ask about booster	_____	5	
b. Took vital signs and recorded	_____	5	
c. Recorded other information	_____	5	
5. Asked patient to remove appropriate clothing if necessary.	_____	10	
6. Assisted patient to treatment table.	_____	5	
a. Into position and draped as necessary	_____	10	
b. Explained procedure	_____	5	
7. Washed hands.	_____	5	
a. Put gloves on	_____	5	
8. Removed bandage/inspected site.	_____	10	
9. Soaked to remove bandage if stuck.	_____	10	
10. Advised physician to check the site.	_____	10	
11. Followed doctor's orders to remove sutures.	_____	15	
a. Opened sterile pack of instruments	_____	15	
b. Used thumb forceps to grasp knot of suture and pull up	_____	15	
c. Placed tip of suture removal scissors next to skin to clip suture	_____	15	
d. Pulled suture toward the incision	_____	15	
e. Continued until all sutures were removed.	_____	15	
12. Applied antiseptic solution to site.	_____	10	
a. Allowed to air dry	_____	5	
b. Applied steri-strips or butterfly closures PRN.	_____	15	

PROCEDURE STEPS	STEP PERFORMED	POINTS POSSIBLE	COMMENTS
c. Bandaged as necessary.	_____	10	
d. Asked patient if allergic to adhesive	_____	10	
13. Removed gloves.	_____	5	
a. Washed hands	_____	5	
14. Provided patient education.	_____	5	
15. Cleaned room.	_____	5	
a. Cared for instruments (gloves PRN)	_____	5	
16. Recorded information on patient's chart.	_____	5	
a. Initialed	_____	5	

EVALUATOR: NOTE TIME COMPLETED _____

ADD POINTS OF STEPS CHECKED   _____ EARNED

TOTAL POINTS POSSIBLE   285 POSSIBLE

Points assigned reflect importance of step to meeting objective: Important = (5)   Essential = (10)   Critical = (15)

Automatic failure results if any of the critical steps are omitted or performed incorrectly.

DETERMINE SCORE (divide points earned by total points possible, multiply results by 100)   _____ SCORE*

Evaluator's Name (print) _____ Signature _____

Comments _____

DOCUMENTATION

Chart the procedure in the patient's medical record.

Date: _____

Charting: _____

_____

_____

_____

Student's Name: _____   Physician's Initials: __(____)__

Name _____

Date _____ Score* _____

PROCEDURE 17-1   Obtain and Administer Oral Medication

PERFORMANCE OBJECTIVE—Demonstrate the steps required to obtain the ordered oral medication and administer it to the patient.

PROCEDURE STEPS	STEP PERFORMED	POINTS POSSIBLE	COMMENTS
EVALUATOR: Place check mark in space following each step performed satisfactorily			
NOTE TIME BEGAN _____			
1. Read order of medication and compared it with medication in storage area.	_____	10	
a. Obtained ordered medication	_____	15	
2. Calculated dosage if necessary.	_____	15	
3. Washed hands.	_____	5	
4. Removed bottle cap.	_____	5	
a. Placed cap inside-up on counter	_____	5	
b. Poured desired amount into cap and then into medicine cup	_____	15	
or			
If liquid; poured desired amount directly into medicine cup at eye level.	_____	15	
5. Placed medicine on tray.	_____	5	
a. Placed cup of water on tray (if medicine is in pill or capsule form)	_____	5	
6. Read label of medicine container again.	_____	10	
a. Took medicine to patient	_____	10	
7. Identified patient.	_____	5	
8. Explained procedure to patient.	_____	15	
9. Observed patient taking medication.	_____	15	
a. Reported any reaction or problem to the physician	_____	10	
10. Read label of medication container again.	_____	10	
11. Discarded disposables.	_____	5	
12. Returned items to proper storage.	_____	5	
13. Recorded medication information on patient's chart.	_____	15	
a. Initialed	_____	5	
EVALUATOR: NOTE TIME COMPLETED _____			

ADD POINTS OF STEPS CHECKED _____ EARNED

TOTAL POINTS POSSIBLE 185 POSSIBLE

Points assigned reflect importance of step to meeting objective: Important = (5)   Essential = (10)   Critical = (15)
Automatic failure results if any of the critical steps are omitted or performed incorrectly.

DETERMINE SCORE (divide points earned by total points possible, multiply results by 100) _____ SCORE*

Evaluator's Name (print) _____ Signature _____

Comments _____

DOCUMENTATION

Chart the procedure in the patient's medical record.

Date: _____

Charting: _____

_____

_____

_____

Student's Name: _____   Physician's Initials: __( )__

Name _____

Date _____ Score* _____

PROCEDURE 17-2   Withdraw Medication from Ampule

PERFORMANCE OBJECTIVE—Demonstrate each of the steps required to withdraw medication from an ampule.

PROCEDURE STEPS	STEP PERFORMED	POINTS POSSIBLE	COMMENTS
EVALUATOR: Place check mark in space following each step performed satisfactorily			
NOTE TIME BEGAN _____			
1. Washed hands.	_____	5	
2. Placed sterile gauze square over middle of ampule.	_____	5	
3. Held ampule between thumb and index finger of one hand.	_____	10	
4. Flicked pointed end of ampule with index finger to release medicine into bottom of ampule.	_____	15	
5. Grasped tip of ampule and snapped off.	_____	15	
a. Discarded tip of ampule	_____	10	
6. Secured needle and syringe by turning barrel to right while holding guard.	_____	10	
7. Expelled air from syringe.	_____	10	
8. Inserted tip of needle below line of liquid in ampule without touching sides.	_____	15	
9. Drew ordered amount of medicine into barrel of syringe.	_____	15	
a. Avoided air from entering by keeping tip of needle below line of liquid	_____	15	
10. Removed needle without touching sides of ampule.	_____	15	
11. Replaced needle guard without contaminating needle (scoop method).	_____	5	
12. Placed filled syringe on medicine tray.	_____	5	
13. Discarded disposables in proper receptacle.	_____	5	
EVALUATOR: NOTE TIME COMPLETED _____			

ADD POINTS OF STEPS CHECKED   _____ EARNED

TOTAL POINTS POSSIBLE   155 POSSIBLE

Points assigned reflect importance of step to meeting objective: Important = (5)   Essential = (10)   Critical = (15)
Automatic failure results if any of the critical steps are omitted or performed incorrectly.

DETERMINE SCORE (divide points earned by total points possible, multiply results by 100)   _____ SCORE*

Evaluator's Name (print) _____ Signature _____

Comments _____

Name _____

Date _____ Score* _____

PROCEDURE 17-3   Withdraw Medication from Vial

PERFORMANCE OBJECTIVE—Demonstrate each of the steps required to withdraw medication from a vial.

PROCEDURE STEPS	STEP PERFORMED	POINTS POSSIBLE	COMMENTS
EVALUATOR: Place check mark in space following each step performed satisfactorily			
NOTE TIME BEGAN _____			
1. Washed hands.	_____	5	
2. Calculated dosage.	_____	15	
3. Cleaned rubber-topped vial with alcohol pad.	_____	10	
4. Secured needle onto syringe by holding needle guard and turning barrel of syringe to the right.	_____	10	
5. Removed needle guard without contaminating the needle.	_____	10	
6. Pulled back on plunger to fill syringe with same amount of air as medication ordered.	_____	10	
7. Held syringe at barrel.	_____	10	
8. Held vial upside down.	_____	10	
9. Inserted needle into rubber top and pushed plunger in, expelling air into vial.	_____	15	
10. Pulled back plunger to allow desired amount of medication to enter syringe.	_____	15	
a. Kept needle below level of medication in vial to avoid air bubbles	_____	15	
b. Flicked barrel of syringe to release air bubbles into hub of syringe and pushed plunger to release	_____	15	
11. Pulled needle out of vial without contaminating it.	_____	10	
12. Replaced needle guard.	_____	5	
13. Placed filled syringe on medicine tray.	_____	5	
a. Placed alcohol on tray	_____	5	
EVALUATOR: NOTE TIME COMPLETED _____			

ADD POINTS OF STEPS CHECKED   _____ EARNED
TOTAL POINTS POSSIBLE   165 POSSIBLE

Points assigned reflect importance of step to meeting objective: Important = (5)   Essential = (10)   Critical = (15)
Automatic failure results if any of the critical steps are omitted or performed incorrectly.

DETERMINE SCORE (divide points earned by total points possible, multiply results by 100)   _____ SCORE*

Evaluator's Name (print) _____ Signature _____

Comments _____

Name _____

Date _____ Score* _____

PROCEDURE 17-4   Administer Intradermal Injection

PERFORMANCE OBJECTIVE—Demonstrate each of the steps required in administering an intradermal injection.

PROCEDURE STEPS	STEP PERFORMED	POINTS POSSIBLE	COMMENTS
EVALUATOR: Place check mark in space following each step performed satisfactorily			
NOTE TIME BEGAN _____			
1. Washed hands.	_____	5	
2. Read order.	_____	5	
3. Prepared syringe with ordered amount of medicine.	_____	15	
4. Replaced needle guard.	_____	10	
5. Placed medicine on tray.	_____	5	
6. Compared medicine order with patient's chart.	_____	15	
7. Identified patient.	_____	5	
8. Explained procedure to patient.	_____	5	
9. Placed medicine tray near patient.	_____	5	
10. Used alcohol pad to clean injection site.	_____	10	
a. Allowed alcohol to air dry	_____	5	
11. Removed needle guard without contaminating it.	_____	15	
12. Held patient's skin taut between thumb and index finger to steady area to be injected.	_____	5	
13. Inserted needle at 10°–15° angle.	_____	10	
a. Held bevel of needle up	_____	15	
14. Expelled medicine from syringe.	_____	15	
a. Caused wheal to develop	_____	15	
15. Removed needle quickly.	_____	10	
a. At same angle as insertion	_____	10	
b. Wiped site with gauze pad	_____	5	
c. Did not massage site	_____	10	
16. Observed patient.	_____	10	
a. Timed reaction	_____	15	
17. Gave patient instructions/answered questions.	_____	5	
18. Applied bandage.	_____	5	
19. Discarded disposables in sharps container including intact syringe and needle.	_____	5	

PROCEDURE 17-4   Administer Intradermal Injection—continued

PROCEDURE STEPS	STEP PERFORMED	POINTS POSSIBLE	COMMENTS
20. Returned items to proper storage.	_____	5	
21. Recorded information on patient's chart.	_____	15	
a. Initialed	_____	5	

EVALUATOR: NOTE TIME COMPLETED _____

ADD POINTS OF STEPS CHECKED   _____ EARNED
TOTAL POINTS POSSIBLE   260 POSSIBLE

Points assigned reflect importance of step to meeting objective: Important = (5)   Essential = (10)   Critical = (15)
Automatic failure results if any of the critical steps are omitted or performed incorrectly.

DETERMINE SCORE (divide points earned by total points possible, multiply results by 100)   _____ SCORE*

Evaluator's Name (print) _____ Signature _____

Comments _____

DOCUMENTATION

Chart the procedure in the patient's medical record.

Date: _____

Charting: _____

_____

_____

_____

Student's Name: _____   Physician's Initials: __(_____)__

Name _____

Date _____ Score* _____

PROCEDURE 17-5   Administer Subcutaneous Injection

PERFORMANCE OBJECTIVE—Demonstrate each of the steps required in administering a subcutaneous injection.

PROCEDURE STEPS	STEP PERFORMED	POINTS POSSIBLE	COMMENTS
EVALUATOR: Place check mark in space following each step performed satisfactorily			
NOTE TIME BEGAN _____			
1. Compared orders with medication.	_____	10	
2. Washed hands.	_____	5	
3. Prepared syringe.	_____	10	
a. Replaced needle guard	_____	5	
4. Placed filled syringe on medicine tray.	_____	10	
5. Compared medication order with patient's chart.	_____	15	
6. Identified patient.	_____	5	
7. Explained procedure to patient.	_____	5	
8. Asked patient to remove necessary clothing.	_____	10	
9. Used alcohol pad to clean injection site.	_____	10	
10. Removed needle guard without contaminating it.	_____	15	
11. Held skin at injection site taut.	_____	5	
12. Held syringe securely with bevel of needle down.	_____	10	
13. Inserted needle at 45° angle.	_____	15	
14. Held barrel of syringe with one hand.	_____	10	
a. Aspirated with other hand	_____	15	
b. Determined if in a blood vessel	_____	15	
15. Pushed plunger of syringe to release medication.	_____	15	
16. Pulled needle out at same angle as insertion.	_____	10	
17. Wiped site with alcohol pad.	_____	5	
18. Placed dry cotton ball on site.	_____	5	
a. Massaged area gently	_____	5	
19. Observed patient for possible reaction.	_____	5	
20. Reported any reaction to physician.	_____	10	
21. Advised patient to remain for 20 minutes.	_____	10	
22. Answered questions from patient.	_____	5	
23. Applied bandage.	_____	5	
24. Discarded disposables including intact syringe and needle in sharps container.	_____	5	

PROCEDURE 17-5 Administer Subcutaneous Injection—continued

PROCEDURE STEPS	STEP PERFORMED	POINTS POSSIBLE	COMMENTS
25. Returned items to proper storage.	_____	5	
26. Recorded information on patient's chart.	_____	5	
a. Initialed	_____	5	

EVALUATOR: NOTE TIME COMPLETED _____

ADD POINTS OF STEPS CHECKED   _____ EARNED
TOTAL POINTS POSSIBLE   265 POSSIBLE

Points assigned reflect importance of step to meeting objective: Important = (5) Essential = (10) Critical = (15)
Automatic failure results if any of the critical steps are omitted or performed incorrectly.

DETERMINE SCORE (divide points earned by total points possible, multiply results by 100)   _____ SCORE*

Evaluator's Name (print) _____ Signature _____

Comments _____

DOCUMENTATION

Chart the procedure in the patient's medical record.

Date: _____

Charting: _____

_____

_____

_____

Student's Name: _____   Physician's Initials: __(____)__

Name _____

Date _____ Score* _____

PROCEDURE 17-6   Administer Intramuscular Injection

PERFORMANCE OBJECTIVE—Demonstrate each of the steps required in administering an intramuscular injection.

PROCEDURE STEPS	STEP PERFORMED	POINTS POSSIBLE	COMMENTS
EVALUATOR: Place check mark in space following each step performed satisfactorily			
NOTE TIME BEGAN _____			
1. Washed hands.	_____	5	
2. Read label of medication.	_____	5	
3. Compared with order.	_____	10	
4. Prepared syringe with ordered amount of medication.	_____	15	
5. Replaced needle guard.	_____	5	
6. Placed filled syringe on medicine tray.	_____	10	
7. Compared medication order with patient's chart.	_____	15	
8. Identified patient.	_____	5	
9. Explained procedure to patient.	_____	5	
10. Asked patient to remove necessary clothing.	_____	5	
11. Cleaned injection site with alcohol pad.	_____	10	
a. Allowed to air dry	_____	5	
12. Removed needle guard.	_____	10	
13. Secured injection site between thumb and index finger.	_____	10	
14. Grasped syringe as a dart.	_____	10	
15. Inserted needle at 90° angle.	_____	15	
16. Aspirated syringe.	_____	15	
a. Determined if in a blood vessel	_____	15	
17. Pushed plunger of syringe to release medication.	_____	15	
18. Pulled needle out at angle of insertion.	_____	10	
19. Wiped injection site with alcohol pads.	_____	5	
20. Gently massaged area with dry cotton ball.	_____	5	
21. Observed patient for reaction.	_____	10	
22. Reported any reaction to physician.	_____	10	
23. Applied bandage.	_____	5	
24. Discarded disposables including intact syringe and needle in sharps container.	_____	5	

PROCEDURE 17-6 Administer Intramuscular Injection—continued

PROCEDURE STEPS	STEP PERFORMED	POINTS POSSIBLE	COMMENTS
25. Washed and sterilized reusable items.	_____	5	
26. Returned items to proper storage.	_____	5	
27. Recorded information on patient's chart.	_____	5	
a. Initialed	_____	5	

EVALUATOR: NOTE TIME COMPLETED _____

ADD POINTS OF STEPS CHECKED   _____ EARNED

TOTAL POINTS POSSIBLE   255 POSSIBLE

Points assigned reflect importance of step to meeting objective: Important = (5) Essential = (10) Critical = (15)

Automatic failure results if any of the critical steps are omitted or performed incorrectly.

DETERMINE SCORE (divide points earned by total points possible, multiply results by 100)   _____ SCORE*

Evaluator's Name (print) _____ Signature _____

Comments _____

DOCUMENTATION

Chart the procedure in the patient's medical record.

Date: _____

Charting: _____

_____

_____

_____

Student's Name: _____   Physician's Initials: __(____)__

Name _____

Date _____ Score* _____

PROCEDURE 17-7   Administer Intramuscular Injection by Z-Tract Method

PERFORMANCE OBJECTIVE—Demonstrate each of the steps required in administering an intramuscular injection by Z-tract method.

PROCEDURE STEPS	STEP PERFORMED	POINTS POSSIBLE	COMMENTS
EVALUATOR: Place check mark in space following each step performed satisfactorily			
NOTE TIME BEGAN _____			
1. Washed hands.	_____	5	
2. Read label of medication.	_____	10	
3. Compared with order.	_____	15	
4. Prepared syringe with ordered amount of medication.	_____	15	
5. Replaced needle guard.	_____	5	
6. Placed filled syringe on medicine tray.	_____	5	
7. Compared medication order with patient's chart.	_____	15	
8. Identified patient.	_____	5	
9. Explained procedure to patient.	_____	5	
10. Asked patient to remove necessary clothing.	_____	10	
11. Cleaned injection site with alcohol pad.	_____	10	
a. Allowed to air dry	_____	5	
12. Removed needle guard.	_____	5	
13. Read package insert instructions of medication.	_____	10	
14. Used sterile gauze square to displace skin/tissues throughout injection.	_____	10	
15. Inserted needle at 90° angle.	_____	15	
16. Used fingers to pull back on plunger to aspirate while holding barrel of syringe with thumb and ring finger.	_____	15	
17. Pushed plunger of syringe to slowly expel medication.	_____	15	
18. Waited a few seconds before withdrawing needle.	_____	15	
19. Removed needle quickly in same path as entered.	_____	10	
20. Let go of displaced skin/tissue immediately after needle is withdrawn to cover needle path.	_____	15	
21. Covered injection site with alcohol pad.	_____	5	
a. Held in place a few seconds	_____	5	
b. Did not massage injection site	_____	10	
22. Observed patient for reaction.	_____	10	

PROCEDURE STEPS	STEP PERFORMED	POINTS POSSIBLE	COMMENTS
23. Reported any reaction to physician.	_____	5	
24. Applied bandage.	_____	5	
25. Discarded disposables including intact syringe and needle in sharps container.	_____	5	
26. Washed and sterilized reusable items.	_____	5	
27. Returned items to proper storage.	_____	5	
28. Recorded information on patient's chart.	_____	5	
a. Initialed	_____	5	

EVALUATOR: NOTE TIME COMPLETED _____

ADD POINTS OF STEPS CHECKED   _____ EARNED

TOTAL POINTS POSSIBLE   280 POSSIBLE

Points assigned reflect importance of step to meeting objective: Important = (5)   Essential = (10)   Critical = (15)
Automatic failure results if any of the critical steps are omitted or performed incorrectly.

DETERMINE SCORE (divide points earned by total points possible, multiply results by 100)   _____ SCORE*

Evaluator's Name (print) _____ Signature _____

Comments _____

DOCUMENTATION

Chart the procedure in the patient's medical record.

Date: _____

Charting: _____

_____

_____

_____

Student's Name: _____   Physician's Initials: __(   )__

Name _____

Date _____ Score* _____

PROCEDURE 18-1   Give Mouth-to-Mouth Resuscitation

PERFORMANCE OBJECTIVE—In a course taught by a certified instructor, using a training mannequin, demonstrate mouth-to-mouth resuscitation. Perform the steps as instructed following recommended standard precautions.

PROCEDURE STEPS	STEP PERFORMED	POINTS POSSIBLE	COMMENTS
EVALUATOR: Place check mark in space following each step performed satisfactorily			
NOTE TIME BEGAN _____			
1. Determined whether unresponsive victim is breathing.	_____	15	
2. Positioned victim on back on firm surface.	_____	5	
3. Rescuer was positioned at victim's side near head and shoulders.	_____	5	
4. Opened airway. If not effective, continued with procedure.	_____	15	
5. Checked for mouth obstruction.	_____	10	
6. Demonstrated procedure to remove obstruction.	_____	15	
7. Used head tilt-chin lift maneuver, thereby moving tongue from back of throat. If not effective, continued with procedure.	_____	15	
8. Pinched victim's nostrils together with fingers of one hand while placing heel of hand on forehead to keep the head tilted.	_____	10	
9. Took a deep breath and then sealed mouth over victim's. Breathed two slow breaths into the victim's mouth. Took a breath after each ventilation.	_____	15	
10. Turned head to one side, felt and listened for return of air. Watched chest for movement. If not effective, lifted chin, tilted head, tried again.	_____	15	
11. If inflation had not occurred, gave cycles of 12 breaths per minute. Watched for return of breathing.	_____	15	
12. Continued cycles until breathing restored, assistance arrived, or resuscitation was no longer possible.	_____	10	
13. Recorded and signed procedure on patient's chart.	_____		
EVALUATOR: NOTE TIME COMPLETED _____			

ADD POINTS OF STEPS CHECKED   _____ EARNED
TOTAL POINTS POSSIBLE   155 POSSIBLE

Points assigned reflect importance of step to meeting objective: Important = (5)   Essential = (10)   Critical = (15)
Automatic failure results if any of the critical steps are omitted or performed incorrectly.

DETERMINE SCORE (divide points earned by total points possible, multiply results by 100)   _____ SCORE*

Evaluator's Name (print) _____ Signature _____

Comments _____

DOCUMENTATION

Chart the procedure in the patient's medical record.

Date: _____

Charting: _____

_____

_____

_____

Student's Name: _____   Physician's Initials: __( )__

Name _____

Date _____ Score* _____

PROCEDURE 18-2   Give Cardiopulmonary Resuscitation (CPR) to Adults

PERFORMANCE OBJECTIVE—In a course taught by a certified instructor, and using a training mannequin, demonstrate the procedure performing each step, following recommended precautions.

PROCEDURE STEPS	STEP PERFORMED	POINTS POSSIBLE	COMMENTS
EVALUATOR: Place check mark in space following each step performed satisfactorily			
NOTE TIME BEGAN _____			
1. Gently shook victim and asked "Are you OK?"	_____	10	
2. If no response, called or sent someone for help.	_____	15	
3. Positioned mannequin on floor.	_____	5	
4. Rescuer was positioned at victim's side near head.	_____	5	
5. Opened airway. If not effective, continued with procedure.	_____	15	
6. Checked for mouth obstruction.	_____	5	
7. Positioned victim to open airway; pinched nostrils together with fingers while placing heel of hand on forehead to maintain head tilt.	_____	10	
8. Took a deep breath, sealed mouth over victim's, and breathed two slow breaths into victim's mouth. Took a breath after each ventilation.	_____	15	
9. Turned head to one side, listened, and felt for return of air. Watched chest for movement.	_____	5	
10. Checked for carotid pulse; allowed up to 10 seconds.	_____	15	
11. If victim had a pulse, continued mouth-to-mouth respiration at rate of one breath every five seconds, if no pulse, began chest compressions.	_____	—	
12. Identified location for chest compressions and positioned hands.			
a. Located lower rib cage	_____	5	
b. Followed up to sternum	_____	5	
c. Placed two index fingers at lower end of sternum	_____	5	
d. Placed heel of hand nearest head next to fingers	_____	5	
e. Positioned other hand over hand on sternum, locked fingers	_____	10	
f. Held fingers away from body	_____	10	
13. Rose on knees, shoulder width apart.	_____	5	
a. Directly over sternum	_____	5	
b. Locked elbows	_____	5	

PROCEDURE STEPS	STEP PERFORMED	POINTS POSSIBLE	COMMENTS
14. Used a smooth, even motion to push straight down on chest and compressed about 1½″ to 2″ for a count of fifteen compressions.	_____	15	
15. Gave two ventilations.	_____	15	
16. Repeated four cycles: Pause, checked for signs of circulation.	_____	15	
17. If no pulse, resumed compressions and ventilations.	_____	—	
18. Paused every few minutes to check for pulse and respirations.	_____	—	
19. Continued CPR until victim recovered, help arrived, victim was pronounced dead, or after 15 minutes, no signs of life have occurred.	_____	—	
20. Cleaned mannequin as instructed.	_____	10	
21. Recorded and signed procedure on patient's chart.	_____	10	

EVALUATOR: NOTE TIME COMPLETED _____

ADD POINTS OF STEPS CHECKED   _____ EARNED
TOTAL POINTS POSSIBLE   220 POSSIBLE

Points assigned reflect importance of step to meeting objective: Important = (5)   Essential = (10)   Critical = (15)
Automatic failure results if any of the critical steps are omitted or performed incorrectly.

DETERMINE SCORE (divide points earned by total points possible, multiply results by 100)   _____ SCORE*

Evaluator's Name (print) _____ Signature _____

Comments _____

DOCUMENTATION

Chart the procedure in the patient's medical record.

Date: _____

Charting: _____

_____

_____

_____

Student's Name: _____   Physician's Initials: __(   )__

PROCEDURE 18-3   Give Cardiopulmonary Resuscitation (CPR) to Infants and Children

PERFORMANCE OBJECTIVE—In a course taught by a certified instructor, using a training mannequin, demonstrate the procedure as instructed, performing each step, and following standard precautions.

PROCEDURE STEPS	STEP PERFORMED	POINTS POSSIBLE	COMMENTS
EVALUATOR: Place check mark in space following each step performed satisfactorily			
NOTE TIME BEGAN _____			
1. Gently shook and called to a child or flicked bottom of foot of an infant to check for consciousness.	_____	5	
2. Called to another person to phone 911 or local emergency service and began resuscitation.	_____	15	
3. Placed infant or child on back on firm surface.	_____	5	
4. Tipped victim's head back and lifted chin to open airway.	_____	15	
5. Listened and watched and felt for breathing.	_____	10	
6. If no breathing was observed, gave two slow breaths, one to two seconds each.	_____	15	
7. Checked carotid pulse and signs of circulation for up to 10 seconds.	_____	15	
a. Child at carotid location	_____	10	
b. Infants at mid upper arm over brachial	_____	10	
8. If pulse, continue one ventilation.	_____	10	
a. Every 3 seconds for infant			
b. Every 4 seconds for child			
9. If no pulse was present, started cardiac compression.			
a. Infant—Two fingers, mid sternum, depress ½"–1"; not less than 100 times per minute.	_____	15	
b. Child—Adult position, one hand, depressed 1 inch to 1½ inches, 100 times per minute.	_____	15	
10. Did ten cycles of compressions and breaths.	_____	15	
11. Checked for pulse and signs of circulation for up to 5 seconds.	_____	5	
12. If alone, summoned help.	_____	15	

PROCEDURE STEPS	STEP PERFORMED	POINTS POSSIBLE	COMMENTS
13. If there was no pulse, gave one breath and continued cycle until help arrived.	_____	10	
14. Sanitized the mannequin.	_____	5	
15. Recorded and signed procedure on patient's chart.	_____	10	

EVALUATOR: NOTE TIME COMPLETED _____

ADD POINTS OF STEPS CHECKED   _____ EARNED
TOTAL POINTS POSSIBLE   200 POSSIBLE

Points assigned reflect importance of step to meeting objective: Important = (5)   Essential = (10)   Critical = (15)
Automatic failure results if any of the critical steps are omitted or performed incorrectly.

DETERMINE SCORE (divide points earned by total points possible, multiply results by 100)   _____ SCORE*

Evaluator's Name (print) _____ Signature _____

Comments _____

DOCUMENTATION

Chart the procedure in the patient's medical record.

Date: _____

Charting: _____

_____

_____

_____

Student's Name: _____   Physician's Initials: __(   )__

Name _____

Date _____ Score* _____

PROCEDURE 18-4   Clean Wound Areas

PERFORMANCE OBJECTIVE—Provided with all necessary equipment and supplies, demonstrate cleaning wounds, following procedure steps and standard precautions.

PROCEDURE STEPS	STEP PERFORMED	POINTS POSSIBLE	COMMENTS
EVALUATOR: Place check mark in space following each step performed satisfactorily			
NOTE TIME BEGAN _____			
1. Assembled equipment and materials.	_____	5	
2. Washed hands and put on gloves.	_____	10	
3. Grasped gauze sponges with sponge forceps.	_____	5	
4. Dipped into warm detergent water.	_____	5	
5. Washed wound and wound area to remove microorganisms and any foreign matter.			
a. Avoided further injury from instrument	_____	10	
b. Worked from inner to outer area, 2″ to 3″ beyond wound	_____	15	
6. Discarded sponges in biohazardous waste container.	_____	10	
7. Irrigated wound thoroughly with sterile water.	_____	15	
8. Blotted wound dry with sterile gauze and discarded gauze in biohazardous waste container.	_____	10	
9. Covered with dry sterile dressing and bandaged in place.	_____	15	
10. Instructed patient to call physician immediately if evidence of infection developed.	_____	15	
Cleaned up work area. Placed all used materials and gloves in the biohazardous waste bag and into 11. proper receptacle for safe disposal.	_____	5	
12. Washed hands.	_____	5	
13. Recorded and signed procedure on patient's chart.	_____	10	
EVALUATOR: NOTE TIME COMPLETED _____			

ADD POINTS OF STEPS CHECKED   _____ EARNED
TOTAL POINTS POSSIBLE   135 POSSIBLE

Points assigned reflect importance of step to meeting objective: Important = (5)   Essential = (10)   Critical = (15)
Automatic failure results if any of the critical steps are omitted or performed incorrectly.

DETERMINE SCORE (divide points earned by total points possible, multiply results by 100)   _____ SCORE*

Evaluator's Name (print) _____ Signature _____

Comments _____

DOCUMENTATION

Chart the procedure in the patient's medical record.

Date: _____

Charting: _____

_____

_____

_____

Student's Name: _____   Physician's Initials: __(____)__

Name _____

Date _____ Score* _____

PROCEDURE 18-5   Apply Bandage in Recurrent Turn to Finger

PERFORMANCE OBJECTIVE—Provided with all necessary equipment and supplies, apply recurrent turn bandage following procedure steps and standard precautions.

PROCEDURE STEPS	STEP PERFORMED	POINTS POSSIBLE	COMMENTS
EVALUATOR: Place check mark in space following each step performed satisfactorily			
NOTE TIME BEGAN _____			
1. Washed hands. Put on gloves if appropriate.	_____	5	
2. Assembled supplies.	_____	5	
3. Covered injury with dressing.	_____	10	
4. Secured dressing with bandage of gauze.			
a. Start at proximal end, palm side	_____	5	
b. Go to proximal end, back of hand	_____	5	
c. Repeat desired times	_____	5	
5. Held recurrent turns in place with spiral turns.	_____	10	
6. Secured by tying off gauze at proximal end of finger.	_____	10	
7. Discarded contaminated materials and gloves, if used, in biohazardous waste bag.	_____	15	
8. Washed hands.	_____	5	
9. Recorded and signed procedure in patient's chart.	_____	10	
EVALUATOR: NOTE TIME COMPLETED _____			

ADD POINTS OF STEPS CHECKED   _____ EARNED
TOTAL POINTS POSSIBLE   85 POSSIBLE

Points assigned reflect importance of step to meeting objective: **Important** = (5)   **Essential** = (10)   **Critical** = (15)
Automatic failure results if any of the critical steps are omitted or performed incorrectly.

DETERMINE SCORE (divide points earned by total points possible, multiply results by 100)   _____ SCORE*

Evaluator's Name (print) _____ Signature _____

Comments _____

DOCUMENTATION

Chart the procedure in the patient's medical record.

Date: _____

Charting: _____

_____

_____

_____

Student's Name: _____   Physician's Initials: __(____)__

Name _____

Date _____ Score* _____

PROCEDURE 18-6   Apply Bandage in Open or Closed Spiral

PERFORMANCE OBJECTIVE—Provided with all necessary equipment and supplies, apply open and closed spiral bandage so dressing is secure, following procedure steps and standard precautions.

PROCEDURE STEPS	STEP PERFORMED	POINTS POSSIBLE	COMMENTS
EVALUATOR: Place check mark in space following each step performed satisfactorily			
NOTE TIME BEGAN _____			
1. Washed hands. Put on gloves if appropriate.	_____	5	
2. Assembled needed supplies.	_____	5	
3. Carefully opened dressing, without contaminating, and placed over wound area.	_____	10	
4. Anchored bandage by placing end of bandage on bias at starting point.	_____	5	
5. Encircled part, allowing corner of bandage end to protrude.	_____	5	
6. Turned down protruding tip of bandage.	_____	5	
7. Encircled part again.	_____	5	
8. Continued to encircle area to be covered with spiral turns spaced so that they do not overlap. *OR* Formed closed spiral by continuing to encircle with overlapping spiral turns until all open spaces were covered.	_____	5	
a. Subtract 10 pts. if wrapped straight around.	_____		
9. Completed bandage by tying off or taping in place.	_____	5	
a. Tape if used, must be in opposite direction to body movement. Subtract 10 pts. if applied incorrectly	_____		
10. Discarded contaminated materials and gloves, if used, in biohazardous waste bag.	_____	15	
11. Washed hands.	_____	5	
12. Recorded and signed procedure on patient's chart.	_____	10	
EVALUATOR: NOTE TIME COMPLETED _____			

ADD POINTS OF STEPS CHECKED   _____ EARNED

TOTAL POINTS POSSIBLE   80 POSSIBLE

Points assigned reflect importance of step to meeting objective: Important = (5)   Essential = (10)   Critical = (15)
Automatic failure results if any of the critical steps are omitted or performed incorrectly.

DETERMINE SCORE (divide points earned by total points possible, multiply results by 100)   _____ SCORE*

Evaluator's Name (print) _____ Signature _____

Comments _____

DOCUMENTATION

Chart the procedure in the patient's medical record.

Date: _____

Charting: _____

_____

_____

_____

Student's Name: _____   Physician's Initials: __(____)__

Name _____

Date _____ Score* _____

PROCEDURE 18-7   Apply Figure-Eight Bandage to Hand and Wrist

PERFORMANCE OBJECTIVE—Provided with all necessary equipment and materials, apply a figure-eight bandage to the hand and wrist neatly to secure dressing following procedure steps and standard precautions.

PROCEDURE STEPS	STEP PERFORMED	POINTS POSSIBLE	COMMENTS
EVALUATOR: Place check mark in space following each step performed satisfactorily			
NOTE TIME BEGAN _____			
1. Washed hands. Put on gloves if appropriate.	_____	5	
2. Assembled needed supplies.	_____	5	
3. Applied dressing. Did not contaminate any part that would touch wound area.	_____	10	
4. Anchored bandage with one or two turns around palm of hand.	_____	5	
5. Rolled gauze diagonally across front of wrist and in figure-eight pattern around the hand.	_____	10	
6. Tied off at the wrist. Avoided constricting circulation.	_____	15	
7. Discarded contaminated materials and gloves, if used, in biohazardous waste bag.	_____	15	
8. Washed hands.	_____	5	
9. Recorded and signed procedure on patient's chart.	_____	10	
EVALUATOR: NOTE TIME COMPLETED _____			

ADD POINTS OF STEPS CHECKED   _____ EARNED
TOTAL POINTS POSSIBLE   80 POSSIBLE

Points assigned reflect importance of step to meeting objective: Important = (5)   Essential = (10)   Critical = (15)
Automatic failure results if any of the critical steps are omitted or performed incorrectly.

DETERMINE SCORE (divide points earned by total points possible, multiply results by 100)   _____ SCORE*

Evaluator's Name (print) _____ Signature _____

Comments _____

DOCUMENTATION

Chart the procedure in the patient's medical record.

Date: _____

Charting: _____

_____

_____

_____

Student's Name: _____   Physician's Initials: __(____)__

508

Name _____

Date _____ Score* _____

PROCEDURE 18-8   Apply Cravat Bandage to Forehead, Ear, or Eyes

PERFORMANCE OBJECTIVE—Provided with all necessary equipment and supplies, apply a cravat bandage to the head following procedure steps and standard precautions.

PROCEDURE STEPS	STEP PERFORMED	POINTS POSSIBLE	COMMENTS
EVALUATOR: Place check mark in space following each step performed satisfactorily			
NOTE TIME BEGAN _____			
1. Washed hands. Put on gloves if appropriate.	_____	5	
2. Assembled needed supplies.	_____	5	
3. Carefully placed dressing over wound, taking care not to contaminate area over wound.	_____	15	
4. Placed center of cravat over dressing.	_____	5	
5. Took ends around to opposite side of head and crossed them. Did not tie.	_____	5	
6. Brought ends back to starting point and tied.	_____	10	
7. Discarded contaminated materials and gloves, if used, in biohazardous waste bag.	_____	15	
8. Washed hands.	_____	5	
9. Recorded and signed procedure on patient's chart.	_____	10	
EVALUATOR: NOTE TIME COMPLETED _____			

ADD POINTS OF STEPS CHECKED   _____ EARNED

TOTAL POINTS POSSIBLE   75 POSSIBLE

Points assigned reflect importance of step to meeting objective: Important = (5)   Essential = (10)   Critical = (15)
Automatic failure results if any of the critical steps are omitted or performed incorrectly.

DETERMINE SCORE (divide points earned by total points possible, multiply results by 100)   _____ SCORE*

Evaluator's Name (print) _____ Signature _____

Comments _____

DOCUMENTATION

Chart the procedure in the patient's medical record.

Date: _____

Charting: _____

_____

_____

_____

Student's Name: _____   Physician's Initials: __(____)__

Name _____

Date _____ Score* _____

PROCEDURE 18-9   Apply Triangular Bandage to Head

PERFORMANCE OBJECTIVE—Provided with all necessary equipment and supplies, apply a triangular bandage to the head following procedure steps and standard precautions so the dressing is neat and secure.

PROCEDURE STEPS	STEP PERFORMED	POINTS POSSIBLE	COMMENTS
EVALUATOR: Place check mark in space following each step performed satisfactorily			
NOTE TIME BEGAN _____			
1. Washed hands. Put on gloves if appropriate.	_____	5	
2. Assembled needed supplies.	_____	5	
3. Carefully placed dressing over wound area without contaminating.	_____	15	
4. Folded a hem about two inches wide along base of bandage.	_____	10	
5. With hem on outside, placed bandage on head so that middle of base was on forehead close to eyebrows and point hangs down back.	_____	10	
6. Brought two ends around head above ears and crossed them just below occipital prominence at back of head.	_____	10	
7. Drew ends snugly around head and tied them in center of forehead.	_____	5	
8. Steadied head with one hand and with other hand drew point down firmly behind to hold dressing securely against head.	_____	10	
9. Grasped point and tucked it into area where bandage ends crossed.	_____	5	
10. Discarded contaminated materials and gloves, if used, in biohazardous waste bag.	_____	15	
11. Washed hands.	_____	5	
12. Recorded and signed procedure on patient's chart.	_____	10	
EVALUATOR: NOTE TIME COMPLETED _____			

ADD POINTS OF STEPS CHECKED   _____ EARNED
TOTAL POINTS POSSIBLE   105 POSSIBLE

Points assigned reflect importance of step to meeting objective: Important = (5)   Essential = (10)   Critical = (15)
Automatic failure results if any of the critical steps are omitted or performed incorrectly.

DETERMINE SCORE (divide points earned by total points possible, multiply results by 100)   _____ SCORE*

Evaluator's Name (print) _____ Signature _____

Comments _____

DOCUMENTATION

Chart the procedure in the patient's medical record.

Date: _____

Charting: _____

_____

_____

_____

Student's Name: _____   Physician's Initials: __(____)__

Name _____

Date _____ Score* _____

PROCEDURE 18-10   Apply Arm Sling

PERFORMANCE OBJECTIVE—Provided with the necessary equipment, demonstrate the steps in the procedure for applying an arm sling so that the arm is supported properly and the sling is correctly tied.

PROCEDURE STEPS	STEP PERFORMED	POINTS POSSIBLE	COMMENTS
EVALUATOR: Place check mark in space following each step performed satisfactorily			
NOTE TIME BEGAN _____			
1. Washed hands.	_____	5	
2. Placed one end of triangle bandage over shoulder on uninjured side and let other end hang down over chest.	_____	15	
3. Pulled point behind elbow of injured arm.	_____	5	
4. Pulled end of bandage which was hanging down up around injured arm and over shoulder.	_____	5	
5. Raised end until hand rested 4" to 5" above elbow.	_____	15	
6. Tied ends at side of neck; checked hand.	_____	15	
7. Closed point end at elbow.	_____	15	
a. Folded neatly and pinned or			
b. Tied knot in cloth to make sling snug at elbow			
8. Extended fingers slightly beyond edge of sling.	_____	15	
9. Recorded and signed procedure on patient's chart.	_____	10	
EVALUATOR: NOTE TIME COMPLETED _____			

ADD POINTS OF STEPS CHECKED   _____ EARNED
TOTAL POINTS POSSIBLE   100 POSSIBLE

Points assigned reflect importance of step to meeting objective: Important = (5)   Essential = (10)   Critical = (15)
Automatic failure results if any of the critical steps are omitted or performed incorrectly.

DETERMINE SCORE (divide points earned by total points possible, multiply results by 100)   _____ SCORE*

Evaluator's Name (print) _____ Signature _____

Comments _____

513

DOCUMENTATION

Chart the procedure in the patient's medical record.

Date: _____

Charting: _____

_____

_____

_____

Student's Name: _____   Physician's Initials: __(____)__

Name _____

Date _____ Score* _____

PROCEDURE 18-11   Use a Cane

PERFORMANCE OBJECTIVE—Provided with a cane, demonstrate adjusting the length of a cane and provide patient with instruction to properly and safely use a cane. The cane will be the appropriate length and the patient will demonstrate correct usage.

PROCEDURE STEPS	STEP PERFORMED	POINTS POSSIBLE	COMMENTS
EVALUATOR: Place check mark in space following each step performed satisfactorily			
NOTE TIME BEGAN _____			
1. Identified patient and confirmed physician's orders.	_____	5	
2. Assembled equipment. Checked cane for intact rubber tip.	_____	10	
3. Adjusted height of cane.			
a. Elbow flexed at 25° to 30° angle	_____	15	
b. Handle just below hip on strong side	_____	15	
4. Demonstrated use of cane—moving cane forward with injured extremity.	_____	15	
5. Allowed patient to practice the procedure.	_____	5	
6. Demonstrated going up stairs and had patient practice (Uninjured extremity up first).	_____	15	
7. Demonstrate going down stairs and had patient practice (Uninjured extremity down first).	_____	15	
8. Rechecked cane height.	_____	5	
9. Ensured correct usage.	_____	15	
10. Recorded and signed procedure on patient's chart.	_____	10	
EVALUATOR: NOTE TIME COMPLETED _____			

ADD POINTS OF STEPS CHECKED   _____ EARNED
TOTAL POINTS POSSIBLE   125 POSSIBLE

Points assigned reflect importance of step to meeting objective: Important = (5)   Essential = (10)   Critical = (15)
Automatic failure results if any of the critical steps are omitted or performed incorrectly.

DETERMINE SCORE (divide points earned by total points possible, multiply results by 100)   _____ SCORE*

Evaluator's Name (print) _____ Signature _____

Comments _____

DOCUMENTATION

Chart the procedure in the patient's medical record.

Date: _____

Charting: _____

_____

_____

_____

Student's Name: _____   Physician's Initials: __( )__

PERFORMANCE EVALUATION CHECKLIST

Name _____

Date _____ Score* _____

PROCEDURE 18-12   Use Crutches

PERFORMANCE OBJECTIVE—Provided with all necessary equipment and supplies, adjust the length of the crutches and
demonstrate the steps of this procedure to instruct a patient in the correct use of crutches. The crutches will be the correct
length and the patient will be able to demonstrate the proper and safe use of crutches.

PROCEDURE STEPS	STEP PERFORMED	POINTS POSSIBLE	COMMENTS
EVALUATOR: Place check mark in space following each step performed satisfactorily			
NOTE TIME BEGAN _____			
1. Identified patient and confirmed physician's orders.	_____	5	
2. Assembled equipment. Made sure crutches were intact (hand pads and rubber tips) and stable.	_____	5	
3. Stabilized patient upright near wall or chair for support.	_____	10	
4. Adjusted length of crutches.			
a. Elbows with 30° bend	_____	15	
b. Pads 2″ below axilla	_____	15	
5. Explained proper usage to patient.			
a. Supported weight on hands	_____	15	
b. Took small steps	_____	10	
c. Stood on uninjured extremity, swung injured extremity with crutches	_____	15	
6. Demonstrated proper use of crutches for gait ordered.	_____	15	
7. Allowed patient to practice the procedure to ensure correct use.	_____	10	
8. Recorded and signed procedure on patient's chart.	_____	10	

EVALUATOR: NOTE TIME COMPLETED _____

ADD POINTS OF STEPS CHECKED   _____ EARNED

TOTAL POINTS POSSIBLE   125 POSSIBLE

Points assigned reflect importance of step to meeting objective: Important = (5)   Essential = (10)   Critical = (15)
Automatic failure results if any of the critical steps are omitted or performed incorrectly.

DETERMINE SCORE (divide points earned by total points possible, multiply results by 100)   _____ SCORE*

Evaluator's Name (print) _____ Signature _____

Comments _____

DOCUMENTATION

Chart the procedure in the patient's medical record.

Date: _____

Charting: _____

_____

_____

_____

Student's Name: _____   Physician's Initials: __(____)__

518

Name _____

Date _____ Score* _____

PROCEDURE 18-13   Use a Walker

PERFORMANCE OBJECTIVE—Provided with a walker, adjust it to the appropriate height and demonstrate the steps in the procedure to instruct a patient in the proper use of a walker. The patient will be able to demonstrate the safe and correct use of a walker.

PROCEDURE STEPS	STEP PERFORMED	POINTS POSSIBLE	COMMENTS
EVALUATOR: Place check mark in space following each step performed satisfactorily			
NOTE TIME BEGAN _____			
1. Identified patient and confirmed physician's orders.	_____	5	
2. Assembled equipment. Checked walker for rubber tips, pads at handles, and stability.	_____	10	
3. Stabilized patient upright near wall or chair for support.	_____	10	
4. Adjusted walker to fit patient.			
a. Handles at hip level	_____	15	
b. Elbows bent 25° to 30°	_____	15	
5. Positioned the walker around the patient.	_____	5	
6. Instructed patient to pick up the walker and move it slightly forward and walk into it.	_____	10	
7. Demonstrated the correct use of a walker.	_____	15	
8. Had patient practice the procedure.	_____	5	
9. Observed patient and was ready to assist in case of possible fall until able to use safely and correctly.	_____	10	
10. Recorded and signed procedure on patient's chart.	_____	10	
EVALUATOR: NOTE TIME COMPLETED _____			

ADD POINTS OF STEPS CHECKED   _____ EARNED
TOTAL POINTS POSSIBLE   110 POSSIBLE

Points assigned reflect importance of step to meeting objective: Important = (5)   Essential = (10)   Critical = (15)
Automatic failure results if any of the critical steps are omitted or performed incorrectly.

DETERMINE SCORE (divide points earned by total points possible, multiply results by 100)   _____ SCORE*

Evaluator's Name (print) _____ Signature _____

Comments _____

DOCUMENTATION

Chart the procedure in the patient's medical record.

Date: _____

Charting: _____

_____

_____

_____

Student's Name: _____   Physician's Initials: __( )__

Name _____

Date _____ Score* _____

PROCEDURE 18-14   Assist Patient from Wheelchair to Examination Table

PERFORMANCE OBJECTIVE—Provided with necessary equipment, demonstrate the steps in the procedure for assisting a patient from wheelchair to examination table in a safe manner.

PROCEDURE STEPS	STEP PERFORMED	POINTS POSSIBLE	COMMENTS
EVALUATOR: Place check mark in space following each step performed satisfactorily			
NOTE TIME BEGAN _____			
1. Unlocked wheels of chair and wheeled patient to examination room.	_____	5	
2. Positioned chair as near as possible to place where patient should sit on table.	_____	5	
3. Lowered table to chair level or provided stool.	_____	5	
4. Locked wheels on chair.	_____	15	
5. Folded footrests back.	_____	10	
6. Assumed stable position in front of patient.	_____	10	
7. Assisted patient to stand; side step or pivot to front of table.	_____	15	
8. Assisted patient to sitting position on table.	_____	10	
9. Helped adjust position and recline for examination.	_____	5	
10. Placed pillow under head.	_____	5	
11. Draped as appropriate.	_____	5	
12. Unlocked chair wheels and moved chair out of way.	_____	5	
EVALUATOR: NOTE TIME COMPLETED _____			

ADD POINTS OF STEPS CHECKED   _____ EARNED
TOTAL POINTS POSSIBLE   95 POSSIBLE

Points assigned reflect importance of step to meeting objective: Important = (5)   Essential = (10)   Critical = (15)
Automatic failure results if any of the critical steps are omitted or performed incorrectly.

DETERMINE SCORE (divide points earned by total points possible, multiply results by 100)   _____ SCORE*

Evaluator's Name (print) _____ Signature _____

Comments _____

PERFORMANCE EVALUATION CHECKLIST

Name _____

Date _____ Score* _____

PROCEDURE 18-15   Assist Patient from Examination Table to Wheelchair

PERFORMANCE OBJECTIVE—Provided with a wheelchair and an examination table, demonstrate the steps in the procedure, in order, to assist the patient from examination table to wheelchair in a safe manner.

PROCEDURE STEPS	STEP PERFORMED	POINTS POSSIBLE	COMMENTS
EVALUATOR: Place check mark in space following each step performed satisfactorily			
NOTE TIME BEGAN _____			
1. Repositioned chair and locked wheels.	_____	15	
2. Assisted patient to sitting position on table.	_____	10	
3. Assisted to redress as needed.	_____	5	
4. Supported patient while assisting to step onto floor or stepstool (if stool—assisted to step onto floor).	_____	15	
5. Side-stepped or pivoted patient to position in front of chair.	_____	15	
6. Instructed patient to reach back to chair arms while helping lower patient into chair.	_____	15	
7. Adjusted footrests.	_____	10	
8. Unlocked wheels and returned patient to consultation or reception room.	_____	5	
EVALUATOR: NOTE TIME COMPLETED _____			

ADD POINTS OF STEPS CHECKED   _____ EARNED

TOTAL POINTS POSSIBLE   90 POSSIBLE

Points assigned reflect importance of step to meeting objective: Important = (5)   Essential = (10)   Critical = (15)
Automatic failure results if any of the critical steps are omitted or performed incorrectly.

DETERMINE SCORE (divide points earned by total points possible, multiply results by 100)   _____ SCORE*

Evaluator's Name (print) _____ Signature _____

Comments _____

523

CERTIFICATE OF COMPLETION

CERTIFIES THAT

_____

NAME

Has successfully completed the study of

MEDICAL ASSISTING

ESSENTIALS OF ADMINISTRATIVE AND CLINICAL COMPETENCIES

_____
SCHOOL

_____
DIRECTOR

_____
DATE

_____
INSTRUCTOR